CONTENTS

understanding health promotion

Edited by
Helen Keleher
Colin MacDougall
Berni Murphy

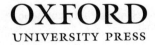

OXFORD
UNIVERSITY PRESS

OXFORD
UNIVERSITY PRESS

253 Normanby Road, South Melbourne, Victoria 3205, Australia

Oxford University Press is a department of the University of Oxford.
It furthers the University's objective of excellence in research, scholarship,
and education by publishing worldwide in

Oxford New York

Auckland Cape Town Dar es Salaam Hong Kong Karachi
Kuala Lumpur Madrid Melbourne Mexico City Nairobi
New Delhi Shanghai Taipei Toronto

With offices in

Argentina Austria Brazil Chile Czech Republic France Greece
Guatemala Hungary Italy Japan Poland Portugal Singapore
South Korea Switzerland Thailand Turkey Ukraine Vietnam

OXFORD is a trade mark of Oxford University Press
in the UK and in certain other countries

National Library of Australia Cataloguing-in-Publication data:

Keleher, Helen, 1950-
Understanding health promotion

Bibliography
For 2nd and 3rd year undergraduate students.
ISBN 9780195552942

ISBN 0 19 555294 6

1. Health promotion - Australia - Textbooks. 2. Health promotion - Study and teaching
(Higher) - Australia. I. Murphy, Berni. II. MacDougall, Colin. III. Title.

613.071194

In accordance with the Copyright Act 1968 a copy of each book published must be lodged with the
National Library. Under relevant State or Territory Legislation a copy must also be lodged with the
appropriate library or libraries in the state of publication. For information about Legal Deposit, see the
website at: http://www.nla.gov.au/services/ldeposit.html or contact the Legal Deposit Unit, National
Library of Australia on 02 6262 1312.

Edited by Liz Filleul
Text and cover design by Kerry Cooke, eggplant communications
Typeset in India by diacriTech, Chennai
Proofread by Greg Alford
Indexed by Russell Brooks
Printed in Australia by Ligare Book Printers.

LIST OF BOXES,
CASE STUDIES,
FIGURES, AND TABLES

BOXES

CASE STUDIES

FIGURES

TABLES

CONTRIBUTORS

Rebecca Armstrong is the Knowledge Translation Research Fellow with the Cochrane Health Promotion and Public Health Field at the Victorian Health Promotion Foundation (VicHealth). Rebecca provides training and support for those undertaking systematic reviews of health promotion and public health interventions. Her research interests include the evaluation and systematic review of complex health promotion and public health interventions and strategies to support knowledge translation. She was previously Research Fellow at the School of Health and Social Development at Deakin University, Melbourne.

Grace Blau is a Research Fellow who joined the Health Impact Assessment (HIA) Research Unit at Deakin University in 2004 to undertake research that explored the positioning and application of HIA in the Victorian local government sector. Prior to this appointment, she worked as a public health planner in several Victorian local governments. Before diverting her career path to the field of population health, Grace developed considerable knowledge and experience in primary health care, having worked as a pharmacist, a dietician, and a diabetes educator in both the private and public sectors.

Iain Butterworth is a community psychologist with an interest in the relationship between urban planning, sense of place and community, and well-being. In 2001 his doctoral research on environmental adult education received the American Psychological Association's 'Emory L. Cowen Dissertation Award for the Promotion of Wellness'. Iain co-produced *Environments for Health*, the Victorian State Government's municipal public health planning policy framework, which drew strongly on the Healthy Cities approach. In 2003–04 Iain was a Fulbright Visiting Scholar, investigating Healthy Cities evaluations with Professor Duhl at UC Berkeley.

Jodie Doyle is a Research Fellow with Deakin University. She has been the Coordinator of the Cochrane Health Promotion and Public Health Field since 2001. Jodie's interests lie in prioritising and enhancing the use of high-quality systematic reviews of health promotion for public health practitioners and decision-makers.

Len Duhl is a psychiatrist who has specialised in urban planning and is a pioneer in associating urban design with mental health. Considered to be the intellectual father of the Healthy Cities concept, Len Duhl has radically changed thinking about urban health, having written about the concept of sick cities as early as 1952. He published *The Urban Condition: People and Policy* in the Metropolis in 1963. For many years, Len Duhl has been Professor of Public Health and Urban Planning at the School of Public Health, University of California at Berkeley. He is also Chair of the International Healthy Cities Foundation.

Anne Johnson is Associate Professor and Deputy Head (Academic) of the Department of Public Health at Flinders University where she teaches in the Master of Primary Health Care and Doctorate of Public Health. Anne has had a particular interest in consumer participation in health services for many years and has undertaken innovative work and research in this area. Anne was the recipient of the Leadership in Health Promotion award from the Australian Health Promotion Association (SA branch) in 2005.

Nerida Joss is a Research Fellow in the School of Primary Health Care at Monash University and the Health Promotion Adviser for the Department of Veterans' Affairs Victorian office. She is a committee member of the Australian Health Promotion Association. Previously, Nerida has worked in community health. Her work centres on community capacity-building and evaluation with particular interest in the mechanics of intersectoral partnerships and alliances.

Helen Keleher is Professor of Health Sciences and Head of the Department of Health Sciences at Monash University. Helen's research and teaching is focused on how health promotion and health services can better respond to vulnerability and disadvantage, the factors that determine health, and the need for policy and practice in health sciences to promote community engagement and intersectoral working. Her research has resulted in studies on mental health promotion, primary health care, building capacity in the workforce, organisational change, and policy to support equity-focused health promotion. Helen holds an appointment to the Women and Gender Equity Knowledge Network of the World Health Organisation's Commission on the Social Determinants of Health. Helen co-edited the OUP text *Understanding Health: A Determinants Approach* with Berni Murphy.

Paul Laris has a background in social work in metropolitan and rural South Australian health services, and in management, planning, and, most recently, evaluation consultancy. During the early 1990s he worked with the then South Australian Health Commission as Senior Planner and later Manager of the Western and Central Region Planning Unit, playing a key role in developing a collaborative process for involving consumers, providers, and the commission in setting health service development priorities. As Principal Social Planner (1996–97) in the Adelaide office of Hassell Pty Ltd, he focused on social planning and social policy development for public sector human services agencies.

Evelyne de Leeuw has been Professor of Health and Social Development, and Head, School of Health and Social Development at Deakin University, Melbourne since early 2005. She has produced several textbooks on health promotion and health policy, and published over 100 articles.

Ian Lowe is Emeritus Professor of Science, Technology, and Society at Griffith University. He directed the Commission for the Future in 1988 and chaired the advisory council that produced the first national report on the state of the environment in 1996. Among many advisory roles, he is a member of EnHealth Council and the Radiation Health and Safety Advisory Council. He is President of the Australian Conservation Foundation and Vice-President of the Queensland Academy of Arts and Sciences.

Colin MacDougall is Associate Professor and Deputy Head (Research) in the Department of Public Health in the School of Medicine at Flinders University and the public health component of the Graduate Entry Medical Program. He convenes the Doctor of Public Health program and has previously coordinated the Master of Health and International Development, the Master of Primary Health Care, and the PhD programs. He was involved in curriculum development in remote Australia, for clinicians moving into population health, and for the reconstruction of post-apartheid South Africa. Currently, he is involved in research on location and health, and participation of children in health promotion, with particular relevance to the relationship between child development, health and well-being, and control over the environment.

Catherine Mackenzie is a PhD student at the Department of Public Health, Flinders University, South Australia. She is currently working as a Research Associate on an Australian Research Council–funded Gender Analysis Project with the University of Adelaide and Office for Women, South Australian Government.

Mary Mahoney is Senior Lecturer in the School of Health and Social Development at Deakin University's Melbourne campus, and coordinates the Family and Society major in the Health Sciences degree. She joined Deakin in 1996, after working at Bath Spa University College, England, as Course Director of Human Ecology. Mary's research interests are focused on the intersection between policy and the health and well-being of people. Her most recent work has focused on the application of health impact assessment (HIA) to policy development and on aspects of rural health. In 1999, Mary was awarded the Vice Chancellor's Outstanding Achievement Award for Outstanding Teaching at Deakin University.

Berni Murphy has lectured in health promotion at Deakin University since 2000. Her research interests focus around the social determinants of health, strategic communication, and promoting health through sport. Berni is an active consultant in the field, particularly with respect to facilitating the development of integrated health promotion planning frameworks at regional and partnership levels. Berni co-edited the Oxford University Press text *Understanding Health: A Determinants Approach* with Helen Keleher.

Lisel O'Dwyer has been advocating geographical approaches to public health since the late 1990s. Her research interests include relationships between housing and health, and the use of Geographical Information Systems in public health. In the past her research has focused on access to different housing tenures and their implications for wealth creation and the supply dynamics of private rental housing.

Jennie Popay has been Professor of Sociology and Public Health at the Institute for Health Research at Lancaster University since January 2002. Her research interests include social and gender inequalities in health, the sociology of knowledge and the evaluation of complex social interventions. She has used a range of methods in her work but has a particular interest in developing the role of qualitative research in public health. She was previously convenor of the Campbell Collaboration Process Implementation Methods Group and is joint convenor of the Cochrane Collaboration Qualitative Research Methods Group.

Christine Putland is Senior Lecturer in the Department of Public Health at Flinders University in South Australia, where she has worked since 2000, teaching in the Master of Primary Health Care and Professional Doctorate in Public Health. She has a background in policy development and managing community services in local government and non-government organisations, including community arts. Her research interests include a focus on citizen participation, health inequities, and gender in public health. An abiding interest in the role of art in promoting health and well-being stems from her undergraduate studies in drama, and is fuelled by continuing involvement in community-building initiatives that work through art and cultural activities.

Frank Teseriero is a qualified social worker. He is Senior Lecturer and Director, Bachelor of Social Work at the University of South Australia. He has thirty-two years' experience working in primary health care, community health and development work in Australia and in South India. He is currently working on a three-year Myer Foundation-funded Healthy Districts Project in rural South India. His experience in public health includes community development practice, management, research, and teaching.

Elizabeth Waters is Professor of Public Health at Deakin University, a VicHealth Public Health Research Fellow, and Co-Director of the Cochrane Health Promotion and Public Health Field. Her research interests are health inequalities, equity, evidence, and public health. Her research focuses on child health areas of high morbidity and inequality, and related domains of knowledge translation, engagement of community, and cultural competence.

INTRODUCTION

Welcome to *Understanding Health Promotion*! We trust that this book will be a valuable resource for you as you learn about the wonderful world of health promotion. The book draws on the research of the editors and contributors who bring a wealth of experience to the chapters and guidebooks that make up this volume.

Ways to engage with this book will be many and varied. We have drawn on the metaphor of health promotion travel for which you need guides, visas, and advice, for planning, getting around, and where to go for further information. Because no book can cover everything there is to know on any given topic, we have included guidebooks to a wide range of topics to get you started. Richly interspersed with key (take-home) messages, case studies to bring theory to life, exercises, key terms, useful websites, further reading and expert summaries, this book is full of practical information to help you discover health promotion and explore the wonderful resources that are now available to support the work of health promotion practitioners.

In many chapters, contributing authors have provided suggestions for further reading at the end of chapters, together with useful websites. Exercises at the end of each section are designed to assist you in reviewing your learning and understanding.

The guidebooks are intended to assist you in getting the most from your journeys into learning about health promotion. The guidebooks refer to resources available on the Internet, with annotations (notes) that contain descriptions of the important sites, pointing out their context. They refer to information that is not always easily accessible, such as the health promotion professional organisations that you can join. The guidebooks cover various elements of health promotion theory, policy, and practice but, of course, you will find some overlap between the guidebooks and content in the book because health promotion cannot be broken down into component parts. Therefore, we have suggested routes between some chapters and guidebooks to help you navigate your journey. Guidebooks are not meant to be a detailed set of infallible or prescriptive instructions! Keep in mind that Internet sites change their information, some get better, some become dated, so you will need a strategy to keep your own guidebooks (or 'favourite sites') refreshed and up-to-date.

To help you navigate the contents of this book, it is organised into three parts.

PART 1: FOUNDATIONS FOR HEALTH PROMOTION

It is fundamentally important to get the foundations and scaffolding right for health promotion as supports for your development. In Part 1, we lay the foundations for understanding health promotion and, in particular, the implications of the knowledge we have about the social determinants of health. We agree with Milio (1987) that health promotion will work best if it is ecological in perspective, multisectoral in scope, and participatory in strategy. To build the scaffold on this foundation, Part 1 is informed by a synthesis of professional evidence and lay knowledge. Part 1 is supported by four guidebooks:

- Guidebook 1: Milestones in the History of Health Promotion
- Guidebook 2: Health Promotion Associations, Alliances, and Advocacy Organisations
- Guidebook 3: Key Resources about the Socio-economic Determinants of Health
- Guidebook 4: Health Promotion as a Gendering Practice

PART 2: HEALTH PROMOTION PRACTICE

Part 2 covers key practice skills for health promotion: healthy public policy, policy analysis, organisational assessment, health impact assessment, strategic thinking and health promotion program planning and evaluation, engaging communities, communication in collaborative environments, health promotion competencies, and reflective practice. To learn about health promotion, there are many details (the nuts and bolts of health promotion) you need to know, and skills you will need to acquire, so this section is packed with information to assist you. Part 2 is supported by seven guidebooks:

- Guidebook 5: Health Promotion Program Planning and Evaluation Resources
- Guidebook 6: Resources on Health Equity
- Guidebook 7: Capacity-building Resources
- Guidebook 8: Preparing for a Media Interview—Ten-point Checklist
- Guidebook 9: Developing Training, Facilitating, and Presenting Skills
- Guidebook 10: Preparing a Press Release—Ten-point Checklist
- Guidebook 11: Cross-cultural Communication

PART 3: MULTISECTORAL ACTIONS

Part 3 is about actions that promote health from different sectors or parts of our society. Some of the work discussed was in partnership with the health sector directly or indirectly, and some were not, but they all demonstrate contributions to promoting health, well-being, and quality of life. They tackle the determinants of health, and identify core skills for effective health advancement and capacity-building.

We trust this book will help you to understand health promotion and that it is a useful resource for your efforts to 'make a difference' through health promotion.

Helen Keleher, Colin MacDougall, and Berni Murphy

PART 1
FOUNDATIONS FOR HEALTH PROMOTION

Part 1 provides an overview of the foundations of health promotion, its principles and guiding frameworks. Following the Introduction, which sets the scene, Chapter 1 sets out a central premise of this book, which is that health promotion must focus on the fairest and most effective ways to improve health for all people and develop more effective strategies to reduce inequalities. Unless the social causes that undermine people's health are addressed, their opportunities for health, well-being and a good quality of life will not be achieved. Because the drivers for health lie outside the health sector, our health promotion gaze must take in much more than the health sector. Chapter 2 sets out the principles for health promotion laid down by World Health Organisation charters and declarations. Chapter 3 sets out elements of a reframed health promotion that is focused on strengthening health equity. Chapter 4 explains the social and economic factors that drive health and well-being, drawing on the social determinants of health literature. This is linked to Chapter 5, which sets out the principles of a rights approach to health. Together these chapters provide the context for conceptualising health promotion as ecological in perspective, multisectoral in scope, and participatory in strategy (Milio 1987).

When we build our health promotion scaffold on these foundations, we are informed by a synthesis of lay knowledge and professional evidence. Chapter 6 explains why lay knowledge is essential for health promotion to be effective, and then Chapter 7 introduces the concept of evidence-informed health promotion and some of the debates that surround the construction of the evidence base that is emerging to support health promotion.

Part 1 is supported by four guidebooks:

- Guidebook 1: Milestones in the History of Health Promotion
- Guidebook 2: Health Promotion Associations, Alliances, and Advocacy Organisations
- Guidebook 3: Key Resources about the Socio-economic Determinants of Health
- Guidebook 4: Health Promotion as a Gendering Practice

APPROACHING HEALTH PROMOTION

1

Helen Keleher, Colin MacDougall & Berni Murphy

Key concepts

- Health promotion is a wide-ranging endeavour with a distinct base of knowledge and skills.
- Health is a primary pathway towards well-being and quality of life.
- Health may be an end in itself but pursuit of such ends may obscure efforts to address underlying social and economic factors that cause poor health.
- The promotion of human rights and reconciliation, and understanding of the determinants of health, are a necessary foundation of health promotion.

Key terms

- Well-being and quality of life
- Health
- Healthism
- Determinants of health and well-being
- Health promotion

OVERVIEW

This book is about understanding health promotion and its mission—to strengthen communities, populations, and individuals so that they can enjoy health, well-being and a good quality of life as a prerequisite for achieving their potential in other facets of their lives. Health promotion works to support healthy environments while simultaneously creating opportunities for people to learn about the things that affect their health and well-being and what they can do about them. Ultimately, health promotion endeavours are about assisting people to live their lives with dignity, and giving them decent life chances whereby all people are accorded the right to education, to opportunity, to employment, to participation and engagement with the decisions that affect them. These are the tenets of a just society, which is one that genuinely strives to enable all people to live a life that they themselves value. Health promotion endeavours are a mirror for the broad values of rights, respect, equity, and social justice that shape this book. This means that healthy communities, healthy cities, and healthy citizens can only be achieved by taking action on the social determinants of health* in order to achieve these outcomes. Broadly, the social determinants of health are the social conditions in which people live and work, reflecting people's differing position in the social hierarchy, their level of resources, and their control and degree of influence over those conditions (WHO 2005b: 1). Decent and equitable life chances and optimal health are also dependent on good government, principles and practices of democracy, sustainable and stable social systems and environments, as well as a guarantee of human rights.

However, increasing proportions of people find such rights and aspirations to be beyond their reach. Health and social inequities have widened and deepened across countries, intensifying social and economic tensions. Health is sensitive to social environments. As our understanding of social and health inequities has increased, we have learnt why traditional approaches to lifestyle health promotion have not universally succeeded. Indeed, they are thought to have increased health inequalities because they impose middle class values, so only those with education and good access to other resources have taken up health promotion messages and improved their overall health (NSW Health 2004). In other words, health promotion efforts have not benefited all groups and communities and the net effect is a widening of the health gap.

Despite the best intentions of health promoters, the narrowly cast versions of health promotion that are focused on expert-led health education and exhortations for behaviour change are frequently culturally inept, lacking in skills to address the causes of poor health, and lacking in capacity to enhance people's agency. People are too often, the passive participants in programs that have little, if any,

---

* The term 'social determinants of health' is used to refer to and include both social and economic determinants of health.

relevance for them. So much health promotion effort has been invested in risk factors and behaviour-change propaganda and so little on the causes of health and social problems from which risk behaviours arise. If communities are suffering from lack of employment and education opportunities, limited access to transport and services, and health-challenging environments, then people's priority for health promotion investment is not likely to be a focus on the usual soft-target culprits of obesity, physical activity, or reduction of smoking rates (Syme 2003). One of the ethical principles guiding health is to 'do no harm', so it is beholden of health promotion practitioners to ensure that their work does not do harm by ignoring people's realities or their need for agency in their own lives.

For example, the deeply entrenched colonialist history of Australia has had profound consequences for Aboriginal Australians. The lack of acknowledgment by white Australia of past injustices towards Aboriginal people is part of the story about the causes of their poor health (Thomson 2003). Australia is shamed by the ongoing failure of governments and services to invest in Aboriginal health and recognise the fundamental rights of Aboriginal people to self-determination, the right to learn about, practise and protect culture, the right to control education, health and social services, and to shape opportunities through the control of those resources. But health promotion has also been part of that story—especially when health promotion is devoid of recognition of culture and fails to recognise Aboriginal people's knowledge and wisdom. This is apparent in the repeated attempts to deliver heath education and behaviour-change programs that have been developed through middle Australia white man's [sic] eyes (Tilmouth 2006). The starting point for health promotion needs to be in the causes, which are much further back than those soft-target culprits of lifestyle and behaviours.

Health promotion must therefore turn its gaze to enabling people and communities to take control over those factors (or determinants) that affect their health and well-being or decisions that have health and well-being consequences. The rising incidence of mental health disorders, unhealthy substance use, the effects of decades of violence particularly against women and children, an ageing demographic, and increasing levels of complex chronic illnesses mean that in health terms we live in times that demand new ways of working, in order to find new solutions to what are becoming entrenched problems. More unequal societies have higher rates of violence and discrimination, lower levels of civic trust and involvement in community life (Berkman & Kawachi 2000). These conditions are strong indicators of the need to rethink how health promotion should operate, in order to create health, well-being and quality of life.

This book is designed to introduce you to health promotion working across societal infrastructure and diverse populations, to make strategic choices about where to direct your efforts, how to work at some of the many levels of health promotion, and to use evidence effectively to support your practice. We encourage you to reflect on the values and assumptions inherent in health promotion— including your own and those of the people with whom you work.

UNDERSTANDING HEALTH AND HEALTH PROMOTION

The content of this book assumes that you have a basic grasp of the determinants of health. Our previous book, *Understanding Health: A Determinants Approach* (Keleher & Murphy 2004), explored the emerging evidence about the extent to which health is socially determined. Seeing health through the 'lens' of its determinants is central to our understanding of how health, well-being and quality of life are created and sustained, founded on the understanding that the drivers for health lie in broader society, and frequently outside the health sector.

The foundations of health are recognised as peace, shelter, adequate economic resources, adequate food, a stable ecosystem and sustainable resource use (WHO 1978; Nutbeam 1998). There are many and varied definitions of health, with no single definition of health that is right for all programs or purposes. Statements of understanding about health must be developed for particular contexts so that they are meaningful for the context, situation, and people involved.

Of course, there are some definitions of health available that are consistent with the ideas of this book. This understanding of health from the WHO is clear about the right to good health:

> The enjoyment of the highest attainable standard of health is one of the fundamental rights of every human being without discrimination (WHO 2005).

Another explanation of health is from the WHO (1986), says that:

> Health is a resource for everyday life, not the object of living. It is a positive concept emphasizing social and personal resources as well as physical capabilities.

Optimal health is a balance of physical, emotional/mental, social, and spiritual well-being. Health Canada (2002) defines health more in terms of outcomes:

> Health is a capacity or resource which corresponds more to the notion of being able to pursue one's goals, to acquire skills and education and to grow—and to be able to respond to life's challenges and changes.

The National Aboriginal Health Strategy (NAHS 1989) sets out the philosophy of Aboriginal community control and the holistic view of health that this entails:

> Aboriginal health is not just the physical well being of an individual but is the social, emotional and cultural well being of the whole community in which each individual is able to achieve their full potential thereby bringing about the total well being of their community. It is a whole-of-life view and includes the cyclical concept of life-death-life.

This definition indicates that Aboriginal health is about identity tied to community, culture, and land, which is not separable from community and individual well-being. You will notice important differences between the NAHS understanding of health and the one put forward by the WHO. While the WHO definition is widely used, it is not the preferred definition of Aboriginal people. It is therefore critical for health promotion practitioners to understand the concept of health embodied by those they work with—whether a community (for example an Aboriginal community) or an organisation. A concept of health can be refined or changed to guide the development of a project or program but it must always be culturally appropriate and agreed by stakeholders. It should also be sufficiently broad to enable the use of various health promotion approaches.

Health promotion practitioners will find it useful to be able to identify different definitions of health that are used to influence the direction of health promotion practice. Use of a critical perspective can explain the purpose of using particular definitions of health. Learn to examine definitions of health against criteria such as:

- orientation to the individual or to populations
- a silo approach to disease or a recognition of the influence of the socio-economic determinants on health
- a predominant biological or behavioural approach or socio-ecological approach
- the approaches to practice implied by the definition.

In other words, how the causes of problems are understood will lead to different ways of understanding them, which in turn lead to the approaches, strategies, and actions that will be taken to address the problem. Conceptual confusion about definitions and understandings of health will lead to sloppy practice. Health promotion definitions do impose values (Tesh 1988; Raphael 2002). For example, an exclusively biomedical or behaviourist orientation towards health will limit the scope of health promotion, and exclude actions that are designed to influence the social determinants of health. In contrast, an approach that is underpinned by an understanding of the social determinants of health can inform and enhance biomedical and behaviourist approaches (Baum 2002; Syme 2003). Whether health promotion is about improving management of illness, or helping people to cope with social conditions, or about changing social conditions, are key value-driven questions for people engaging in health promotion (Raphael 2002).

A key point here is that people in the health sector have a tendency to construct definitions of health that make sense to them, but not to others. It is as if you are travelling to another country that does not have the same currency. Lots of organisations and collaborations are working to create more just, more equal, stable, more democratic, stronger, and healthier communities. These are highly valued ends that, incidentally, are the same ends as good health. It is highly likely that the principal goal of such work is not expressed in terms of health does not have to be, and nor should health promoters try to make it so. For you to get your travel documents approved to work alongside sectors outside your own, you need their approval and an entry visa—make sure that you show appreciation for how they work and of their culture(s), and a willingness to listen and learn from their wisdom and experiences.

The alternative is to try to convert other countries to your language, customs, and currencies—which is known in politics as imperialism. The health equivalent of this is 'healthism', a term that refers to the questionable assumption that everyone should work and live to maximise their health (Metcalfe 1993), an orientation which can recast health as a moral value (Peterson 1994). In practice this could have health promotion practitioners asking everyone else to rewrite and reframe their agenda in terms of health. Robertson and Minkler (1994: 297–299) express the means–end debate very nicely:

> Should the goal be improved health status (individual and collective)–health as an end? Or should the goal be social justice—health as a means? If health becomes the analytical lens through which all social issues are seen, it may dilute and obfuscate not only health related efforts but other social and political efforts as well.

In other words, health promotion gets caught between the means–ends debates. Labonte and Laverack (2001a) point out Sen's (1999) explanation of the difference between constitutive and instrumental elements of human development.

> Constitutive elements are ends in themselves. They may function instrumentally to achieve other goals but this is where politically charged confusion begins to arise. A popular defense of early childhood development programs that improve educational attainment is that they increase labour market participation which then increases income which then increases lifetime health expectancy and which, as a whole, may increase economic growth … [an] instrumental pathway, in which economic growth is positioned as the ultimate goal … Sen would argue it is inconsequential to the defence of healthy childhood development and educational attainment, and the increased human agency this brings, as constitutive ends of human development itself, regardless of their distal effects on economic development (Labonte & Laverack 2001a: 111–12).

Nonetheless, health is essential to the overcoming of other social disadvantages (Braverman & Gruskin 2002). Seeing health through a social determinants of health 'lens' leads towards understanding its ends, which are about human agency, social justice, and community well-being.

Definitions of health promotion, then, need to be consistent with the values and principles of definitions and understandings of health. The Ottawa Charter for Health Promotion (WHO 1986) definition of health promotion has stood the test of time:

> Health promotion is the process of enabling people to increase the control over, and to improve, their health.

The key word here is 'process'—health promotion is a process of enablement and empowerment for which the Ottawa Charter provides an empowering discourse. If actions are not enabling and empowering, then they are not health promotion (Macdonald & Davies 1998). These concepts are discussed in more detail in Chapters 2 and 3. However, there are significant differences of opinion about the strategies and research methods for health promotion—differences that run deeper than technical nuances over the best way to achieve a mutually agreed goal. These differences reflect deep-seated beliefs and values about health—as a means or an end, which is reflected in understandings of health, technical approaches to health promotion, and the way we go about planning, conducting, and evaluating health promotion strategies.

EVIDENCE FOR HEALTH PROMOTION

Interest in health promotion evidence is rapidly increasing in response to demands by funding bodies for health promotion to increase its effectiveness. There is an associated need to build evidence about what works in health promotion, from the perspective of the social determinants of health, to guide practitioners and decision-makers. Health promotion needs a strong and easily accessible evidence base about the most effective health promotion approaches to influence the social determinants of health (Raphael 2002). Health promotion evidence has been primarily focused on health promotion coming out of the health sector and on broad public health issues such as prevention of cardiovascular disease, diabetes, or smoking, which are likely to have only limited success in improving health and well-being, particularly among people living in difficult circumstances.

It is clear that we have to derive ways of working across health promotion approaches and with a wide range of sectors (Syme 2003) so that actions are set up in a determinants framework, and with sound evaluation about 'what works' in reducing the negative impacts of one or more of the determinants of the issue—whether health, social, or environmental. For example, tobacco policy, transport policy, child care, and employment are all determinants of health. Health promotion practitioners therefore need to evaluate interventions such as local strategies to increase affordable child care, or access to affordable public transport, and not just evaluate those programs that are based on disease. Local child care, and access to public transport, and tobacco policy are important for local communities, and even though they are driven by sectors outside health, their impact is on the same people who have, or are at risk of, cardiovascular disease, for example. Child care is a determinant of employment opportunities, particularly for mothers. Transport is a determinant of access to health and social services, as well as employment. Tobacco policy is essential for minimising the harms associated with smoking rates, particularly among the young.

There is, therefore, a need to share the evidence about the determinants with other sectors, work with them to develop strong partnerships and collaborative ways of working to find evidence about how the determinants of health are played out at local levels, and disseminate the findings effectively. We suggest that health promoters need three levels of knowledge:

- interactively derived knowledge (from sharing lived experiences)
- critical knowledge—derived from reflection and action on what is right and just, raising consciousness about the causes of problems and what would alleviate them
- instrumental knowledge—drawn from scientific and technical approaches (Raphael 2002).

You will find that these three types of knowledge are developed consistently through this book. A more formal discussion of health promotion evidence is explored in Chapter 7, but is a recurring theme throughout.

VALUES

Health promotion is a movement with a strong values base, and references to values are made throughout this book. Of course, no bunch of editors and authors can or should impose their values on others so it is not our intention to be prescriptive about what health promotion values you should espouse. It is critical that health promotion practitioners are aware of their own values and those of the discipline(s) to which they belong, and of their organisations, of colleagues, and especially of those with whom they work in health promotion. Exploring our own values and understanding the purposes of health promotion is part of the process of building a better world.

Australia is a diverse population with many Aboriginal cultures and more than 140 new cultural groups who have arrived in the last 100 years, all of whom have strongly held values. Therefore, we are prepared to say that core values for every health promotion practitioner are respect for the values of others, respect for their rights, and a desire for social justice and equity across all groups that make up our population. Equity is explained and discussed further in Chapter 4, while Chapter 5 explains human rights in relation to health and health promotion.

A useful (brief) definition of social justice is 'a vision of society where rules are just and fair and resources are shared equitably among the members of the community, in the interests of the common good' (Health Promotion Forum of New Zealand 2000). Social justice will, of course, be understood and defined in different ways by different population groups and societies. For organisations working with Aboriginal Australians, a good understanding of the principles of self-determination and reconciliation with Australia's Aboriginal people are also necessary (see NACCHO: <www.naccho.org.au/>).

The failure of traditional approaches to health promotion to engage with Aboriginal health issues suggests that deeper value systems within health promotion and the health system require critical reflection. Having good intentions and being well-meaning are not a sufficient value base on which to build the promotion of health with Aboriginal Australians or Australians from diverse ethnic backgrounds. So much of health promotion is based on a traditional medical model that is expert-led, focused on behaviours, planned through the dominant culture ('white-man's eyes' [sic]), and is lacking in respect for Aboriginal cultures. These practices can promote oppression and inequity. Values about who defines the problems and needs, rights, the role of communities, roles of individuals in those communities, the sources of knowledge, the place of professionals as a resource not an expert, the sharing of responsibility, and acknowledgement of history need to be explored by professionals involved in health promotion. Knowledge does not result from experts infusing others with their information. Knowledge comes from individuals, groups, and communities working together to understand the social influences that affect their lives (Patterson 2006).

Both cultural imperialism and healthism are destructive forces for health promotion and are often fatal in their effect—communities, individuals, and organisations become understandably hostile to the efforts of perhaps well-meaning practitioners who are not sensitive to their own values base and come across as both ignorant and lacking in respect of the values of others.

THE APPROACH OF THIS BOOK

Health promotion is multifaceted, so practitioners need to be able to work with complexity, and that requires a diverse skill set. As health promotion evolves, there are imperatives to advance the knowledge, understanding, and skill base of health promotion in the pursuit of more effective health promotion actions. The extent to which health promotion should be positioned in the health sector, or whether it should be diffused through a range of other sectors, is a central question for the health promotion movement. Health promotion may be characterised as either as attempting to direct traffic from the centre of an intersection of complex intersectoral activities, or as a partner in the mobilising of activities aimed at improving health alongside a range of sectors such as justice, community arts, local government, education, the environment, and a host of others. These different but nonetheless critical characterisations are central to this book.

Effective health promotion practitioners can work across models and approaches, using critical reflection to draw on the best features of each and to reach and engage those with whom the work is being done. Improving population health is not as simple as fixing a broken leg, and the more we know about population health, the less anyone can do in isolation from other strategies. Health promotion work is about doing the right thing, based on good process, with sound values, and necessarily involves engaging people in those processes. This is understood as people-centred health promotion practice (Springett 2001).

In preparing this book, we acknowledge that our readership comes from many disciplines with a variety of perspectives and existing knowledge, beliefs, and practices. In the health sector, many practitioners may be required to work primarily within a biomedical model. In the community arts sector, there will be a strong focus on arts practice and community development, and so on. We seek to increase your desire to explore and consider health promotion practices in new ways. In this book, we are reframing health promotion as grounded in practices that address the social determinants of health. By taking them in to account wherever possible, practitioners will be enabling more effective and sustainable change. And by integrating health and well-being outcomes into the work of community arts or sport, for example, the programs themselves are able to demonstrate their contribution not just to health and well-being but also to the higher order issues of tackling inequities and social justice. The mental health promotion outcomes of a Women's Circus, established for women who have experienced extreme forms of violence, and a sports participation program for young sole mothers, which has a focus on social connectedness and inclusion, are examples of health promotion practice that seeks to influence determinants of health. Such projects are responding to the unambiguous evidence about the need for broadened conceptions of health, wellness, and quality of life and the evidence that in order to make a difference, our programs must tackle the determinants of health and incorporate equity approaches.

This book is for a variety of audiences including:

■ experienced and budding practitioners from a wide range of disciplines that contribute to rights, community practice, health, well-being and quality of life
■ lifelong learners, including those taking up postgraduate study or professional development courses, taking up the challenges of change and innovation
■ policy-makers and managers who wish to increase their understanding of the changing landscape in which the work of health advancement is conceived and developed in order to plan and manage services
■ academics, teachers, and students in any course concerned with health, well-being and quality of life.

Many books have been written about health promotion. It is not the intention of this book to repeat or restate all theories, models, and approaches to health promotion, as no single book can cover the literature on the myriad content that has developed in the twenty years since the Ottawa Charter for Health Promotion (WHO 1986). Some of that content is outdated and we see little point in reviewing it. Other material is narrowly cast, from our perspective, and has little in common with the intentions of this book. For example, lifestyle theories from behaviourist approaches and social marketing are not covered in this book. Nonetheless, our approaches in this book are extremely relevant for lifestyle health promotion in order to reframe from individualism to more integrated conceptions of people, their social environments, and well-being and for incorporation of lay understandings of health and well-being.

This is not to dismiss medical and behaviourist approaches to the promotion of health. For someone who has had a health crisis, there are excellent opportunities for one-to-one health education. But will that form of health promotion change the health of populations and address underlying causal pathways to the health issue? The answer is 'no'. And no matter how good you are at that type of intervention, the answer will always be 'no'. It might be a good thing to do for the individual at the time, but it will not make a difference in the long term, or at the population level (Syme 2003).

At the behavioural level, it is very attractive to believe that interventions to change risky behaviours in particular groups will make a difference. Sadly, the evidence doesn't support this—it would be terrific if this were the case because health promotion would be much easier than the social determinants-focused health promotion for which we argue in this book. Our stance is that medical and behavioural approaches have their place and can contribute to the health jigsaw if, and only if, health promotion is driven by actions that reflect an understanding of the power of social determinants. Social determinants work directly on well-being and quality of life. They do not have to be mediated by behaviours, risk factors, or lifestyle (see Chapter 22 on physical activity for example). Health professionals do have very important roles to play in facilitating decision-making for behaviour change, but one of the premises of this book is that behaviourist and lifestyle health promotion need to be reframed through the lens of the social determinants of the lifestyle issues of concern.

SUMMARY

The values we hold about people, their history, their present, and their future are critical for how we approach our work in partnership with them. Effective health promotion is driven by principles and actions that are designed to allow people to take control over the determinants of their health—to facilitate learning, to overcome powerlessness and tackle the social and structural barriers to good health. Unhealthy behaviours reflect deep structural inequities, which is why health promotion must be essentially a social and political process.

2 HEALTH PROMOTION PRINCIPLES

Helen Keleher

Key concepts

- Health promotion is a global movement supported by World Health Organisation charters.
- The principles derived from those charters are a solid guide to health promotion practices.
- Health promotion has narrowed its focus from the WHO charters but a stronger focus on equity-driven health promotion and a reframing from health education and behaviour change to socio-ecological models are both necessary and well overdue.
- The values that underpin health promotion actions and the processes used are as important as the actions themselves.

Key terms

- Health promotion
- Health promotion principles
- Health promotion approaches and models

OVERVIEW

This chapter discusses the core principles of health promotion from the World Health Organisation Charters for Health Promotion. The range of health promotion approaches are outlined, and key practices explored and illustrated in relation to real-world issues. The value base outlined in Chapter 1 provides the context for this chapter. Those values include equity and the socio-economic determinants of health, respect for all those with whom we work and their cultures, a rights framework, and reconciliation with Aboriginal and Torres Strait Islander people. Because the determinants of health primarily lie outside the health sector, partnerships and collaborations that are essential for community practice and multisector working are explained as core skills for health promotion practitioners. Consistent with the philosophy of this book, my intention in this chapter is to facilitate your learning rather than trying to cover everything there is to know about health promotion, so this chapter is supported by two guidebooks (see the end of Part 1):

- Guidebook 1: Milestones in the History of Health Promotion
- Guidebook 2: Health Promotion Associations, Alliances, and Advocacy Organisations

In addition, you will find that health promotion is supported by an enormous knowledge base, with published literature in books, journals, reports, and websites. This chapter and the guidebooks will enable you, as a learner, to engage with the discipline of health promotion, and to develop your own professional growth and capabilities.

DEFINING HEALTH PROMOTION

The achievement of good health is becoming increasingly precarious for growing numbers of people amid changing and unpredictable environments. Health promotion is a field that has the potential to support and sustain better health but that potential is dependent on the approaches taken in programs and their theoretical foundations, and clear understanding of the intentions and outcomes of those programs. Explicit explanations of the values base of approaches, theories, and programs are necessary for clear statements of vision and purpose, to guide the direction and implementation of health promotion. Social justice and strategies to address inequities can only be achieved through sustained advocacy and the genuine participation and engagement of people and their communities, and other stakeholders.

Numerous definitions of health promotion are available, but the Ottawa Charter definition is now a classic:

> Health promotion is the process of enabling people to increase control over, and to improve, their health. To reach a state of complete physical, mental and

social wellbeing, an individual or group must be able to identify and to realise aspirations, to satisfy needs, and to change or cope with the environment. Health is, therefore, seen as a resource for everyday life, not the objective of living. Health is a positive concept emphasising social and personal resources, as well as physical capacities. Therefore, health promotion is not just the responsibility of the health sector, but goes beyond healthy life-styles to wellbeing (World Health Organisation 1986).

More recently, health promotion is understood in terms of determinants of health, as Nutbeam (1998: 1–2) explains:

Health promotion represents a comprehensive social and political process, it not only embraces actions directed at strengthening the skills and capabilities of individuals, but also action directed towards changing social, environmental and economic conditions so as to alleviate their impact on public and individual health. Health promotion is the process of enabling people to take control over the determinants of their health and thereby improve their health.

Health promotion has many levels so the concept of health promotion represents both social and political processes and is understood in terms of both art and science. Contemporary health promotion places emphasis on social change, environmental development, development of capacities and opportunities for communities, and behaviour change of individuals, organisations, and society.

For people to take control of the factors and determinants of their health, health promotion practitioners need to use methods consistent with rights and empowerment.

Empowerment is an ethic that arises from the Ottawa Charter concept of 'enabling'. In other words, health promotion is about assisting people to take control of the factors influencing their health; and for that to be possible practitioners need a solid understanding of people's experiences of everyday life, of the social factors that contribute to those experiences, including the systemic influences. For example, a systemic influence on the incidence of sexually transmitted infections is the quality and dissemination of sexual and reproductive health programs for young people, and social factors include attitudes towards, and the use of, condoms.

Alongside determinants of health approaches, health promotion practitioners are increasingly aware of the need for strategies that have an equity focus. To achieve this, health promotion is based upon principles of:

- Equity and the redress of inequity
- Respect for culture and rights to self-determination
- Social change
- Physical and environmental change
- Policy development
- Empowerment
- Community participation and active community engagement

■ Accountability
■ Building of capacity for partnerships, collaborations, and alliances between organisations, sectors, and groups.

Health promotion is a core strategy for health development, which is the process of continuous, progressive improvement of the social and health status of populations and communities (WHO 1998). The foundations of health development were first laid out in the Declaration of Alma Ata for Primary Health Care (WHO 1978). Several of Australia's Indigenous people were part of the Alma Ata conference in Russia, to contribute their experience and knowledge about health development and the prerequisites for health.

That Declaration articulates the essential prerequisites for health as peace, shelter, education, food, income, a stable ecosystem, sustainable resources, social justice, social and economic support, safety from violence, and reliable, affordable food supplies. This is the basis of the social model of health, whereby health is understood as contingent on, and emerging from, social conditions and environments. The social model of health is based on understandings that in order for health gain to occur, people's basic needs must first be met (WHO 1978). Health promotion must be practised from these understandings.

The concept of health promotion was conceived and articulated in World Health Organisation Charters for Health Promotion, beginning with the First Global Conference on Health Promotion held in Ottawa in 1986. The strategic intent of the five principles of the Ottawa Charter (WHO 1986) is to mobilise action for health development, and provide key action domains to improve health outcomes for individuals, communities, and wider populations. The charter conceptualises health as:

■ a fundamental right
■ both an individual and collective responsibility
■ an opportunity that should be equally available
■ an essential element of social and economic development.

Based on these understandings of health, the Ottawa Charter conceptualises health promotion in terms of health development and expresses the need for health promotion to positively address the social, economic, environmental, and political determinants that support health development.

PRINCIPLES AND PRACTICES OF HEALTH PROMOTION

Guidebook 1, Milestones in the History of Health Promotion, sets out the pioneering events in health promotion history that have shaped the principles of contemporary health promotion. Understanding the history of the health promotion movement assists in understanding what directions are being taken and why. Box 2.1 details ten major health promotion action areas that are widely used to guide policy and

Box 2.1: Ten health promotion action areas

The prerequisites of health in the Ottawa Charter (WHO 1986) are reiterated from the Alma Ata Declaration for Primary Health Care (WHO 1978) as peace, shelter, education, food, income, a stable ecosystem, sustainable resources, social justice, and equity. From this foundation of prerequisites for health, the following five action areas were put forward by the Ottawa Charter.

1 Build healthy public policy

Health promotion goes beyond health care. It puts health on the agenda of policy-makers in all sectors and at all levels, directing them to be aware of the health consequences of their decisions and to accept their responsibilities for health. Healthy public policy combines diverse but complementary approaches, including legislation, fiscal measures, taxation, and organisational change. Healthy public policy is coordinated action that leads to health, income, and social policies that foster greater equity. Joint action is necessary to ensure safer and healthier goods and services, healthier public services, and cleaner and more enjoyable environments. Health promotion policy requires the identification of obstacles to the adoption of healthy public policies across all sectors and ways of removing those obstacles. The aim must be to make the healthier choice the easier choice for people and for policy-makers as well.

2 Create supportive environments

Any health promotion strategy must address the protection of the natural and built environments and the conservation of natural resources. The inextricable links between people and their environment constitute the basis for a socio-ecological approach to health. The overall guiding principle for the world, nations, regions, and communities alike is the need to encourage reciprocal maintenance—that is, to take care of each other, our communities, and our natural environment. The conservation of natural resources throughout the world should be emphasised as a global responsibility. Changing patterns of life, work, and leisure have a significant impact on health. Work and leisure should be a source of health for people. And the way in which society organises work should help create a healthy society. Health promotion generates living and working conditions that are safe, stimulating, satisfying, and enjoyable. Therefore, systematic assessment of the health impacts of rapidly changing environments, particularly in areas of technology, work, energy production, and urbanisation, is essential and must be followed by action to ensure a positive benefit to public health.

3   Strengthen community action

Health promotion works through concrete and effective community action in setting priorities, making decisions, planning strategies and implementing them to achieve better health. At the heart of this process is the empowerment of communities, whereby all people are enabled to own and control their own endeavours and destinies. Community development draws on existing human and material resources in the community to enhance self-help and social support, and to develop flexible systems for strengthening public participation and direction of health matters. This process requires full and continual access to information, learning opportunities for health, and funding support.

4   Develop personal skills

Health promotion supports personal and social development of people and communities by providing information, educating about health and enhancing life skills. By doing so, it increases the options available to people to exercise more control over their own health and environments, and to make choices conducive to health. Enabling people to learn throughout life, to prepare themselves for all of its stages and to cope with chronic illness and injuries, is essential. This enablement has to be facilitated in school, home, work, and community settings. Action is required through educational, professional, commercial, and voluntary bodies, and within institutions.

5   Reorient health services towards primary health care

Individuals, community groups, health professionals, health service institutions, and governments share the responsibility for health promotion in health services. They must work together towards a health care system that contributes to the pursuit of health. The role of the health sector must move increasingly in a health promotion direction, beyond its responsibility for providing clinical and curative services. Health services also need to embrace an expanded mandate that is sensitive and respects cultural needs. This mandate should support the needs of individuals and communities for a healthier life, and open channels between the health sector and broader social, political, economic, and physical environments.

Then in the 1990s, the Jakarta Declaration (WHO 1997) added five more action areas to the Ottawa Charter to further strengthen the work of health promotion.

6   Promote social responsibility for health

Policies and practices should be pursued that: avoid harming the health of other individuals; protect the environment and ensure sustainable use of resources; restrict production and trade in inherently harmful goods and substances; safeguard both the citizen in the marketplace and the individual in the workplace; and include equity-focused health impact assessments as an integral part of policy development.

7 Increase investments for health development to address health and social inequities

Increasing investment for health development requires a truly multisectoral approach, including additional resources for education and housing as well as the health sector. Investments for health should reflect the need to address health and social inequities, focusing on groups such as women, children, older people, Indigenous people, those in poverty, and marginalised populations.

8 Consolidate and expand partnerships for health

Health promotion requires health and social development partnerships among the different sectors at all levels of governance and society. Existing partnerships need to be strengthened and the potential for new partnerships must be explored. Partnerships offer mutual benefit for health through the sharing of expertise, skills, and resources.

9 Strengthen communities and increase community capacity to empower the individual

Key strategies at a community level are:

- strengthening advocacy through community action, particularly through groups organised by women
- enabling communities and individuals to take control over their health and environment through education and empowerment
- building alliances for health and supportive environments to strengthen the cooperation between health and environmental campaigns and strategies
- mediating between conflicting interests in society to ensure equitable access to supportive environments for health
- improving the capacity of communities for health promotion, which requires practical education, leadership training, and access to resources
- empowering individuals, which demands more consistent, reliable access to the decision-making process and the skills and knowledge essential to effect change
- reorienting health services, which requires stronger attention to health research and changes in professional education and training. This must lead to a change of attitude and organisation of health services, refocusing on the total needs of the individual as a whole person.

10   Secure an infrastructure for health promotion

Governments are the stewards of the health of populations. They have a responsibility to establish a strong infrastructure for public health that includes a funded commitment to health promotion. 'Settings for health' represent the organisational base of the infrastructure required for health promotion. New health challenges mean that health and non-health organisations need to be able to respond effectively, so new and diverse networks need to be created to achieve multisectoral collaboration. Training in, and practice of, local leadership skills should be encouraged to support health promotion activities.

practice, and which have arisen from two of those milestone events: the Ottawa Charter for Health Promotion and the Jakarta Declaration on Health Promotion.

The early twenty-first century of health promotion is being guided by the charters of both Ottawa and Jakarta as well as the more recent Bangkok Charter (WHO 2005). This newest Charter for Health Promotion reiterates efforts to increase the effectiveness of health promotion by affirming the place of health promotion in global development, and the ongoing need to tackle threats to health from trade, products, and services, and marketing practices. This indicates the importance of a wider social development agenda that is necessary to achieve social justice and equity underpinning health promotion. That agenda is about:

- redistributive justice to overcome unfairness in the distribution of resources
- acknowledgment and action to ensure rights to health
- reconciliation with Indigenous people
- achievement of equity of access to appropriate health care for all to reduce or eliminate factors that are unavoidable or unfair.

These agendas require greater alignment across health and social policy than has been addressed to date, so opportunities to promote good health really do sit alongside efforts to reduce health differentials (see Chapter 4) to the lowest levels possible. In other words, partnerships between health promotion policy and social policy are necessary to address health inequities.

An equity-focused approach to health promotion recognises that the social, environmental, and economic determinants of health are necessary foundations for practice, and it follows that understanding and knowledge of the social determinants of health among populations underpins the ability of government, organisations, and their programs to deliver effective health promotion. The tying together of equity and health promotion is integral to the reduction of health inequities, as is the need for policy and practice to be both intersectoral and multidisciplinary (Health Inequalities Research Collaboration 2002). The value base of the Declaration of Primary Health Care (WHO 1978) and the WHO Charters for Health Promotion (WHO 1986, 1997, 2000, 2005) are clear that

Box 2.2: The Mexico Statement (WHO 2000)

The participants in this conference pledge:

- to move into the arena of healthy public policy, and to advocate a clear political commitment to health and equity in all sectors
- to counteract the pressures towards harmful products, resource depletion, unhealthy living conditions and environments, and bad nutrition; and to focus attention on public health issues such as pollution, occupational hazards, housing, and settlements
- to respond to the health gap within and between societies, and to tackle the inequities in health produced by the rules and practices of these societies
- to acknowledge people as the main health resource; to support and enable them to keep themselves, their families and friends healthy through financial and other means, and to accept the community as the essential voice in matters of its health, living conditions, and well-being
- to reorient health services and their resources towards the promotion of health; and to share power with other sectors, other disciplines and, most importantly, with people themselves
- to recognise health and its maintenance as a major social investment and challenge; and to address the overall ecological issue of our ways of living.

The Conference urges all concerned to join them in their commitment to a strong public health alliance.

success in health promotion is dependent on a reframing of health promotion from lifestyle and behavioural strategies towards social and health development.

PUBLIC HEALTH AND HEALTH PROMOTION

You will notice that health promotion documents often refer to public health concepts and frameworks. Public health is about the prevention of disease or injury from occurring or recurring, the promotion of health, and the restoration of health to populations and communities following health breakdown such as occurs following natural or man-made disasters. Public health fields include epidemiology, biostatistics, health economics, policy, population health, environmental health, and health promotion. The wider field of public health focuses on populations at greatest risk of disease or injury, and aims to preserve, promote, and improve health across whole populations. Key steps in designing a public health response to any threat to well-being include:

- defining and monitoring the extent of the problem
- identifying the causes of the problem
- formulating and testing ways of dealing with the problem
- applying widely the measures that are found to work.

In the design and implementation of large community interventions, there is often overlap of public health and health promotion strategies and approaches. For example, public health methods may be used to develop the research to establish the problem and understand its significance, and then health promotion approaches (such as community/health development) and strategies such as social marketing (media campaigns), health education, skills training, organisational change (schools, workplaces), and policy development will be developed and implemented. Health promotion methods will be used particularly to measure process and impact of individual or perhaps a mix of interventions but for large multilevel programs, public health research designs may be used to measure the effectiveness of the overall community intervention.

Public health interventions are often described in three levels explained in the following, which are illustrated using examples:

- **Universal interventions**—approaches aimed at large groups or the general population, and often focused on risk factors. Examples might include violence prevention curricula delivered to all pupils in a school or community-wide media campaigns such as quit smoking.
- **Selected or targeted interventions**—approaches aimed at those considered to be at a heightened risk of perpetrating violence (having one or more risk factors for violence). An example of such an intervention is parenting skills training provided to low-income single parents (AIC 2003). Selected or targeted interventions usually pay attention to social, economic, and environmental factors and may include strategies to increase access to services (NSW Health 2004).
- **Indicated interventions**—approaches aimed at those who have a demonstrated problem. Examples are programs for perpetrators of domestic violence, or specifically for people with unstable diabetes or other chronic illnesses. Generally, indicated interventions are more downstream than selected or universal interventions.

Understanding the relationship and intersections between health promotion and public health policies, approaches, and levels of interventions is a core skill for health promotion practitioners.

CORE PRACTICES

A core skill for all health promotion practitioners is to turn concepts and strategies into practical actions that are effective in creating change and tackling inequity. This may seem a challenging task, so in order to help health promotion practitioners understand how to make it happen, the Ottawa Charter set out three foundation practices that are just as relevant today as they were in 1986: *advocacy*, *enabling*, and *mediating*:

■ **Advocacy in health promotion** is the process of defending or promoting a cause. It involves active participation in public debate and activity to gain political commitment, social acceptance, and policy support for a particular issue or change (Health Promotion Forum of New Zealand 2000). Advocacy is also a combination of individual and social actions designed to gain political commitment, policy support, social acceptance, and systems support for a particular health goal or program (WHO 1998). In other words, health promotion advocacy aims at making conditions favourable for health, which is a core responsibility of all health professionals.

■ **Enabling in health promotion**: Enabling means that health promotion practitioners take action in partnership with individuals or groups with the intention of empowerment. This will require the mobilisation of human and material resources (WHO 1998) and, very often, encompasses facilitation skills such as the facilitation of learning or skill development in others. Health promotion practitioners are catalysts for the development of appropriate health resources in the community, and assisting people to increase their health knowledge and skills. Practitioners enable access to political processes that shape public policies affecting people's health; they assist people to identify the determinants of their own health; and to identify actions through partnerships to increase health, and improve the conditions for health.

■ **Mediating in health promotion** is the process through which competing interests are reconciled in ways that promote and protect health (WHO 1998). Competing interests include personal, social, political, and economic interests, in the pursuit of better health outcomes for individuals, communities, and populations.

COMMUNITIES AND 'TARGETING'

We keep talking about communities, but what is a community? Is there a community of people that health promotion should target? First, let us debunk the notion of targeting—it is a personal preference but we prefer to not use the language of targeting in relation to people because it carries connotations of guns and war, as well as suggesting that we are doing something to people who are embattled or besieged. We can (and do) target things but not people because it is antithetical to the language and intentions of health promotion. We prefer to work *with* people and not direct things at them or try to do things to them, like change their behaviours or empower them, because people can only do those things for themselves. Health promotion folk are facilitators of change, activists, and advocates but should always work alongside people in their community. So are there communities of low income earners, or communities of young mums, or isolated elderly, or people with disabilities? Perhaps, but people are only a community if they have a shared identity (Labonte 1997: 30). As Labonte explains, when people come together to share their own reality, they are 'empowering themselves to act more effectively upon it' (Labonte 1997: 30). This is about shared consciousness, a feeling of belonging that carries with it trust and bonds of shared experience. Knowledge alone is insufficient for health or social change—people need to feel that the conditions of their lives can also be changed so that those conditions are enabling and supportive of their goals. Empowerment in health promotion is discussed in more detail in Chapter 10.

HEALTH PROMOTION APPROACHES AND MODELS

Health promotion approaches range from those grounded in a primary care paradigm such as health counselling and health education towards community-based practices such as capacity-building for health promotion including organisational change, community development, and policy. As explained in Chapter 1, our purpose in this book is not to replicate the high-quality information provided in other texts, but to identify those approaches needed to develop and be sustained in collaborative, multisectoral, and multimethod health promotion.

Table 2.1, 'Summary of health promotion approaches', sets out differing approaches to health promotion action with their corresponding theoretical base, the aims of the approach, the methods likely to be used within that approach, and the level and type of action intended.

The principles and action areas for health promotion suggest those approaches that are necessary for effective health promotion work, indicating that single level (working only with individuals), single sector (i.e. health), single action approaches (i.e. behaviour change) to health promotion are unlikely to have much effect. For health promotion work to have more impact than single level approaches, there is a need to use an integration of approaches and to work across sectors. Take the example again of sexual and reproductive health. A program that combines the expertise of the health and education sectors, which is focused on individuals within the context of the school community (i.e. a whole school approach to sexual and reproductive health) and that uses behaviour change strategies plus empowerment approaches will be much more effective than sexual and reproductive health counselling to individual adolescents. Integrated approaches are dependent on solid partnerships and collaborations (addressed in Chapter 3). And practitioners will find their work more coherent if they have developed a clear understanding of the theories and intentions of the models being developed for programs and actions with which they are involved. Programs must make sense locally, so some developmental work is always required even for established programs such as a health education program for sexual and reproductive health. It must be acceptable to the schools involved, be appropriate to the audience, and take account of local contexts and situations in its delivery. Involvement of local stakeholders is critical to both the success of the program delivery and for its ultimate effectiveness (these concepts are explored further in Chapter 12). Participation and engagement are necessary, as is flexibility (for example in adapting programs to fit with the context and audience and being able to respond to emerging needs). We need time frames that allow for program adaptation or design, as well as testing of the feasibility of strategies (NSW Health 2004: 10).

Health promotion approaches are commonly conceived in functional terms—achieving behaviour change or delivering health education to people—more as a means to an end, rather than seeing health as a means, or a resource for well-being. Measurement of success is very often on the number of people who attended a program, rather than whether the program achieved any lasting change.

Health promotion practices range widely but very few practitioners are skilled across the range of practices from prevention to behaviour change through to socio-ecological models (Naidoo & Wills 2000). Table 2.2 sets out more details about the principles and characteristics of socio-ecological approaches, which show a strong focus on communities and organisations rather than on individuals.

Table 2.1 Summary of health promotion approaches

APPROACH	THEORY	AIMS	METHODS	LEVEL AND TYPE OF ACTION
Primary care/Disease prevention	Biomedical Treatment and diagnosis; Prevention and management of conditions	Improve physiological risk factors (e.g. high blood pressure, early detection, immunisation) and personal behaviours	Takes advantage of a person's point of entry to health system through GP, nurse or allied health consultation Screening Advice	Individuals Expert-led Passive client
Health education and behaviour change	Behaviour change theories: Reasoned Action; Health Belief; Health Action; Stages of Change	Psychosocial and behavioural risk factors (e.g. smoking, poor nutrition, physical inactivity)	Health information One-to-one or group education sessions Development of personal skills	Individuals or groups Expert-led Passive clients

APPROACH	THEORY	AIMS	METHODS	LEVEL AND TYPE OF ACTION
Participatory health education	Participation Empowerment	Provision of information e.g.: Healthy choices Social support Development of personal skills via empowerment	Integrated methods Health development One-to-one or group education sessions Social marketing Settings approaches	Individual or groups Active clients Facilitation
Community action	Community development Community engagement	Action on determinants of health Sustainable social change Strengthening community capacity Empowerment	Intersectoral partnerships and collaborations Community capacity-building Building social capital Community control Policy and organisational change Enabling Advocacy Mediating	Intersectoral partnerships and collaborations Community action Community leadership Organisational change
Socio-ecological health promotion	Determinants of health Health and social development Primary health care Empowerment Community engagement	Redress of inequities Works from health determinants: social, political, environmental	Primary health care Community engagement Creating supportive environments Advocacy Enabling Mediating Organisational development to reorient health services Build healthy local policy	Active clients and communities Changes in communities and organisations

Table 2.2 Socio-ecological approach for community interventions

CORE SOCIAL AND ECOLOGICAL PRINCIPLES	OPERATING GUIDELINES FOR INTERVENTION, DESIGN AND IMPLEMENTATION
Physical, mental, and social well-being are influenced by a variety of environmental factors	Encompass multiple settings and life domains Reinforce health-promoting social norms through existing social networks
Personal characteristics and environmental conditions often have interactive as well as direct effects on well-being	Target changes in the community or organisational environment
The degree of fit between people's biological, behavioural, and socio-cultural needs and the environmental resources available to them is a key determinant of well-being	Tailor programs to fit the setting through participation of the community and communities of interest Empower individuals to make changes
Within the context of structured community settings, certain behaviours and roles exert pivotal influences on well-being	Identify influential points in the community for promoting health Utilise multiple delivery points and methods over an extended time period
Examine the links between physical and social conditions within particular settings and the joint influences of multiple settings and life domains on persons' health over extended periods	Address social conditions and recognise the social context of health behaviours in interventions Implement coordinated interventions across multiple life domains
Interdisciplinary research, linking the perspectives of public health, medicine, the behavioural and social sciences, and policy, is essential for developing comprehensive and effective health promotion programs	Establish a collaborative, interdisciplinary research team Link results of epidemiological research, intervention research, and policy analysis

Source: Sorenson, Emmons, Hunt & Johnston 1998

SUMMARY

As health promotion knowledge, skills, and evidence have developed since the 1970s and in response to the interventions of the WHO Charters for Health Promotion, a wide range of health promotion practices have developed. However, the funding for health promotion and the dominance of medical approaches have resulted in a narrowing of health promotion approaches. The fixation in Western health promotion programs with health education and behaviour change has not benefited all people, and is likely to have impacted negatively on many groups, especially the poorest and more vulnerable. Health promotion will benefit from a more developed theory of community practice that is soundly based on socio-ecological values and principles that are consistent with the WHO Charters for Health Promotion.

REFRAMING HEALTH PROMOTION 3

Helen Keleher

Key concepts

- Reframing health promotion is about moving from lifestyle and behaviour change methods of health promotion to more empowering approaches.
- Contemporary health promotion integrates approaches to address individual, social, and environmental determinants of health.
- Upstream health promotion requires good understanding of health equity, capacity-building for health promotion, partnerships and collaborations, and leadership.
- Community development is a necessary knowledge and skill base for all health promotion practitioners.

Key terms

- Health promotion
- Health promotion interventions
- Integrated health promotion
- Intersectoral collaboration
- Multisectoral collaboration
- Partnership and collaboration
- Community development
- Health promotion leadership

OVERVIEW

This chapter builds on the definitions and foundations of health promotion discussed in Chapter 2. It now sets out the elements of reframing of health promotion, which involves a shift from traditional medical and lifestyle approaches towards socio-ecological and environmental approaches, as they are articulated in the WHO Charters for Health Promotion. The elements of reframing discussed in this chapter are levels and types of interventions, integrated health promotion, health equity approaches, capacity-building, partnerships and collaboration, and health promotion leadership.

INTERVENTION TYPES

Modelling interventions in a framework is commonly used in health promotion to assist in understanding the range of health promotion practices available. A more comprehensive approach to integrated health promotion is to understand interventions in relation to levels of action that are designed to influence the determinants of health. Levels of action are upstream–downstream, and move away from the concept of 'intervention' with its connotations of doing something to people. Delivering interventions to people is a term more consistent with a medical/primary care approach than with the empowerment intentions of equity and determinants-focused health promotion, while the term 'action area' is consistent with the WHO Charters for Health Promotion. Thinking in upstream–downstream terms enables planning to develop multiple levels of action as Figure 3.1 illustrates.

This Framework identifies categories of actions, and where they fit in with health promotion approaches. Their linear approach is not meant to suggest that health promotion begins with screening and health education and finishes somewhere more upstream. The risk with this is that socio-ecological approaches are more complex and difficult to implement so we find that some practitioners and their organisations find it easier to keep doing screening and health education. This is especially the case for clinicians who have no specific health promotion skills and for whom screening and health education sit comfortably with disease prevention approaches (i.e. those targeted to a disease such as cardiovascular disease or diabetes). Narrowly focused funding programs for disease prevention are still more common than funding for socio-ecological health promotion work. The point is that health promotion intervention or action frameworks are merely a tool for 'modelling' the range of approaches being undertaken, either in a particular project or across the practices of an organisation or partnership, and as such are a useful tool for the development of integrated health promotion. So use intervention or action frameworks of health promotion with care, because they may be used to justify single-level practices rather than reflect or respond to

Figure 3.1 Framework for health promotion actions

Framework for Health Promotion Action				

INTERVENTIONS

Downstream ⟵⟶ Upstream

Disease Prevention	Communication Strategies	Health Education & Empowerment	Community & Health Development	Infrastructure & Systems Change
Primary	Health Information	Knowledge	Engagement	Policy
Secondary	Behaviour Change Campaigns	Understanding		Legislation
Tertiary		Skill Development	Community Action	Organisational Change

Primary Care — Lifestyle/Behaviourist Approaches — Socio-ecological Approaches

Source: Keleher & Murphy 2004: 160

the more complex values and intentions of health promotion that reside in the WHO charters.

The Framework of Health Promotion Actions maps the levels of downstream–upstream action (explained further in Chapter 4) from determinants of health approaches onto the health promotion approaches. In other words, the Framework demonstrates the range of actions that can be taken and the level at which they are likely to have an effect. Chapter 4 discusses the social and economic factors that affect health, and explains them in relation to the upstream–midstream–downstream continuum. Chapter 12 discusses the selection of actions and approaches in relation to the evidence. Briefly though, in order to address inequalities, interventions must identify and target social, economic, and environmental factors leading to poor health.

Figure 3.2 is an expanded Framework that provides examples of actions that can be taken at upstream–downstream levels, to influence change in the social determinants of health. The landscape of health promotion is moving upstream because downstream approaches have done little to change the health status of the poorest and most vulnerable people. Indeed, lifestyle health promotion is thought to have actually increased inequities as people with education, financial resources, and good social support have taken up health messages to increase their health status. Health promotion is therefore in transition, with a focus on the consolidation of practices that will create social change and tackle inequities so that all people have opportunities in their lives to develop the personal skills required for good health, and to manage change and the challenges of everyday living.

Table 3.1 Determinants framework of health promotion actions

APPROACHES				
PRIMARY CARE LIFESTYLE/BEHAVIOURIST			*SOCIO-ECOLOGICAL*	
Disease-prevention Primary Secondary Tertiary	Communication strategies Health information Behaviour-change campaigns	Health education Knowledge Facilitation Skill development	Community & health development Engagement Community action Advocacy	Infrastructure & systems change Organisational change Policy Legislation

LEVELS OF ACTION		
DOWNSTREAM	*MIDSTREAM*	*UPSTREAM*
Access to health services Disease self-management Screening Provision of appropriate health information Development of culturally competent health providers	Programs to address: Smoking Alcohol misuse Drug addiction Physical activity Weight control Diet/nutrition Provision of appropriate health information Development of personal coping skills and individual capacity	Programs to address determinants of health: Inequities and poverty reduction Healthy public policy Strengthen community action Social exclusion Gender equity Racism and discrimination Universal high-quality education Lifelong learning, including work programs Access to affordable and secure housing Local employment programs Training Enhancement of work conditions Neighbourhood renewal programs Local leadership development Capacity building of health services to ensure cultural competence Tobacco control Universal child-care

INTEGRATED HEALTH PROMOTION

Integrated health promotion is a response to traditional patterns of single platform services or programs run by agencies and 'delivered' to unsuspecting people out there in the general community. Integration requires a considerable shift in the practice of practitioners, organisations, and systems—a reframing of health promotion—to achieve greater planning and program coordination across sectors and health promotion approaches (i.e. medical/preventive-behavioural/socio-environmental), across action areas and at different levels (see Figure 3.2).

The most effective and equitable disease prevention and health promotion strategies are those that address the individual, social, and environmental determinants of health (Nutbeam 1998). This requires an integrated or multilevel approach that has two main prongs:

(i)   integrated health promotion works across relevant sectors (e.g. housing, health, welfare, transport, urban planning, environment, sport and recreation, food policy and regulation, education), and simultaneously

(ii) integrated health promotion adopts multiple-level strategies implemented concurrently.

Another way to think of integration is in terms of integrating resources, programs, and expertise that could be called 'ways of knowing'. Practitioners find that the principles, foundation practices, and approaches outlined above work in different ways with different people, communities, organisations, and populations. Many communities and populations have their own 'ways of knowing' about health, and what creates it or destroys it, which is a critical foundation for developing programs that will be both effective and sustainable. To understand those ways of knowing, health promotion practitioners need a few essentials in the toolbox: values about respect, rights, and reconciliation, and partnerships with expertise to guide everyone into those ways of knowing and doing. The 'Pallert Tooree Larr' Case Study 3.1 further on in this chapter illustrates the importance of shared values, principles, and practices. The multilevel strategies used included:

■   government working with the supported accommodation sector and women's workers in a domestic violence service
■   community development approaches with outreach
■   organisational change with a focus on equity and sustainable change.

The case study demonstrates that an integrated approach offers the greatest potential for impacting on a population with unmet needs, addressing health inequities in a sustainable model. These learnings have relevance for the integration of health promotion which also seeks to:

■   impact on the health of the population as a whole
■   address health inequities
■   sustain change over the long term.

Integrated health promotion will only be able to address health inequalities if it is planned strategically to do so, with an obvious incorporation of conceptualisations of the determinants of health from the earliest stages of planning (see Chapter 12).

INTERSECTORAL OR MULTISECTORAL COLLABORATION

Intersectoral or multisectoral collaboration is defined as 'a recognized relationship between part or parts of different sectors of society which has been formed to take action on an issue to achieve health outcomes or intermediate health outcomes in a way which is more effective, efficient or sustainable, than might be achieved by the health sector alone' (WHO 1998: 24).

Understanding of the concept of intersectoralism is dependent on the context in which it is used or operationalised. The embedded verb within intersectoralism is *to intersect*—to work with and create connections across dual or multiple sectors. In the context of the promotion of health and well-being, intersectoralism incorporates notions of cooperation and collaboration, integration. and interdisciplinarity. Work that intersects with that of others enhances opportunities and maximises available resources to achieve outcomes that are compatible for partners and stakeholders. Working intersectorally in health promotion suggests that the knowledge, skills, and experience of partners is combined, to reach desired outcomes for the advancement of health among groups, populations, or communities. Intersectoralism increases capacity and opportunities for sharing of expertise.

Questions that arise from a focus on intersectoral health promotion include:

- whether insectoralism is more than the sum of different perspectives to address the social determinants of health
- how intersectoralism creates a health promotion imagination
- what factors promote or hinder the development of intersectoralism
- identification of the barriers and enablers of intersectoralism
- the evidence and policy base for intersectoral health promotion theory and practice
- in what ways intersectoral health promotion theory and practice can influence healthy public policy and health promotion practice.

Many sectors are influential in the promotion and, conversely, the demotion of health. Decisions that affect health are made in taxation, welfare, education, agriculture, transport, and the environment, for example. Achieving greater awareness of the impact of decisions made in these sectors is one aspect of taking an intersectoral—or multisector—approach. Working across sectors provides opportunities for cooperation and collaboration between different sectors including civil society and the public and private sectors, and requires skills of mediating, enabling, and advocacy.

EQUITY/INEQUITY

Health promotion from a determinants approach is founded on a values base of social justice and equity, and the need, therefore, for health promotion to tackle health and social inequities. Social justice is 'a vision of society where rules are just and fair and resources are shared equitably among the members of the community, in the interests of the common good' (Health Promotion Forum of New Zealand 2004).

The concepts of equity and inequity, equality and inequality, require some careful unpacking. Kawachi, Subramanian, and Almeida-Filho (2002) define inequality and equality as dimensional concepts that refer simply to measurable quantities—they are descriptive terms that designate disparities, or observed differences, among and between groups (Hayward & Colman 2003). Inequity and equity, on the other hand, are political concepts because they express a moral commitment to social justice and human rights (Hayward & Colman 2003; Kawachi et al. 2002). Equity and inequity in health are defined in terms of the presence or absence of 'systematic and potentially remediable differences in one or more aspects of health across populations or population groups defined socially, economically, demographically, or geographically' (International Society for Equity in Health ISEqH 2005). When inequities and social and economic inequalities are beyond the control of individuals and communities, or are the result of inadequate distribution of material factors, discrimination, and gender or racial disparity, they are considered unfair and unjust.

> Equality in health is not about eliminating all health differences so that everyone has the same level of health, but rather to reduce or eliminate those which result from factors which are considered to be both avoidable and unfair. Equity is therefore concerned with creating equal opportunities for health and with bringing differentials in health down to the lowest levels possible (Whitehead 1990).

Inequity can occur in relation to access to economic resources, race, gender, and health. The work of equity-focused health promotion is towards achieving social justice and equity through strong commitment to the prerequisites and determinants of health. Health equity is a key concept for health promotion. Inequities are explored further in Chapter 4 in discussion of the social and economic factors that affect health; and the significance for health promotion of equity approaches is visited throughout the book as we argue, as does NSW Health (2004), that changes to practice are necessary if health promotion is to address health inequity.

Health equity

Equity approaches in policy, health actions, and research are about making visible the sources and characteristics of inequity and actively taking policy decisions and programmatic actions directed at improving equity in health or in reducing or eliminating inequities in health (ISEqH 2005). These are steps that any organisation can take to ensure it is addressing inequities but surprisingly few actually do incorporate specific health equity steps into health promotion planning.

The UK Health Development Agency (Hamer et al. 2003) defines health equity as the process by which partners:

■ systematically review inequities in the causes of ill health and in access to effective services and their outcomes, for a defined population
■ ensure that action required is agreed and incorporated into local plans, services, and practice
■ evaluate the impact of actions on reducing inequity.

To meet tests of fairness, planning needs to be transparent about the distribution of resources in relation to the health needs of different groups. The greater allocation of resources to those whose needs are greater is necessary to reduce avoidable health inequalities and promote equal opportunity to the determinants of good health, access to health, and other services.

NSW Health (2004) identify three important aspects of a health equity approach:

1   the organisation should expressly incorporate a commitment addressing health equity in its health promotion principles
2   the organisation needs to have the capacity to support health equity
3   the organisation should incorporate equity strategies into the planning cycle.

Health equity approaches will be more likely at the level of organisations if governments providing the funding have a health equity policy statement and guidelines for its implementation through identified health promotion and public health programs.

CAPACITY-BUILDING

Capacity for health promotion or public health is understood at the level of organisations and systems. The capacity for 'systems-thinking' is a necessary attribute of competent practitioners, and should be purposefully developed by beginning practitioners to enable the achievement of the higher levels of competence that mark an experienced practitioner. All health promotion practitioners should have developed understanding of capacity-building and its various dimensions, be able to access theories and evidence that support capacity-building as a strategy of health promotion, and identify tools and resources to assist with capacity-building

In terms of organisations and systems, capacity-building has three components necessary for the development of effective health promotion work: a mandate to act; a framework for action; and the capacity to act (Bowen et al 2001).

Once labelled the 'invisible work of health promotion', capacity-building is now understood as a set of strategies or series of actions that can be applied both within programs and across systems to lead to greater capacity of people, organisations, and communities to promote health (Heward, Hutchins & Keleher 2006). Five key action areas for capacity-building have been identified by NSW Health (2001):

- *Organisational change and development*: 'the structures, policies, procedures and practices that contribute to fulfilling an organisation's vision through a managed process of change. The description of this action area explicitly incorporates the factors from organisational change highlighting the importance of the external, internal (described as domains) context, vision, roles and responsibilities and organisational structures to support change' (Heward, Hutchins & Keleher 2006: 3). These are addressed further in Chapter 10.
- *Workforce development*: the deliberate processes of upskilling people to assist them to develop the skills and abilities to realise the organisational visions and responsibilities with regard to health promotion and addressing inequalities and determinants of health. For example, staff and board members can undertake training and development in health promotion.
- *Resource allocation*: the material things needed for health promotion work: people, financial and information resources, physical space, planning, and planning tools.
- *Leadership*: this refers to visioning and direction setting, engagement with the challenges of advocacy, and strategy in the context of critical health promotion issues. All staff can provide leadership for health promotion but managers have particular responsibilities to ensure that planning frameworks are focused on multisector partnerships, population health, and inequities. Leadership is addressed further in Chapter 18.
- *Partnerships*: 'refers to the characteristics of systems thinking and critical analysis essential for working in collaboration, particularly to address the underlying determinants of health' (Heward, Hutchins & Keleher 2006: 3) and addressed in more detail below.

In addition, capacity-building involves the development of:

- sustainable skills and the capacity to retain experienced staff
- organisational infrastructure and policy (both statewide and organisational) for health promotion
- strategic organisational planning processes
- the capacity to build networks and desirable organisational structures
- the capacity to draw additional income to supplement core funding
- the capacity to find resources to fund capital works
- the capacity to develop social infrastructure
- the capacity to promote social citizenship
- health improvement infrastructure to prolong and multiply health gains many times over.

■ strengthened agency/system infrastructure to respond to population growth, infrastructure gaps, and issues of isolation
■ strengthened problem-solving capability of organisations and communities to develop innovative solutions to chronic illness, vulnerability, and disadvantage
■ learning through experience
■ the capacity to link development funds to program sustainability
■ increased problem solving strategies across organisations.

A search on the Internet about capacity-building in health promotion will quickly provide many sites from government and non-government agencies that explain the various elements of capacity-building in detail, provide frameworks for the application of capacity-building particularly in organisations and through systems, and illustrate how those frameworks have been applied. Chapter 10 discusses empowerment in terms of community capacity-building.

COMMUNITY DEVELOPMENT

Capacity-building, empowerment, and the creation of enabling environments are closely connected to community development approaches to health promotion. Community involvement in health action is critical for both capacity-building and the mobilisation of communities to enable stronger levels of participation, which is a pathway to empowerment. As identified in Chapter 1, empowerment is an approach that helps people to understand and identify their own health or social issues and concerns and gain the skills and confidence to take action to deal with them. Community empowerment works through the skills of community development and advocacy. The intention of these strategies is to create active participating communities that are able to challenge and change those things about them that they feel are contributing to poor health in some way.

The Alma Ata Declaration for Primary Health Care (WHO 1978) and the Ottawa Charter for Health Promotion (WHO 1986) provide the foundations for community development in health, drawing on Paolo Freire's (1970) seminal work on empowerment and participatory approaches to education and health development.

Community development means there is an active involvement of people sharing in the issues that affect their lives, by drawing on existing human and material resources to enhance self-help and social support (WHO 1986). For many communities, social well-being needs to occur before health outcomes can be improved. This is because powerlessness, lack of opportunity, low income, and stress are key determinants of illness and disease (Keleher 2006). Empowerment, a sense of control, and hope are linked to better health, while loss of meaning or value in life underpins much self-destructive behaviour (Labonte & Laverack 2001a; Syme 2003).

Health promotion and community development have much in common, sharing commitment to participatory research and learning for empowerment, based on the premise that a community's insights into their own problems, and community involvement in solution-building, are critical for sustainable social change. The same principles apply to individuals—for a person to feel empowered, he or she must have insight into his or her own problem(s), and be involved in solution-building.

Community development is a term applied to a range of ways of 'doing' health promotion but much of that activity actually has the genuine characteristics of community development in health promotion (Raeburn & Corbett 2001). Raeburn and Corbett identify the distinct characteristics of health promotion involving community:

Level A: Community-based health promotion

Community-based health promotion uses a settings approach to conduct health in a community setting such as a school or workplace. Little effort is made to engage the people of the community other than expecting them to be cooperative consumers of the activity.

Level B: Community participation

Community participation models are often an instrumental approach to requirements for community involvement in a health program or research project. There are four subcategories of community participation (Keleher 2006: 240):

(a) consultation, discussion, and needs assessment that involves staff from locally based organisations
(b) consultation, discussion, and needs assessment that includes community representatives on working or advisory groups
(c) local organisations and community people are given decision-making power over the design of some elements of the program
(d) partnership where the balance of power and decision-making is shared and is based on a deep respect for culture which drives the program design and implementation.

Understanding these levels of community participation is useful when developing programs or models for community development, helping to clarify the power relations between professionals and consumers, and what outcomes might be expected from the model developed.

Level C: Community development

The third level incorporates community development principles that explicitly arrange for the balance of power to be held by the community, and where everyone involved is explicitly engaged in community capacity-building. Professionals are co-facilitators of a process where goals are about empowerment.

In reality, the boundaries between the different levels may be blurred but the principles of empowerment (see Chapter 10 for further discussion

Table 3.2 Attributes and barriers to community development in health

TEN CORE ATTRIBUTES NEEDED BY WORKERS FOR COMMUNITY DEVELOPMENT IN HEALTH		TEN BARRIERS TO COMMUNITY DEVELOPMENT IN HEALTH	
1	Ability to see a bigger picture of actions needed to create healthy communities	1	Lack of consultation or true participatory mechanisms
2	Ability to give up personal and professional power	2	Community expectations of service deliverers
3	Ability to work effectively in teams	3	Short-term funding allowing insufficient time for due processes
4	Knowledge of the broad social, economic, and political determinants of health	4	Lack of identification and understanding of the community of interest
5	Understanding of local, prioritised determinants of health	5	Needs and wishes not well understood
6	Skills in community organising	6	Active opposition from groups with unhealthy investments
7	Advocacy at the level of communities	7	Inadequate skills in managing people and conflict
8	Respect for communities	8	Inability to deal with the 'you're paid and I'm not' comments from community members
9	Negotiation and mediation	9	Hijacking of the project
10	Flexibility and responsiveness	10	Long-term outcomes not funded

of empowerment) are fundamental to genuine health promotion that is transformative in its intent and its outcomes.

Table 3.2 summarises core attributes of successful health workers and barriers that thwart community development in health (Keleher 2006: 246).

PARTNERSHIP AND COLLABORATION

You can work in partnerships for some projects some of the time.
You can work in partnerships with some health promoters and projects all of the time.
But you can't work in partnerships for all health promotion all of the time.

The incorporation of strong and sustainable partnerships is a core skill for equity-focused, integrated health promotion and for health development. However, notions of partnership mean different things to different people under different circumstances and health promotion practitioners need to have a good understanding of the different levels of partnership, what each is likely to achieve, and the responsibilities of partners for the level of work involved in the partnership. Certainly, partnerships can achieve goals that individual agencies cannot achieve by themselves (Wildridge et al. 2004), but only if all stakeholders are committed to working together.

Box 3.1: Levels of partnership

- Isolation: agencies separate from others with little or no communication
- Networking: a loose arrangement of contact for the purposes of information-sharing
- Cooperation: exchange of information; altering activities for a common purpose; communication is marginal to organisational goals
- Coordination: time-limited activities with some joint responsibility and shared outcomes that require only enough trust to give and receive help from one another
- Collaborative practice: longer term and more deliberate efforts of organisations and groups to undertake shared planning and take joint responsibility with equal commitment for joint activities and shared vision of the outcomes, with high level of trust and power-sharing based on knowledge and expertise
- Integrated health promotion: separate identities of the partners or agencies no longer as significant as the outcome.

Broadly, a partnership is defined as a voluntary arrangement developed between parties who agree to work cooperatively towards shared and/or compatible objectives, and that does not compromise the principles of the partners. The term 'partnership' carries responsibilities about sharing of resources, risks and decision-making, trust, cooperation towards shared and/or compatible objectives, and negotiation of shared goals towards interests in a shared future (Torjman 1998).

A series of levels of partnership can be defined (Carnwall & Carson 2003; Labonte 2003; VicHealth 2003b) as a continuum from isolated service providers to those working collaboratively.

Partners will typically move across these levels as they establish working relationships. The strength of the partnership is dependent on factors such as trust, which facilitates the development of effective collaboration, but it is also useful to identify barriers to collaboration, such as conflict and competition. If these barriers are not understood and dealt with, then the partnership will flounder and become unsustainable.

Collaboration in broad terms is defined as 'a recognized relationship between part or parts of different sectors of society which has been formed to take action on an issue to achieve health outcomes or intermediate health outcomes in a way which is more effective, efficient or sustainable, than might be achieved by the health sector alone' (WHO 1998: 24). However, there is an important and useful conceptual difference between partnership and collaboration. Partnership is about identity and characteristics—partnership is about 'who we are', while collaboration, on the other hand, is about 'what we do' (Carnwall & Carson 2003, 8). And the critical success factor for a successful and effective partnership is that it needs to be in place organisationally at three levels—those of policy, management, and service delivery.

Labonte (2003) provides this schema of preconditions, processes, and outcomes of effective partnerships:

Table 3.3 Effective partnerships

PRECONDITIONS FOR EFFECTIVE PARTNERSHIPS	PROCESSES FOR DEVELOPING EFFECTIVE PARTNERSHIPS	OUTCOMES OF EFFECTIVE PARTNERSHIPS
■ A problem we can't fix on our own ■ A problem no one else can fix on their own ■ Partners out there with enough overlap in values and attitudes towards the problem that we can work together ■ Partners out there with resources (skills, knowledge—both 'expert', technical, and 'lived experience'—materials, finances) necessary to address the problem	■ Creating a common purpose or intent ■ Hiring neutral facilitators or 'midwives' whom all can trust ■ Building trust by sharing differing beliefs or analyses of the problem (why it exists, what can be done about it) ■ Being open about one's own (personal and organisational) interests or agendas about acting on the problem	■ Endurance (lasts for several years) ■ Shared resources (partners contribute towards a common resource pool) ■ Multiple new activities generated ■ Partners demonstrate willingness to put some individual organisational objectives (their own interests) on hold to achieve partnership goals ■ Partners demonstrate understanding that injuring other partners is not in their own interest

Source: Labonte 2003

Labonte's schema (above) is a useful tool to assess when and whether a partnership is needed, what processes will establish a productive partnership, and the outcomes that partners could expect from their involvement. It is also useful to be able to appraise your own organisation's characteristics and ability to perform in partnerships and collaborations. The following scale that shows levels of capacity for collaboration from reactive, through to proactive, and then to high-performing:

Because many sectors are influential in the promotion and demotion of health, collaboration between sectors is critical for health promotion actions.

Figure 3.2 Organisational characteristics of partnerships and collaborations

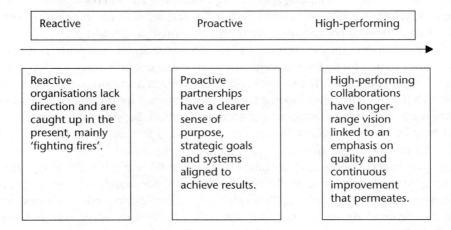

As mentioned earlier, decisions that affect health are made in many different sectors. Achieving greater awareness of the impact of decisions made in these sectors is one aspect of multisectoral practice. Therefore, key to the effectiveness of health promotion are the opportunities for cooperation and collaboration between different sectors, including civil society and the public and private sectors. Multisectoral partnership work requires skills of mediating, enabling, and advocacy. It also requires organisational change which is a key component of capacity-building frameworks (Heward, Hutchins & Keleher 2006).

Case Study 3.1 illustrates the values behind a partnership and its collaborative ways of working, and the characteristics of high-performing organisations.

Case Study 3.1: The Pallert Tooree Larr Program

Pallert Tooree Larr is Dja Dja Wrung language for Strong Black Women's Camp or Home and is an Australian Indigenous domestic and family violence program. Pallert Tooree Larr models non-Indigenous services and workers in the Indigenous community working together, and rests on a statement of apology and reconciliation. The people involved in the development of the Pallert Tooree Larr model believe that the processes used, and the values and philosophy underpinning the model, are every bit as important as the work they do on a day-to-day basis with the women and children they supported.

The program is a unique partnership between a women's refuge, a Transitional Housing Manager and the local Indigenous community. It draws on community strengths, links, relationships, networks and supports, mentoring, role modelling, education and skills, raising awareness, an innovative use of existing resources along with strengthening resources within the community, art work and cultural symbolism, empowerment processes, openness and respect. The program originally emerged because two non-Indigenous specific organisations, a women's refuge and a housing service, who were seeking ways to better provide services for Indigenous women and children, formed a collaborative partnership to provide the program.

In its most simple terms, Pallert Tooree Larr is supported medium-term accommodation for Indigenous women with or without children, in a designated Koori safe house, supported by domestic violence workers and housing services workers. It aims to provide intensive, flexible support for however long the family needs it before they move on to more independent accommodation. Support doesn't necessarily stop when they leave the Pallert Tooree Larr house, and families don't have to be living in it to be part of the program.

The Pallert Tooree Larr program is trying to fill a much needed gap for women whose lives, health, and well-being have been damaged by their experiences of domestic and family violence. Many women were leaving crisis services with some of their immediate issues met, but still suffered in many ways, which impacted on how well they were able to live independently and achieve personal well-being. For example, many women still experienced lengthy and drawn-out court processes, not only with the family court over child contact and residency issues, but also with Child Protection involvement which was an added complication. Many of them needed ongoing support with their children, because of the damage to them from the violence and the abuse. Many women need ongoing access to appropriate health, welfare, and housing services but are not linked in, or services are inappropriate. Many women suffer ongoing physical and mental ill health because of the combined impact of violence and abuse and their Aboriginality, and they were struggling in the community. Sometimes they surfaced to crisis agencies when there was a crisis, but it was obvious that they were not healing or recovering well from their experiences. The problems were repeating with their children and their grandchildren.

With limited resources to work with individual families, the workers were aware that along with supporting these women and children, the program had to have a strong role in community development, so as to ensure a stronger and more lasting impact.

Pallert Tooree Larr rests solidly on community consultation and contribution, knowledge, respect, trust, collaboration, hope that things can change, and excitement that our joint effort of developing the model was a good experience. Many others are interested in adapting the model for their own areas.

Source: Charles, Warren & Oberin 2005

HEALTH PROMOTION LEADERSHIP

Leadership, of course, comes from within communities as well as within organisations, as the Pallert Tooree Larr story illustrates. Working with and learning from local community leadership are core skills in community and health development.

Understanding the sources of leadership and being able to mentor, nurture, and role model leadership are attributes of high-performing practitioners, both young and more experienced. Leadership in its many forms is essential for community practice and multisectoral working. Students of health promotion will find it useful to explore leadership styles, their own capabilities, and those of others. Chapter 17 explores the concept of leadership in more detail. Topics that health promotion practitioners might wish to explore further include: leadership styles and strategies for leadership development; developing visions for healthier futures with communities and other stakeholders; knowledge of ethics and values in public health; advocacy and strategy for health development; partnerships for effective action; and local, national, and global challenges in public health. For practical examples of health promotion leadership in action, refer to Guidebook 2: Health Promotion Associations, Alliances, and Advocacy Organisations at the end of Part 1. Any one of the organisations profiled in this guidebook is an exemplar of leadership and collaborative working by people who see that partnerships have a multiplier effect on health development

HEALTH PROMOTION ASSOCIATIONS, ALLIANCES, AND ORGANISATIONS

The health promotion associations, alliances, and organisations introduced in Guidebook 2 have many benefits for members, and many have reduced rates for students. Many practitioners find that belonging to one or more associations or organisations is invaluable for professional support and development. Getting newsletters, emails, and journals, and attending conferences and seminars, keeps everyone up-to-date and provides opportunities for members to have input to the directions of policy and funding programs that affect health promotion.

SUMMARY

Reframing of health promotion is about shifting practice from a focus on individual health towards understanding health in the context of people's lives and the determinants of their health and well-being, because good health and well-being are a resource for living not just for individuals, but also for communities and populations. It is time for the fixation in Western health promotion programs with health education and behaviour change to be reframed to increase the effectiveness of health promotion. More developed approaches that take an integrated approach that are founded on socio-ecological health promotion will result in more developed theories of community practice. Only when those practices are integrated with the hopes of those we work with, and on a shared vision for what can be achieved together, can health promotion start to create meaningful change. The principles and values of respect and reconciliation embodied in the Pallert Tooree Larr Case Study are surely principles and values that apply to working with all people, communities, and populations, from whatever culture.

Equity-focused health promotion has a values orientation towards the creation of healthy environments for populations that are a prerequisite for individual behaviour change. The strategies of equity-focused health promotion are intended to facilitate change to the social and structural barriers that impede or demote good health (Keleher 2001). Of course, not all health promotion will be focused on the creation of healthy environments, but single-level health promotion activities that are not developed and implemented in the context of the real world and that do not address any social, economic, or environmental factors will have little effectiveness or sustainability. Investments in health promotion are always welcome but it is beholden of organisations and practitioners to ensure that the use of available resources is in health promotion efforts that are evidence-based, planned, and implemented purposely towards intermediate and longer-term outcomes. To achieve effective and sustainable change, necessary health promotion skills and strategies include integrated practice, multisectoral actions, partnerships and collaborations, and capacity-building. These are central concepts for health promotion that require practitioners to acquire appropriate core competencies (see Chapter 16) so you will find that they are revisited in other chapters of this book.

THE DRIVERS FOR HEALTH LIE OUTSIDE THE HEALTH SECTOR

4

Helen Keleher

Key concepts

- Health and well-being are influenced by a wide range of factors, most of which lie outside the health sector.
- Social and economic factors are more influential in shaping people's health status than lifestyles or health care.
- People in disadvantaged circumstances are unduly influenced by exposure to health hazards, which creates a vulnerability to poor health.
- Levels of health promotion action are connected with the drivers of health.

Key terms

- Social determinants of health
- Health equity
- Socio-economic drivers of health
- Upstream–midstream factors
- Gender equity

OVERVIEW

The knowledge base about determinants of health shows that most of the drivers for health lie outside the health sector, in, for example, education, employment and work conditions, social, physical, and natural environments, families and communities, housing, and the 'old' public health services of water and sanitation. Understanding the drivers for health and the unequal social conditions in which they are situated, is critical for the creation of health promotion road maps—or action plans. The aim of this chapter is to overview the social contexts and conditions that are the drivers for health, and connect them with health promotion principles and practices. Given the rising inequities in every society, health promotion actions need to be increasingly directed towards the determinants of the problem around which programs are designed. This chapter is supported by two guidebooks:

- Guidebook 3: Key Resources about the Socio-economic Determinants of Health
- Guidebook 4: Health Promotion as a Gendering Practice

DISCOVER THE HISTORY OF PUBLIC HEALTH

The history of public health is rich and fascinating, and worthy of your attention. Practitioners from all health disciplines will benefit from some understanding of public health history because by understanding past contexts, you are enabled to have a better grasp of contemporary developments and a sense of their future direction. The history of health promotion as a discipline is more recent than public health, which has been traced in every major civilisation. This book cannot do justice to either histories of public health or health promotion but there are many books that do capture their richness, and draw out the lessons we have, or should have, learned from the past. All books mentioned here are available in university libraries.

Australian histories of public health include that of the first Director-General of Health, Dr J.H.L. Cumpston, whose manuscripts were brought together and published some decades after his death by Lewis (1989). Gillespie (1991) examined relationships between the state and the medical profession between 1910–60, while the two-volume history of public health in Australia by Lewis (2003) is the most comprehensive Australian history of public health to date. Roe's (1984) volume is a valuable biography of influential Australian thinkers, their ideologies, and their effect on the development of public services designed to improve people's health. A good summary of the 'old' public health movement and its transition to the 'new' public health and the contemporary health promotion movement is in Baum (2002), and you can follow the rise of the community health movement and primary health care in Baum, Fry, and Lennie (1993).

Volumes about public health in other countries make for fascinating reading. Rosenkrantz (1972), writing about the particularities of public health in Massachusetts, is a classic, as is the American George Rosen's *A History of Public Health* (1958). The political exposition by Friedrich Engels (1844) described the social and economic conditions affecting the dreadful health of mid-eighteenth century British workers, drawing attention to poverty and extreme inequality in British society and government inaction regarding the state of health of the poor. Smith's (1979) volume is a social history of 'the people's health' in the United Kingdom from 1830–1910 while Navarro (1976) analyses the rise of medicine under capitalism in the USA. In all of these books you will find recognition of the social and economic conditions related to health and the need for them to be addressed in order to protect and promote the health of the public.

THE 'NEW' SOCIAL DETERMINANTS OF HEALTH

The term 'social determinants of health' became popular through the 1990s although the social determinants themselves are not new as history has shown us. What is new is the strengthening research-evidence base about the causes of poor health. Again, that is a growing and vast body of literature to which I make some references here that cannot do it justice. You will become increasingly familiar with the literature in your health promotion journeys, and Guidebook 3, Key Resources about the Socio-economic Determinants of Health, includes some good places to start your journey and make some stopovers.

One of your stopovers could be to the website from the United Kingdom Acheson Inquiry, which was a 2002 Treasury-led review of existing programs to identify how government spending could be applied to have the greatest effect on health inequalities. Based on this evidence, actions identified as likely to have greatest impact over the long term were identified in terms of improvements in early years support for children and families; improved social housing; improved educational attainment and skills development among disadvantaged populations; improved access to public services in disadvantaged communities; reduced unemployment; and improved income among the poorest. These were reflected in programs of action to address the underlying determinants of health that were designed to tackle the long-term underlying causes of health inequalities.

Another stopover you could make is to Health Canada's comprehensive website on the social determinants of health. Another stopover should be to the Swedish public health strategy, which is not defined in terms of either risk or morbidity and mortality figures but is based on a social determinants of health model (Swedish National Institute of Public Health 2003). The Swedish strategy aims to alter the social stratification that produces health inequities and produce good health, on equal terms, for the whole population.

An essential stopover must be to the website of the World Health Organisation WHO) to the webpages for the Commission on the Social Determinants of

Health (CSDH) established in 2005. At the time of publication of this book, the Commission was midway through its work. If you bookmark their website, you will be able to follow developments in the knowledge base they are generating. The Commission's background paper includes a very good historical overview of the social determinants of health (SDH), the WHO's commitment to dealing with the social roots of health problems, and the evolution of major programs to address health inequalities. The paper also provides acknowledgment that WHO actions have not always been effective in this regard. For example, the paper discusses 'the proliferation of "vertical" programs—narrowly focused, technology-driven campaigns targeting specific diseases such as malaria, smallpox, TB, and yaws. Such programs were seen as highly efficient, but by their very nature they tended to ignore the social context and its role in producing well-being or disease ... they tended to leave the most serious health challenges of the bulk of the population unaddressed' (WHO 2005b: 9). The paper goes on to discuss the Health for All and (Alma Ata) Primary Health Care strategies, which sought to address 'the underlying *social, economic and political causes of poor health*' (original emphasis) (WHO 2005b: 11) but which were narrowed and effectively sidelined in the 1980s and 1990s.

In that paper, the Commission described the SDH as 'the social conditions in which people live and work ... SDH point to both specific features of the social context that affect health and to the pathways by which social conditions translate in health impacts. The SDH that merit attention are those that can potentially by altered by informed action' (WHO 2005b: 4).

The CSDH papers make clear that understanding health programs in terms of risk is insufficient because actions to enhance health must be framed within a population focus. Thus, our work in health promotion must refocus from individuals and their lifestyles to upstream social patterns and structures that shape people's chances and opportunities to be healthy. In other words, says the Commission, medical and health care are not the main driver of people's health (WHO 2005b: 5), as Figure 4.1 illustrates.

The much-quoted 'rainbow' from Dahlgren and Whitehead (1991) in Figure 4.1, makes it clear that health is created in the social, economic, and political conditions of life. If follows then, that health equity should be a core value for, and foundation of, this work.

HEALTH EQUITY

As identified in Chapter 1, health promotion from a determinants approach is founded on a values base of social justice and equity, raising the responsibility for health promotion to make concerted efforts to tackle health and social inequities. Explanations of the causes of health inequity show that inequity is primarily social and economic.

Figure 4.1 Determinants of health

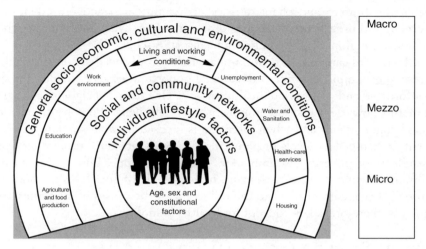

Source: Dahlgren & Whitehead 1991

Equity and inequity in health are defined in terms of the presence or absence of 'systematic and potentially remediable differences in one or more aspects of health across populations or population groups defined socially, economically, demographically, or geographically' (ISEqH 2005). When inequities and social and economic inequalities are beyond the control of individuals and communities, or are the result of inadequate distribution of material factors, discrimination, gender or racial disparity, they are considered unfair and unjust (Victora et al. 2003).

Equality in health is not about eliminating all health differences so that everyone has the same level of health, but rather to reduce or eliminate those that result from factors considered to be both avoidable and unfair. Equity is therefore concerned with creating equal opportunities for health and with bringing differentials in health down to the lowest levels possible (Whitehead 1990). More precisely, Braverman and Gruskin (2002) conceptualise health equity for the purposes of measurement and accountability, and in doing so, link equity to human rights:

> Equity in health is the absence of systematic discrepancies in health (or in the social determinants of health) between groups with different levels of underlying social advantage/disadvantage, that is, wealth, power or prestige. Equity is an ethical principal; it is also consonant with and closely related to human rights principles … Assessing health equity requires comparing health and its social determinants between more and less advantaged social groups (Braverman & Gruskin 2002: 254).

Equity approaches in policy, health actions, and research are about making visible the sources and characteristics of inequity, and actively taking 'policy decisions and programmatic actions directed at improving equity in health or in reducing or eliminating' inequities in health (ISEqH 2005).

Inequities can arise in relation to a whole raft of social conditions, including access to economic resources, educational opportunities, race, gender, and access to affordable and appropriate health services. Health and social inequalities arise from the powerlessness and impoverishment brought about by the widening socio-economic gulf and when attention is focused on high smoking rates, poor nutrition habits, low levels of parenting skill, and substance use, rather than on the effects of poverty, discrimination, and loss of hope. Equity-focused health promotion works towards achieving higher levels of social justice and equity through strong commitment to the redressing of the causes of inequities. Health equity is, therefore, a key concept for health promotion.

SOCIO-ECONOMIC DRIVERS OF HEALTH

Research has shown convincingly that the level of income inequality in any society has a direct relationship to life expectancy and quality of life. Income disparities have grown substantially, despite globalisation and income growth in developing nations. Income ratios of the world's richest 20% of the population to the poorest 20% are now at 82:1 compared to 30:1 in 1960 (Wallerstein 2006). Gaps in health status are widening both between and within countries (Victora et al. 2003).

Income equality influences mortality rates independently of the absolute mean income of that society (Wilkinson 1996; Wilkinson & Marmot 2001). For example, relative income levels and social inequality are strongly associated with heart disease, which is the most common illness associated with low income and poverty (Wilkinson & Marmot 2001). Sub-optimal or adverse early childhood experiences are reliable predictors of heart disease in adult life, regardless of one's adult income status. People in the lower half of income groups are also more likely to die of cancers, diabetes, and respiratory diseases (Wilkinson 1996). Rising rates of obesity and associated rates of Type II diabetes are associated with depression and cardiovascular (CVD) and, in turn, these are associated with increasing social inequality (Everson et al. 2002). The effects of economic disadvantage are cumulative—sustained hardship over time produces the greatest risk of poor mental and physical health. Biomedical and lifestyle factors account for only small proportions of differences of CVD and diabetes rates among populations.

The social determinants of cardiovascular disease are likely to be similar to those of Type II diabetes. These are explained in terms of material deprivation, which creates psychosocial stress, through to the adoption of health-threatening behaviours (Raphael et al. 2003) (Figure 4.2). Material deprivation is explained in terms of clustering of disadvantaged circumstances such as poverty, as well as differential exposures to factors such as housing, education, racism, discrimination, and social exclusion. People who suffer from material deprivation (both relative and absolute poverty) have greater exposures to negative events such as hunger and lack of quality food, poor quality housing, inadequate clothing, and poor environmental conditions at home and work (Raphael et al. 2003: xiii). People suffering from material deprivation have particular susceptibility to inadequate public health infrastructure, less access to social networks and other forms of social support, fewer opportunities for recreation, leisure and physical activity, reduced access to resources such as education, books, newspapers, and the Internet, less exposure or participation in arts and culture—all of which contribute to human development over the lifespan (Raphael et al. 2003: xiii; Wallerstein 2006: 7).

Economic development alone is unable to address the negative effects of such exposures, or to bring about social and distributive justice (Baum 2002). Conservative economic theories, which have dominated the political landscapes of developed countries over the last 100 years, have promoted market-driven economies and individualism based on laissez-faire economic theories. In simple terms, this is about creating an economic environment that is intended to allow people do for themselves what they know how to do and pursue their own ends without particular regard for wider social responsibilities (<www.en.wikipedia.org/wiki/Laissez-faire_economics>). Beliefs that market-driven economies will benefit all members of society via trickle-down effects of the wealth generation of individuals, are based on the economic theory that flourishing business-based economies and unfettered markets will eventually bring benefits to middle- and lower-income people in the form of increased economic activity and reduced unemployment. However, trickle-down effect theory is now considered to be mistaken in light of the evidence that rates of growth in inequality have not abated despite rampant markets and individualism. Now, the enormous social costs of growing inequalities threaten the health of whole societies through decaying social fabric, and increasing levels of crime and social instability (Kawachi & Kennedy 1997). So often, we criminalise the poor, rather than criminalising the poverty. We focus on the behaviours rather than the causes. There is growing understanding that we must do better at supporting people who are deriving least benefit from societies driven by market economics, which spawn individualistic belief systems that decry socio-economic interventions such as Medicare, Australia's universal health insurance scheme. Because everyone pays a percentage of their income, Medicare is widely understood as a very effective wealth-redistribution mechanism because it ensures that all Australians contribute according to their wealth, and all Australians have access to high-quality medical and hospital care systems. Compared to the 40 million+ Americans who are not covered by any form of health insurance, Australia's social redistribution of wealth via Medicare is very effective. People's survival and quality of life are affected when they do not have the security of affordable health care because quality health care is a key determinant of health. But quality can be compromised in economically deprived areas, even when health care is generally available. Victora et al. (2003) report that in many counties, not only are poor children more likely to become sick, but they are not as likely as their better-off peers to receive the quality of care available to people living in wealthier communities.

Socioeconomic inequities in child survival thus exist at every step along the path from exposure and resistance to infectious disease, through careseeking, to the probability that the child will receive prompt treatment with effective therapeutic agents. The odds are stacked against the poorest children at every one of these steps (Victoria et al. 2003: 234–5).

Economic reform of health sectors has been intended to create greater efficiency and address systems management by increasing the private sector presence in the health sector. However, such reforms have failed to remedy the problems of inequality and inadequate access to services for low income people (WHO 2005b: 19). The effect of reforms has been the cutting of human and financial resources from the health sector and contracting of services through the separation of the functions of financing, purchasing, and service delivery. Privatisation has been lucrative for the private sector but has done little to address inequities—indeed, in some cases there have been 'negative impacts on equity' (WHO 2005b: 20).

UPSTREAM–MIDSTREAM FACTORS

Health promotion actions are often discussed in terms of upstream, midstream, and downstream factors. Upstream factors are related to the distal determinants of health—those that that are distant either in time or place, from any change in health status.

This layer of health promotion action is sometimes referred to as socio-ecological health where health is understood as an outcome of the complexity of interactions between people, and their social and physical environments. Proximal determinants or 'downstream factors' are those that are readily and directly associated with a change in health status.

As demonstrated in Figures 4.1 and 4.2, distal determinants operate as a background to the more proximal determinants of health. For example, proximal psychosocial factors (stress, social isolation, lack of quality social support, depression, anxiety and panic disorder, self-esteem, anger, coping, attachment, hostility) are micro-level mechanisms that are related to the social networks at the mezzo level. But they are both influenced by social-structural conditions at the macro level. Berkman and Glass (2000) describe these as intermediate mechanisms that work on psychosocial risk factors, which are consistent with the layer of social and community networks of the Dahlgren and Whitehead diagram (Figure 4.1)

■ social support: instrumental and financial, informational, appraisal, emotional
■ social influence: constraining/enabling influences on health behaviours; norms towards help-seeking; peer pressure
■ social engagement: physical/cognitive exercise; reinforcement of meaningful social roles; bonding/interpersonal attachment; 'handling' effects (children); 'grooming' effects (adults)
■ person-to-person contact: close personal contact; intimate contact.

Figure 4.2 Pathways for CVD-diabetes: determinants and interventions

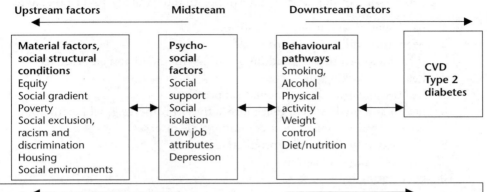

Upstream factors   Midstream   Downstream factors

| **Material factors, social structural conditions** Equity Social gradient Poverty Social exclusion, racism and discrimination Housing Social environments | **Psycho-social factors** Social support Social isolation Low job attributes Depression | **Behavioural pathways** Smoking, Alcohol Physical activity Weight control Diet/nutrition | **CVD Type 2 diabetes** |

Population (Macro)	**Psychosocial (Meso)**	**Individual (Micro)**
Upstream determinants: Inequities and poverty Racism and discrimination Violence Access to economic resources Gender inequity Unemployment Homelessness **Actions:** Develop healthy public policy Develop gendered policy frameworks Strengthen community action Education systems Income and social status Gender and culture Comprehensive primary health care policy and funding programs Reconciliation with Aboriginal and Torres Strait Islander people Enhance access to affordable and secure housing Poverty reduction, especially for single parents Wealth redistribution Capacity-build health services to ensure cultural competence Local employment programs, training and enhancement of work conditions Neighbourhood renewal programs Improve community resource mobilisation	Midstream determinants: Healthy child development Gender inequity Parenting programs Social support networks Create supportive physical, built, natural environments **Actions:** Focus on disadvantage and most vulnerable Strengthening neighbourhoods and networks focusing on disadvantage Early childhood programs Understand gender equity and raise awareness Support for mothers, including creation of physical activity and leisure opportunities to increase networks and connections Parenting programs Food access programs Community-based child-care centres to ensure affordability Develop local leadership	Downstream determinants: Access to appropriate, affordable, cultural-sensitive health care Personal coping skills and individual capacity **Actions:** Health services based on primary health care principles/practices Timely and affordable treatment Culturally competent health services Disease management Prevention Screening Health information Empowerment through health learning and literacy

Source: Dahlgren & Whitehead 1991

The use of determinants as a basis for the Swedish Public Health Strategy is a useful expression of the determinants of health into strategy. Its 11 objectives are:

1 participation and influence in society
2 economic and social security
3 secure and favourable conditions during childhood and adolescence
4 healthier working life
5 healthy and safe environments and products
6 health and medical care that more actively promotes good health
7 effective protection against communicable diseases
8 safe sexuality and good reproductive health
9 increased physical activity
10 good eating habits and safe food
11 reduced use of tobacco and alcohol, a society free from illicit drugs, and a reduction in the harmful effects of excessive gambling.

You will notice that the first six objectives relate to social-structural conditions, while the other five are about lifestyle choices people can make, but the Strategy recognises that social environment is a major influence on those lifestyle choices. Social-structural conditions influence both the intermediate and proximal determinants. Social structural conditions include access to resources needed for daily life and material goods; jobs/economic opportunity and work environments; access to decent housing; clean water and good sanitation; and access to education and health services.

For health promotion, it is important to understand the differences between psychosocial and material factors because they are related to levels of action (see Figure 3.2 in chapter 2 and Figure 4.2 in this chapter) for health promotion. Conceptual looseness about the difference between psychosocial and social-structural drivers for health serve to weaken understandings of what outcomes might be expected of health promotion actions designed to address conditions that impact negatively on health status. So it is important to understand not just which determinants of health a given program is seeking to influence but also their level, in order to identify outcomes that are consistent with the level (or levels) of action (micro–mezzo–macro).

The rising influence of the social determinants of health raises questions about the value of reliance on medical and lifestyle approaches. Policy and funding for these is often through narrow entry points of disease prevention with little evidence of recognition of the social determinants of health. Where policy and funding is still narrowly cast, health promotion practitioners have an advocacy agenda to mediate or influence those policies and funding programs, in order to address the negative impacts of the socio-economic drivers of poor health and well-being.

GENDER EQUITY

Gender is a determinant of health that influences health at all levels. Gender is a system of social relations that are embedded with values and social norms at all levels of society. As a social construct, gender discrimination is classified along with racism, ethnocentrism, and discrimination based on sexuality (Kreiger 2001). In the taxonomy of prevalent types of discrimination, gender inequity occurs where the dominant social groups are male, the subordinate groups are women and girls, and the dominant ideology is sexism.

Gender is a determinant of social experiences and has many dimensions that are interrelated. There is a responsibility for anyone using the concept of gender not to use it selectively or narrowly to only mean biological or psychological differences but to use it comprehensively—to recognise and take responsibility for the stereotypes, societal expectations, discriminations, power relationships, and social and sexual norms that shape so much social experience, and the social, cultural, and economic environment that shapes women's and men's opportunities.

Women's particular health issues, their social position, reduced income and long-term financial security, and their vulnerability to stereotypical attitudes and assumptions about their roles in society are different to those of men, and are frequently disempowering. The 1997 UNDP Report, cited by Astbury and Cabral (2000) states that no society treats its women as well as its men. Key areas where inequities persist include:

- women's financial security
- reproductive and sexual health
- emotional and mental health, including eating disorders and depressive disorders
- violence against women
- caring and the care economy
- ageing and its intersections with poverty.

Women are disproportionately affected by poverty, which diminishes their opportunities to enjoy their rights and entitlements to full citizenship and political participation. Gender roles and relationships shape decision-making and sexual practices, in condom use for example (Theobald, Elsey & Tolhurst 2004). Gender permeates health care, health-seeking behaviour, and treatment.

To address gender equity, health promotion practitioners will find Guidebook 4, Health Promotion as a Gendering Practice, to be useful. In addition, gender-disaggregated data and information can inform planning and evaluation, clarify directions, and guide the development of appropriate approaches (for example, see www.whv.org.au for a range of gendered data and policy analysis).

As new evidence about gender equity and health is made available, there are indications that the needs of special population groups, including Aboriginal and Torres Strait Islander women, migrant women, and refugee women, need to be addressed in a coordinated way, using gender equity frameworks. A new approach would provide an opportunity, through the processes of its development, to engage a wide range of community groups and interests. Recognising the importance of a social view of health and the need to include a gendered perspective, especially gender-sensitive indicators across all health strategies and issues, could provide a unifying theme.

Major health issues such as tobacco, alcohol, violence, mental health, and other priority areas are not isolated issues in the lives of women or men, and a social view of health can underpin a successful and connected approach to prevention. The prevalence of these issues highlight the need for a coordinated, equity-focused and gendered approach as a means of addressing the following issues, focusing on the reality of women's and men's lives.

SO, WHAT'S HEALTH GOT TO DO WITH IT?

The notion of health equity is about the equal right to be healthy and is closely linked to human rights (Braverman & Gruskin 2002). One of the implications of understanding health disparities is that health should not just be measured by assessing its distribution, but also by what social conditions provide pathways into those disparities and distribution across different social groups. The determinants of health are central to our understanding of how health is created and sustained, founded on the understanding that the drivers for health lie outside the health sector. Therefore, there are imperatives to advance our skills, strengthen organisations, and reorient policy, towards multilevel and multisectoral health promotion actions. This leads us to question the nature of traditional health promotion approaches, and the activities or actions on which policy-makers, politicians, and practitioners are focused. The extent to which health promotion should be positioned in the health sector, or whether it should be diffused through a range of other sectors, is a central question for the health promotion movement. Health promotion may be characterised as attempting to direct traffic from the centre of an intersection of complex partnerships and multisectoral activities, or health promotion can be characterised as a partner in the mobilising of activities aimed at improving health alongside a range of sectors such as justice, community arts, local government, education, the environment, and a host of others.

Health services and health care are a determinant of health in relation to the allocation of resources, the funding of health care (i.e. Medicare), and the quality and appropriateness of services (Braverman & Gruskin 2002). The less we care collectively about these elements of the health system, the steeper the price that society will pay for such neglect. A more complete accounting of the costs of inequality might renew interest in collective action (Lewis 1999). As Lewis (1999) reminds us, the successful pay a steep price for inequality: gated communities, private schools and hospitals that ensure that those who can afford it do not have to confront the real problems across society that present as troublesome kids, drug-addicted youth, and adults with multiple social and health problems and insufficient income, education, or resilience to overcome them. Yet, 'it is impossible to quarantine despair' (Lewis 1999: 2) and as the WHO's Commission for the Social Determinants of Health has highlighted, only some governments have realised the need to act.

Health professionals have a wide array of resources available to them. They are health literate, can see the problems first-hand, understand causal pathways, have access to information about the social determinants of health and what to do about them, can act collectively, advocate, enable, and mediate. Victora et al. (2003) argue that we now know enough to move ahead to reduce health inequalities in children and that policy-makers have choices available to them to increase access to government health services. 'Complacency is not an option' (Victora et al. 2003: 236). If you could do one thing about health inequities, what would you do?

SUMMARY

Making the connections between the social determinants of health, and health promotion policy, organisational change, planning, actions, and evaluation will be ongoing challenges. At government levels, there is good guidance on what the social determinants mean, for example, for policy (see for example, the WHO Solid Facts document, and the Swedish National Public Health Strategy). They indicate that social spending on building communities, child care, affordable housing, access to affordable health services, schools and post-school education, employment and working conditions, healthy and safe environments, and so on, are essential. And there is plenty of evidence that indicates the need for health equity and gender equity approaches that target resources where they are most needed.

Evidence about the translation of the social determinants of health into health promotion planning and practice is an emerging knowledge base. The evidence is very strong and clear that social and economic factors are more influential in shaping people's behaviours than lifestyles and risk factor approaches. Yet, that is where so much of our health promotion resources are focused—on midstream approaches devoid of frameworks that link the midstream to the upstream. And such health promotion work will continue to be ineffective for those who most need assistance to take control over those things that make them unhealthy, unless action is taken to increase health equity by addressing relevant socio-economic factors.

The WHO Commission on the Social Determinants of Health and the growing literature that is now being published on these topics are of great importance to health promotion as their findings will influence directions for funding and policy. Guidebook 3, Key Resources about the Socio-economic Determinants of Health, includes some early papers from the Commission but its substantive body of work will not be released until after the publication of this book. I suggest you bookmark the site to keep abreast of the Commission's work.

USEFUL WEBSITES

Canadian National Network on Environments and Women's Health: <www.yorku.ca/gmcr/>

Health Canada's information on the Social Determinants of Health is found at: <www.phac-aspc.gc.ca/ph-sp/phdd/determinants/index.html>

International Society for Equity in Health: <www.iseqh.org>

People's Health Movement (PHM):

Swedish Gender and Health Equity Network: <www.ids.ac.uk/ghen/>

Swedish Public Health Strategy: <www.fhi.se>

World Health Organisation Commission on the Social Determinants of Health: <www.who.int/social_determinants>

PROMOTING HUMAN RIGHTS FOR HEALTH

5

Frank Tesoriero

Key concept

■ A rights perspective on health is a foundation for equity in health services and health promotion.

Key terms

■ Health and human rights
■ People's Health Movement

OVERVIEW

This chapter examines the contributions made to human rights discourse and health and well-being and identifies the intersections between health and the potential for a human rights perspective, through reflective practice, to interrupt traditional professional, disciplinary, and sector boundaries. The argument draws on debates located within the discipline of social work, but is valid for all other health and social service professions.

HUMAN RIGHTS DISCOURSE IN HEALTH

Contemporary public health discourses privilege the notions of equity and rights; and this is in response to the realisation that health approaches up to the 1970s had no or little effect on lessening the gap in health status between rich and poor, both between countries and within countries, as discussed in Chapter 4.

As explained in Chapter 2, the WHO Alma Ata Declaration (WHO 1978) and its comprehensive primary health care principles asserted health as a human right and a global social issue. These assertions represented a view that health was a fundamental component of the human condition and a necessary aspect of human dignity, and that this was the responsibility of agents beyond the health sector—it was a responsibility shared socially, culturally, and politically. This view of health has been significantly eroded since 1978, both by the blunt weapons of economic globalisation as well as the more subtle discourses such as selective primary health care. However, alternative voices have continued to challenge forces hostile to health as a human right. These voices have been in the form of broad social movements, such as the People's Health Movement, which has been driven by health activists across the globe, and which culminated in People's Health Assemblies in Bangladesh in 2000 and in Ecuador in 2005. The People's Health Movement (PHM) <www.phmovement.org> is as much a political movement and a social movement as it is a health movement. While its concern is with heath as a human right, its processes, activities, and aspirations aim to change both the way power is distributed and its use. The PHM aims to enable ordinary citizens to participate in decisions and in democratic processes, and aims to harness power for the benefit of all rather than for the accumulation of wealth for a few.

The PHM's People's Charter for Health (see their website) captures the essence of the discourse that social, economic, and political factors influence health and that it is the poor and marginalised who are affected most by the factors influencing ill health; and that it ought to be governments, international organisations, and corporations that are the targets of social action and advocacy for health. The preamble states:

> Health is a social, economic and political issue and above all a fundamental human right. Inequality, poverty, exploitation, violence and injustice are at the root of ill-health and the deaths of poor and marginalised people. Health For All means that powerful interests have to be challenged, that globalisation has to be opposed, and that political and economic priorities have to be drastically changed (People's Health Assembly 2000: 1)

The People's Health Movement is one example of health activists fighting collectively for health as a human right. The PHM and other movements and campaigns, including the World Social Forum (www.wsfindia.org), represent a sustained attempt to ensure that, at the most, health as a human right achieves dominance and becomes more widely accepted and, at the very least, challenges those discourses that erode health and exposes them for their contraventions of human rights and destroying of human dignity.

If it is accepted that the rights discourse of health resonates strongly with the value base of public health and health promotion and, conversely, the forces that lead to the privatisation and commodification of health disrupt that discourse, then the issue becomes one of how health promotion can engage with the rights discourse in action. It is this question that this chapter will examine.

SIGNIFICANCE OF THE RIGHTS DISCOURSE IN HEALTH AND HUMAN WELL-BEING

While health as a human need is an important perspective on health, because this implies action is required to meet unmet human needs, in the contemporary neoliberal and globalised world, health by itself is an insufficient driver for change. 'Need' has been transformed in this current context from a useful concept to a potentially dangerous one. This may seem a somewhat outrageous claim, but 'need' can be met by the private sector, which is driven by profit and may have little concern with issues of ethics and morality. For example, water was once a social resource, but is now a private commodity. This can mean the death of infants in Africa and other developing countries, when mothers, with no money to feed prepaid water meters, search for free water for their babies, to find that it is generally contaminated. Commodification of such essential and life-sustaining services is an illustration of the critical nature of a human rights perspective.

Beyond such illustrations, it can be more generally argued that 'human rights' is critical. If we examine the notion of human need, then we are referring to 'must haves', such as food, clothing, shelter, water, safety, health, and so on. Needs can be provided by the private, for-profit sector. From the 1980s many governments opened their countries to the global market. The accompanying deregulation of economies, the privatisation of public resources, and the demands of structural adjustment programs all represented a neoliberal paradigm, where economics became dominant and the world was constructed as a marketplace. Within this global marketplace, more and more needs were placed on the market to be bought and sold. As part of the expansion of the goods available to be purchased in the marketplace, we have seen the privatisation of such things as education, water, transport, and health. This represents a transformation of public resources into private goods. The core critique of neoliberalism from a social justice perspective is that neoliberalism and the marketplace paradigm increase inequities. The divide between the rich and the poor becomes greater. Only a few benefit from the movement of money and capital. There is no trickle-down effect to benefit all. Those who can least afford to pay for services miss out. In one African country where water has been privatised and prepaid meters are used to buy water, poor families soon run out of money and are forced to search for free drinking water, which is generally unclean. Their babies contract diarrhoeal diseases and die. This is a stark example of the hostility of neoliberalism towards meeting human needs and towards humane values.

The drivers of neoliberalism have not encouraged debates on issues of human rights, social well-being, and health. Many decisions that affect people's health and welfare are made by transnational corporations. The World Bank provides the most funding for health of any organisation on earth, and the WHO is now more marginalised in determining health outcomes. Health has been colonised by the economic sector. Questions of morality and ethics are replaced by a drive for profit. The great Indian leader, Mahatma Gandhi, warned of the dangers in separating our actions from their moral base. Needs continue to be met, but within a more inequitable system. If 'needs' concern what people must have, then 'rights' concern what people should have. Every human need can imply a human right, and if a human right refers to what people should have, then it is normative—human rights brings the morality and ethics back onto the centre stage of health and its promotion.

HARNESSING HUMAN RIGHTS TO CHALLENGE CONTEMPORARY FORCES OF INEQUITY AND INJUSTICE

'Human rights' has ancient beginnings. Early religions stressed such things as fairness and dignified treatment, things that we now call human rights. Very early philosophers wrote about equality and justice, there is an honourable and long history to modern expressions of human rights. 'Human rights' easily and quickly evokes a sense of decency, and so for professions that serve humanity it can be readily adopted as a guiding framework for thinking and acting. However, 'human rights' is itself a contested discourse with a somewhat contradictory history. At times, the champions of human rights, those who are dominant and privileged, have silenced those less able to find a voice.

Adopting human rights, simply as they appear in the many charters of rights, would represent a grossly inadequate framework for health promotion. This is so for several reasons. Firstly, a narrow legalistic view of human rights, while necessary, is insufficient for a realisation of human rights. Legal prescriptions of human rights will help to ensure minimum standards are adhered to, but will not lead to an optimum standard of rights. Anti-discrimination legislation, for example, will not address racism. Secondly, a legal framework favours those rights that are more amenable to protection in courts and because court processes are often expensive, may marginalise claims of rights of those more vulnerable in society.

It can be argued that many statements of human rights appear as if rights are unchanging truths. Many of these statements have been criticised because they were formulated in forums that were dominated by Western world leaders, and so in their individualism do not take account of human rights, as they may be expressed in non-Western, more collectivist societies. The Asian critiques of human rights declarations challenge rights as absolute truths. If we reject the notion of rights as something objective that exists apart from human agency, then we must acknowledge that human rights are constructed by humans, and that this construction is a dynamic process and must be open to scrutiny and debate. We must also acknowledge that, given power structures and inequalities, the voices of the powerful may often dominate. So, the way in which the process of dialogue, discussion, and debate to identify and construct human rights occurs is critical. Whose voice will be heard in the debates? Whose will not? What claims will be privileged?

If health promotion engages with and adopts a human rights discourse, then it must be much more than the list of actions that appear in Health Promotion Declarations. To embrace human rights as an effective framework, it is necessary for proactive building of a strong culture of human rights. This task cannot be legislated for. Building culture is a pervasive and long-term change process, requiring many of the skills of working in partnership with citizens and communities, and necessarily being interdisciplinary. The process of building a human rights culture is as complex as it is long.

To replace a legalistic and somewhat static list of rights with a process of building a rights culture, we need criteria to guide the dialogue and the endeavour of articulating human rights. It is this work that Australian social work has been struggling with. One of the products of this struggle and the debates in social work has been a set of criteria for establishing what claims are human rights claims. Ife (2000) proposes the following set of criteria:

- **That realising the claimed right is necessary for people to achieve their full humanity, in common with others.** In other words, the claims and demands that are made by people need to be congruent with what would be considered human and personal development and with sustainable strengthening of communities, where people live in common with each other.
- **That the claimed right should apply to all humanity, or at least to groups who are disadvantaged and marginalised.** This criterion is closely aligned with the concept of social justice, where, if the claim were to be realised, there would be some common benefit or advantage to humanity; or there would be some liberatory change for those who are oppressed and in exploitative relationships.
- **That there is widespread support for the claimed right, across cultures.** The importance of wide acceptance is related to the notion of common good and a collectivist view of what will progress human rights. It is akin to a population approach to health rather than an individualistic perspective.
- **That all claimants can reasonably realise the right.** The assertion in the traditional, modernisation approaches to development that economic growth will 'trickle down' to all is a clear example of a claim that, in reality, had no chance of being realised. Such a claim that all would benefit disguised something quite opposite, that inequities between the rich and poor would, in fact, increase.
- **That the claimed right does not contradict other human rights.** This criterion introduces the central and critical relationship between rights and responsibilities: that one set of rights will necessarily carry with it a set of

responsibilities for others to fulfil and a set of responsibilities for the claimants towards others.

The use of these criteria exposes the fact that many rights claims cannot be called claims to human rights. The right of every American to carry a gun is a strong and dominant claim to rights, but is not a human right according to the above criteria. On the other hand, can 'health' be considered a human right? Equally importantly, the criteria expose many views of health as outside the parameters of human rights. The claim of an individual to the right to have an organ transplant does not comply with the criteria outlined above. The criteria then, provide a somewhat sharp set of tools for discriminating against competing discourses within health.

The processes involved in achieving human rights are what Ife (2000) refers to as building a culture of human rights. Such a culture would include a high level of citizen participation. It would have a commitment and set of actions to redress oppression. It would act to change power relationships that were exploitative. It would be inclusive of difference. It would have capacity to act collectively, to advocate, to strengthen supports and to ensure access to societal resources. The path to achieving a culture of human rights is akin to health practice within the principles of comprehensive primary health care. It involves working in partnership with affected groups and communities.

Both the use of the criteria above and the processes of working in partnership invite professionals to ask questions. Are these criteria being satisfied in relation to a particular claim? Who may benefit and who may lose? Who will be the partners? What is their lived experience? What is the expertise they bring to the partnership and to the process of building a culture of rights where their right to health is both respected and achieved? What respective roles do the partners play? What strategies are used? How effective are they? How might things be done differently to increase effectiveness? What are the assumptions underlying how issues are problematised and how they are addressed? Where do these assumptions come from, are they relevant to the issue, and are they shared among partners? These are just some of the questions that may arise from an approach that discounts static declarations of rights as 'the truth' and seeks to engage diverse others in the process of promoting health. This is reflective practice. The process means that knowledge-building is continuous and learning is ongoing, as questions lead to answers that lead to actions that lead to further questions. This iterative process invites the engagement of many others.

Reflective practice is a powerful tool for interrupting the traditional and somewhat entrenched boundaries between disciplines and professions (see Chapter 17), thus enabling truly interdisciplinary, rather than multidisciplinary, work to occur. Boundaries are interrupted because reflective practice implies a view of knowledge that departs from the traditional view of each discipline having its own knowledge base. Reflective practice leads to knowledge biases, rather than knowledge bases.

INTERSECTIONS AND INTERRUPTING TRADITIONAL BOUNDARIES: BUILDING KNOWLEDGE

Interrogating practice through reflection serves to question knowledge. Because reflective practice is a cyclical and iterative process, new knowledge is being generated, or at least, the knowledge already held is being somewhat reshaped, in every new situation, in every different context. In this sense, there are no longer any static knowledge bases. Rather, knowledge is one resource in a process of meaning-making, where every situation may yield different meanings. Here, knowledge is given a different and dynamic bias; and it is this knowledge bias that is most powerful in its respective contexts, because it is this bias that gives meaning to particular situations. This is knowing for doing; knowledge generation for action.

The criteria for human rights claims become tools for working reflectively within a human rights framework, because they become questions that must be asked. Responses to claims to rights must be interrogated. Practice must be questioned. Questions must be asked and, in asking questions, others are engaged in processes of moral and ethical activity. So not only must a claim be interrogated through reflective questioning, but the response to such claims must be continually reflected upon. The outcomes of this reflection, new insights, lead to new knowledge and improved practice.

SUMMARY

Enabling knowledge generation through allowing biases to emerge from particular contexts requires working in partnership with affected groups. This corresponds to notions of empowerment, anti-oppressive practice, and a moral-based practice. In this there are resonances with Primary Health Care principles and health promotion strategies.

'Partnership' becomes a central concept in reflective practice, ongoing knowledge generation, and building a culture of human rights. Promoting health, enabling people and communities to have control over factors that affect them, requires particular kinds of relationships. The acceptance by professionals of their knowledge as useful but partial, and their acceptance that groups or communities they serve also have knowledge and expertise, again useful but partial, leads to partnership work. Acknowledging that people's participation is the practice of citizenship, and that fully participating as a citizen meets the criteria of a human right, working to promote health necessarily entails the negotiation (and continual renegotiation) of relationships that enable participation. Partnership does not imply shared goals and equal power. Indeed, it is clear that within partnerships power is unequal and circulates dynamically as an energy; and there are many different agendas that partners bring with them. The challenge, then, is to work effectively with difference, not as a threat to partnerships, but as a positive resource. The challenge is also to use dynamic power as a positive force.

USEFUL WEBSITES

United Nations Declaration of Human Rights: <www.un.org/Overview/rights.htm>

World Social Forum: <www.wsfindia.org>

LAY KNOWLEDGE

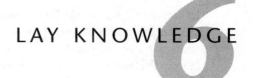

Jennie Popay & Colin MacDougall

Key concepts

- Quantitative research using a biomedically derived definition of health implicitly or explicitly separates individuals from their complex social, physical and economic environments.
- We can improve the theoretical base in health promotion by conducting research that attributes greater validation to lay knowledge.
- Professional dominance and theories discount lay knowledge as subjective.
- Lay knowledge about heath inequalities involves complex and multifactorial theorising about the meaning of place and direct and indirect pathways to health and illness.
- Lay knowledge does not locate the drivers of health in the health sector—rather, lay knowledge focuses on environment, place, social relationships, and ontological resources.
- Lay knowledge contributes to culturally relevant theories of health promotion that in turn leads to new ways to develop policy and practice in response to growing health inequalities.

Key terms

- Lay knowledge
- Professional, codified theories
- Professional dominance
- Qualitative research
- Meaning, environment, place, and ontological resources
- Health inequalities
- Policy and health promotion interventions

PREFACE

In October 2005 Jennie Popay visited South Australia as a guest of the Australian Health Inequities Project (AHIP) and the South Australian government. AHIP is an initiative of Flinders University and Melbourne University, funded by the National Health and Medical Research Council under a scheme to increase the capacity of the Australian workforce. While in South Australia Jennie spoke to a meeting of people interested in health promotion about lay knowledge. This chapter combines an edited version of her talk with explanatory notes about theory and practice.

OVERVIEW

When research uses a biomedically derived definition of health to explore people's attitudes and behaviours implicitly, if not explicitly, individuals are separated from the complex social physical and economic environments in which they live (Milburn 1996). To overcome this problem, Milburn argues:

> questioning of the derivation of the existing theoretical base in health promotion could begin with the process of attributing greater validation to lay theorising as an essential feature in the development of culturally relevant theory and practice (Milburn 1996: 42).

New theories in health promotion should not just come from the minds and pens of professionals. This chapter explores the contribution of research validating lay knowledge that is centrally concerned with social and health inequalities.

WHAT IS LAY KNOWLEDGE?

Lay knowledge is something we all have. This isn't them and us. We are all lay people some of the time, we all wear different hats, but there is a tendency for professionals to think of lay knowledge as something that other people have.

Over the last decade there has been a shift from conversations about lay beliefs to conversations about lay knowledge: and that's a profound and really interesting shift. It's both a research shift and a shift within the public sector. Lay knowledge comprises the ideas and perspectives that people use to interpret their experience—it's experiential, it's drawn out of the experience of everyday life and, in the context of today's presentation, their experience of health and illness. But over the last thirty years, this knowledge has been seen as a primitive, residual, left over from some bygone age. It is as if these 'beliefs' don't really belong to today's world of science and rationality, but remain an interesting curiosity that we should study to understand peculiar behaviours, why people damage themselves; why people get involved in things that damage their health.

Box 6.1: Definitions, terms, and understandings of lay knowledge

Various terms describe the views of people in the community about health and illness: for example, lay epidemiology (Davison et al. 1992; Frankel et al. 1991); lay theorising (Milburn, 1996); lay constructions (Pawluch et al. 2000), and practical logic (Craig 2000).

Pierre Bourdieu also uses the term *practical logic* to describe the way popular medical knowledge exists in ways that help ordinary people to remember, manipulate, and apply their theories to everyday life (Bourdieu 1990).

Abrums (2000) deliberately uses the term *theory* to describe what others have called lay or popular beliefs in order to acknowledge that both experts and ordinary people go through a process of testing their explanations. The difference is that ordinary people do not just test explanations historically and empirically, but by reference to their own everyday experiences (Abrums 2000). In the process, ordinary people may give more weight to what is reasonable for them and people like themselves, than what is defined by experts as rational.

The decision by people about what is reasonable takes more account of the person's personal and social contexts than does the decision for people about what is rational (Backett & Davison 1992).

The shift from talking about lay beliefs to lay knowledge is a sign of the increasing status of experiential wisdom, no longer a primitive leftover, but now a key part of what it is to be a human being in society. Lay knowledge reflects how we make sense of our world at any particular time and in any particular place. And I think the shifting language reflects an increasing understanding of the sophistication of this experiential wisdom and a growing recognition that this wisdom, this knowledge, has important implications for the way policy and practice get done.

So let me say something about crucial ways in which the content and form of lay knowledge differs from professional, codified knowledge. It is an approach to explanation. This knowledge does seek to identify causes in everyday life that lead to experiences of positive health or negative health, so there are causal explanations—lay theories—embedded in this knowledge. But the key issue is that lay knowledge is also about attributing meaning to experience. When we talk about our experiences we are trying to make sense of that experience in terms of morality, politics, and what we call cosmologies—a kind of *who am I?* question. This subjectivity can be the problem for professionals because we've all been trained to be wary of the subjective, adding to the problematic nature of the interface between lay knowledge, policy, and practice.

Box 6.2: Professional dominance and lay knowledge

The following example shows how the tendency for professional dominance can colour the way architects of health promotion campaigns consider and act on opinions from the community:

If you have talked informally to people about physical activity, you have no doubt heard lists of reasons for not being active. The all-time winner is 'I don't have the time.' ... although that is difficult to take seriously when the average US adult watches three hours of television each day. It is not clear whether these lists referred to true reasons or convenient 'excuses' but the ubiquity of these reasons makes them important to study (Sallis & Owen 1999: 119).

Here, the authors do not appraise whether this reason for inactivity is reasonable, rational, or representative, rather they describe it as: '... the all time winner ... difficult to take seriously ... true reasons or convenient excuses'.

MacDougall 2003: 382

LAY KNOWLEDGE AND INEQUALITIES: RATIONALE AND METHODS

So, how might lay knowledge help us develop more effective approaches to improving population health and reducing health inequalities? I want to explore this by looking at two different strands of a large study that I conducted with colleagues in the United Kingdom (UK). The study was looking at four places in the north-west of England. There were two very advantaged and two very disadvantaged places. All four were at the extreme ends of the continuum of advantage and disadvantage in the UK. In those four areas we took routine data and did geographical information mapping, looking at the availability of amenities, access to amenities, health care, mortality data, and incidence of diseases. Then we came down to a smaller area and surveyed around 2000 people and then down again to an even smaller area and did in-depth interviews with some of the people from the survey. The findings I'm going to talk about now are based on the qualitative research because the bottom line is that you can't access lay knowledge unless you use qualitative methodologies. Surveys just won't get you into the stories and won't give you access to the meaning, so these data are based on in-depth interviews with around twenty people in each of these four areas at two points in time over a year (see Popay et al. 2003).

THE CENTRALITY OF MEANING: PEOPLE, PLACE, ENVIRONMENT, AND ONTOLOGY

The data showed how lay knowledge explored what it means to live in a particular place, at a particular time, and how this links with health-related action or agency. Places are simultaneously physical, social, and normative entities that led us to develop the idea of a *proper place*. One respondent described where she was living as *not being a proper place to bring up children*, a very clear normative aspect of place. The powerful strand running through all the advantaged and the disadvantaged people's narratives was about the normative aspects of place, by which we mean socially shared frameworks that provide an idealised notion of this proper place. These normative ideas were shared across very wealthy areas and very disadvantaged areas.

What would define a proper place? Overwhelmingly the *people* who lived there and the *social relationships between people*; for example:

> I have neighbours who are always willing to make themselves known to each other and to help each other, I mean you have your own life, your own friends, your own family but it's like an extension of that when you feel comfortable with the people around you and that's what I feel here.

Another is *respecting people and respecting property*. Property was not just the house and car, it was public property such as bus stops, parks, and schools, for example:

> 'It's quiet here, not as rough. In Salford (which is the rough area), you see the kids effing and blinding at their mothers. It's the people of Salford that make it so bad. They've no respect for people at all.'

This is a very clear statement that it's the people that make the place bad. This place was physically a really difficult place to live but the focus of the narratives was on the people.

> 'And whereas years ago people had pride, you'd see people scrubbing the steps outside. I'd have to say you wouldn't have seen me scrubbing the steps outside.'
>
> 'And all this lot but nobody's got any pride in the place anymore.'

Respect for people and pride about the place was really important from a normative point of view.

Then there was the *ontological element* that in a place that's proper you have to feel like you belong there, like you've got an affinity with other people who live there. For example, somebody who had a strong sense of identity with their really disadvantaged area said:

> 'I still like the area. I've spent thirty years around here. It's hard, isn't it, looking at it. It's not much to look about but well it's like yourself, you know, wherever you were brought up you see it declining and it's a problem isn't it? You feel sorry for the area.'

A final element was the *environment*, the physicality of space, a proper place where you felt safe, where the shops were convenient, where you had access to health care, to libraries, where it was clean. Those elements of the environment were important in their own right and because they had normative significance. People were discussing living in a place that was convenient, which had parks, which had play spaces, which had local shops, and therefore allowed children and young people to develop acceptable behaviour and values and people to socialise with each other. So the place had normative salience in that sense and it also promoted and maintained social relationships. The environment was both physical and normative.

MANAGING DISSONANCE BETWEEN ONTOLOGICAL AND NORMATIVE ASPECTS OF PLACE

This research shows us that in disadvantaged areas there's considerable dissonance between people's lived reality and the normative contours of place. People had a norm about a proper place to live but had to live and bring up their children in improper places that have direct health consequences. Resources to manage discordance in these places included the obvious one of material resources. People in the poorer areas who had cars could travel, move out of the place. People talked about social resources a lot, about families and friends, providing support, emotional support, practical support but some people also talked about an ontological resource. What seemed to be happening was that those people who identified with this place (even though they recognised it wasn't a 'proper place') were better able to cope with the place than those people who couldn't identify with it. So the guy who talked about feeling sorry for the place seemed to be managing living in this place better than some of the respondents who distanced themselves from it.

So we began to look at what we referred to as an *ontological resource*, which is people's sense of belonging or not belonging to a place and the extent to which they saw their identity as linked to a particular place. To do this we began to think about the meanings that people assigned to the place and how that linked to health in their stories, in their narratives. So our question then became *how does this experience of dissonance in place link to the causes of ill health?* In these stories we identified two equally important pathways. The first was this very strong sense that what a lot of people did in order to cope with the dissonance was to construct subtle cartographies of place, so they made distinctions at a really micro level between *us here* and *them there*. So they created other people who were different from them in order to retain a sense of their own properness. For example, '*That over there…we call it hell over there, …where all the houses are derelict sort of thing, but this, this is Langworthy over this side. It's just like it's them and us, isn't it, we're all in the same area but*'. And that was across a couple of little northern English streets, so it's really subtle social division.

But then the other powerful thing that was happening, particularly among older people, was the privatisation of everyday life. People were closing in on themselves in order to cope with this dissonance between the normative contours of a place that would be a good place to live and this place where they were living.

The consequences for health are a result of what I would refer to as an indirect pathway. This dissonance reduces trust and reciprocity between people and from a public health point of view there was a lack of a shared story, a shared narrative about place. We know from social research that to get collective action, engagement to change things, people need a shared understanding about the problem. Privatisation of life undermined the possibility for collective action in these poor places. While there was a lot of reciprocity between neighbours in small areas, there were few groups such as tenants groups, community groups or self-help groups. So collective social action just wasn't there and you can argue these coping mechanisms at the individual level undermined people's ability to cope with really difficult circumstances at the collective level.

The other familiar and plausible pathway is the direct link between experience of place and health-damaging behaviour. This is from a lone mother with a child of three who didn't feel she belonged to the place. She'd been moved into public housing just when her child was born and it wasn't very far from where her parents lived. But she found that she had no sense of belonging in this place so she hadn't let her son out of the house, or let him play in the garden, She said:

> I don't want him out there, I don't want him mixing with them people, we're different.

So there are social divisions going on. But then she went on to note:

> The doctor put me on Prozac a few months back for living here because it's depressing. You get up, you look around and all you see is junkies. I know one day I will come off, I'll get off here, I mean I started drinking a hell of a lot more since I've been here. I drink every night. I have a drink every night just to get to sleep. I smoke more as well. There's a lot of things.

Her story contrasted with a man a few doors down who wasn't a lot older than her, and who had children, but he also had a sense of belonging to this place. He knew the place so he didn't find it so difficult to live there. This shows how people feel a deeply subjective sense of belonging that cannot be measured objectively. If you don't belong there are both indirect and direct links to health-related behaviour.

CAUSES OF HEALTH INEQUALITIES

We now turn to an area about which there is a lot of academic theorising: *what causes health inequalities?* There's very little work actually speaking to people experiencing the inequalities, asking *what do you think about them, what do you think causes these inequalities?* We went back to people in wealthy and poorer areas and asked what they thought about the quantitative data showing different health experiences between areas. Now remember we'd already been to these people a year earlier so we weren't going over old ground and we had kept in contact.

At the beginning of the conversations the people living in the poorer areas disputed the evidence, every single one of them. They would say *'I don't believe that, that puzzles me, I can't believe that.'* There were really sharp differences in deaths from accidents among children, deaths in men aged 50 from heart failure and stroke, big differences. But the people in the affluent area had no problem with these figures. They went straight into discussions about why this might be the case. What became clear very soon in these conversations was that people in poorer areas were rejecting these data because they were rejecting the labelling and the inevitability that if they accepted this it meant that they, their family, their children, almost certainly were at risk of premature death and injury. For example:

> You know I don't believe it. They look at Salford as being a dump. They think nobody lives there. They're seen as outcasts. Yes there's pollution but other than that it's attitudes. They're making out that it's all like scum and they're all dying. It doesn't make sense.

So there's a real kind of moral outrage that these data are stigmatising people.

Previous quantitative research has described poor people as victim blaming, not understanding the social determinants agenda, and tending to have very individualistic views about health and illness. However qualitative research shows that things are much more complicated than that. As our conversations developed from the initial rejection of the data, people began to tell stories about how living in these places illustrated how social and material inequalities became embodied, how they affected their lives and their children's lives. So these were accounts of inequalities and causal pathways to ill health, which were as complex and multifactorial as the academic theories.

An example of complexity is one of the people who said *'I don't believe (the inequality data)'*. Not very long into the interview we were talking about living in this place again and he says:

> I'm a strong person. I can deal with a lot of things but this particular area and living in this area has made me ill. At the end of the day you've got to feel happy in the place you're living in because that's your source, it's where you're based and I can't deal with it.

So he may have rejected the abstract data, but at the same time made a very clear statement that living here is not very good for his health. The theories people offered also emphasised indirect pathways to ill health, focusing in particular on how living in this place was stressful. In other words, despite possible direct

Box 6.3: The complexity of lay knowledge

A qualitative study in Adelaide, South Australia asked, 'How do ordinary people theorise about health, physical activity and constraints on choices to increase physical activity? How do ordinary theories differ from expert theories? What are the implications of these differences for the promotion of physical activity?' The sample of 121 in focus groups and field visits was drawn from existing networks and organisations with varying experiences of factors associated with lower levels of physical activity in that area.

The study demonstrated a number of ways in which ordinary people theorise about health, physical activity, and constraints on choices to increase physical activity. Much ordinary theorising is heavily influenced by, even a response to, expert theories. However, given the opportunity to reflect on their developing ideas (via paraphrasing in focus groups), participants qualified and added to what initially appeared to be close copies of expert theories. Here is evidence of people contextualising expert theory, discussing what such theory means for people like them, and considering how expert theories need to be modified to influence their personal health and physical activity.

Experts use social marketing to distil information into brief messages, sometimes as literal prescriptions by general practitioners specifying the amount of physical activity recommended for an individual patient. A prescriptive approach contrasts with scaffolded learning, which is ' … an approach to teaching and learning that, while careful to provide an initial framework, leaves it to the learner to establish long term structures'.

This study suggests that ordinary theory used expert theory as scaffolds, as a basis to construct their own theories by personalising and contextualising health education messages. They acknowledged specific health benefits of physical activity, then broadened the debate.

Summarised from MacDougall 2003

effects such as living on very low income, in terrible housing, without a job, their primary focus was on how stressful it was to live in these places. The second most common focus was social comparisons, which is also a stress pathway, where you see other people that are better off than you and conclude:

> It's only obvious that we would not feel health wise as someone would who has all the comforts and luxuries around them. You know they go on holidays three times a year whereas we can't afford to go on one holiday. So that's the difference. Their outlook on life is more relaxed at ease and comfortable whereas we're struggling day to day with pressure and to keep up with things.

A really important strand was strength of character, which could in quantitative or less in-depth research, be framed as victim blaming. Everybody in our sample in the poor areas talked about the importance of having the strength of character to overcome these difficulties, for example:

> The first thing you do when you get up is see the graffiti, the vandalism and it doesn't help, but at the end of the day if you let it get to you it just causes ill health. I mean I just lock the door and forget about it—it's how the individual deals with it all. If you let it get you down you're going to have the health problems.

So the notion is that you have to rise above these difficult circumstances. Complexity comes in because people simultaneously talked about how to deal with stress through strength of character, all the while understanding the social determinants of ill health. All of the people living in disadvantageous circumstances at some point acknowledged those aspects of the environment over which they had no control and that those would affect their health, for example:

> I mean everybody has a bit of worry but it's our own worry brought on by ourselves, but outside worries that you haven't got any influence on changing that has a bigger effect on you I think. You can't sit down and think well I've got this problem and how can I solve it because you can't solve it if it's outside your house. It's an outside influence that you can't control, you can't change it. You haven't the power to change it and it takes over your life.

Now in the wealthy areas, people went straight into accounts that highlighted both social determinants and individual behaviour to explain the poor health of those in poor areas with little focus on stress and none on strength of character. One determinant was housing, employment, income and the other that poor people smoke and eat poor quality foods. People in the wealthy areas felt guilty about conversations about inequalities so they tended not to talk about how it made them feel.

PUBLIC HEALTH AND LAY KNOWLEDGE

From a public health perspective, it is really important to understand the purpose of these theories for lay people because it will help us to develop more appropriate ways of intervening. Lay knowledge attaches meaning to the experience of factors that epidemiology has causally related to health inequalities. People recognise complexity, talk about social determinants, talk about stress, so they have multifactorial pathways.

There are three critical and profound ways in which these theories help people cope with life's circumstances. First, they were ways of reconstructing moral worth in a situation in which to be poor and/or to be in poor health is often judged to be unworthy. Lay theories enable people to cope with the view that, individually and collectively, they are not 'proper' parents, 'proper' carers, or just 'proper'. And so they attach meaning to their experience that gives them back some sense of their moral worth through the denial of the inequality data and the emphasis on strength of character. Second, they were reasserting that despite these circumstances, I can control something: that's where stress pathways and strength of character comes from. Third, lay theories allow people to reconcile their understanding and knowledge of the social determinants with their need to have a sense of moral worth and a sense of control.

The problem for health professionals is that policy and practice can do a lot of damage if it unpicks all of this without being aware of the fundamental social purpose of these theories. I believe that in some of these communities, decades of practitioners and policy-makers with the best will in the world have been undermining the coping mechanisms at a normative and knowledge level of many of these communities.

So why should the health sector take lay knowledge seriously?

- Lay knowledge will improve the effectiveness of treatment and control of disease.
- We will also get more appropriate and accessible services by hearing, responding to lay knowledge.
- We'll get a better understanding of health-related behaviour, an understanding who those behaviours are embedded in social context and that only people who can control their social context will heed the health promotion message.
- Athough listening, hearing, understanding the meanings of lay theories about the causes of ill health are more complicated, they will help us to think about more appropriate and effective ways of intervening to do something about population health and inequalities in health experience between different groups.
- And then the bottom line is that this is also about democratic accountability. Lay people are increasingly challenging the professionals' right to define problems—community engagement is a democratic renewal issue.

SUMMARY

There are at least four barriers and enablers to taking ordinary theories seriously in the dominant structures that shape day-to-day research, system design, and professional practice (MacDougall 2001):

1   Researchers and practitioners who adopt a positivist paradigm are less likely to use results or methods that take the time to distil ordinary theories from in-depth interviews or focus groups (Baum 1998). We need research methods that can explore ordinary theorising in hectic and messy practice structures.

2   Bureaucratic structures frequently do not value community knowledge and seem impenetrable to community members (Putland et al. 1997). We need

research on how to influence organisational structure and culture that values and uses community knowledge.

3   In many countries health promotion approaches operate within free-market-inspired policy settings that require evidence-based practice in organisations that either charge a fee for service or that have won a contract to provide a service at the lowest price (Wise & Signal 2000; Ziglio et al. 2000). We need research on whether it is possible to build in use of ordinary theory as best practice within evidence-based and tendering-out policy milieux.

4   Professional training is more likely to prepare workers for a role of professional dominance than one of enhancing community participation (Baum 1998). We need research on curriculum design and teaching and learning methodologies that will critique professional dominance and promote the values and skills in a range of professions that promote community participation.

EVIDENCE TO INFORM MULTISECTORAL APPROACHES IN HEALTH PROMOTION

Elizabeth Waters, Rebecca Armstrong & Jodie Doyle

Key concepts

- There is an evidence base in health promotion that needs to be employed for effective decision-making.
- Given that health promotion covers a wide range of interventions across population groups and contexts, the development and use of evidence to guide decision-making is not straightforward.
- Different sectors define, generate, and use evidence in comparable and contrasting ways.
- Success in health promotion interventions that require multisectoral cooperation depends on a collaborative approach to gathering and using evidence.
- Systematic reviews are a useful method for gathering and synthesising available evidence.
- Research evidence for inclusion in systematic reviews can be derived from a range of sources and should not be restricted by sectoral boundaries.

Key terms

- Evidence
- Evidence-informed decision-making
- Intervention effectiveness
- Systematic reviews

OVERVIEW

Different types of evidence are required to make decisions that impact on health outcomes. Understanding these differences is important in trying to influence them.

This chapter explores how an evidence-informed approach can be utilised in health promotion decision-making, especially where the evidence needs to be drawn from sectors outside health. It draws on the value of systematic reviews as a way of summarising and synthesising any form of evidence, and introduces knowledge-transfer and knowledge-brokering as concepts that support the generation and use of evidence. The process of addressing health issues that require multisectoral input requires partners to engage to identify partners' language around 'evidence', how evidence is perceived and how it is used to make decisions. This chapter highlights and describes how evidence is derived and generated from the sectors in which health promotion aims to affect change, and how health promotion can contribute to the evidence base of other sectors.

INTRODUCTION

Evidence-informed health promotion is an emerging and evolving field of research and practice. It is founded on the argument that interventions need to be based on sound theoretical principles and the knowledge gained through previous experiences. Examples of well-meaning health promotion interventions that are ineffective or have adverse effects suggest that good intentions and perceived wisdom are not a sufficient basis for policy and programs (MacIntyre & Petticrew 2000). But the complexity of health promotion has challenged the existing frameworks that have been developed in clinical medicine. Arguably, the challenges for health promotion are not isolated to health promotion, and the issues raised by the debates to date have also emerged in other areas of health care. However, given the diversity of background contexts and population groups within which health promotion interventions take place, it is important that health promotion practitioners seek to understand 'what works for whom and in what circumstances' rather than overly focusing on study design issues.

Integrating qualitative and quantitative data derived from the health sector and combining this with information derived from other sectors involved in the particular question or decision, including transport, housing, education, economics, or the environment, is likely to appear a daunting task at first glance. In order to meaningfully translate knowledge or evidence into changes in practice or policy a distinct pathway is often followed (either consciously or unconsciously). This pathway, sometimes referred to as *knowledge transfer*, involves several stages and begins with an idea followed by sourcing the evidence, using the evidence, and considering capacity to implement the interventions as recommended by the evidence (see Figure 1) (Bowen & Zwi 2005). Decision-making processes need to occur to see the progression from evidence-gathering to knowledge transfer; these can be termed 'adopt, adapt, and act'. Each of these stages will be influenced by the individuals, organisations, and system-level values that exist within the decision-making context (Bowen & Zwi 2005). 'Knowledge brokers' often play an important role in this process and are individuals who may facilitate the movement between adopt, adapt, and act. Perhaps without realising, health promotion practitioners often act as knowledge brokers. As such they may act as a catalyst in strengthening the relationships between researchers, policy-makers, and other practitioners. This can assist to ensure researchers are conducting research that matches the needs of decision-makers and that decision-makers in turn use such research in their decision-making processes (Choi et al. 2005).

There is considerable rhetoric about the need for health practitioners to work across sectors in policy and in practice. In order to strengthen their capacity to be evidence-informed, health promotion practitioners need to develop partnerships with academics not only in 'traditional' areas of public health and health promotion, but across additional sectors such as geography, social sciences, and information sciences. Increasing these links at the academic level is likely to increase the level of good quality evidence in these other sectors and will also increase the likelihood of population health outcomes in the research sectors outside health (Wanless 2004).

The move towards an evidence-based or evidence-informed approach has a number of advantages. Not only can evidence be used to guide practice and policy, it can also be used to illuminate areas of concern where a *lack* of good quality evidence exists. Decision-makers can examine the evidence base to identify areas where the evidence is particularly poor or non-existent. Similarly, reviews of the evidence base can have a profound impact on the quality and utility of new research and evaluations, particularly if the focus is widened to include study design and all other aspects of study conduct that are core to the needs of users. For example, while sound *methods* for evaluating strategies to improve health outcomes are required, we also need to consider *context* (including rules and regulations) within which interventions may operate—both within and external to health. Understanding what works as well as what doesn't work, in what circumstances, and where the evidence gaps lie, are more powerful applications of the evidence base than simply exploring which interventions have been shown to be effective.

EVIDENCE TO INFORM HEALTH PROMOTION—WHAT DOES IT MEAN?

Health promotion practitioners are increasingly being asked to base their work on evidence. But what does this mean, and does it mean something different to those sectors health promotion practitioners seek to work with to improve health?

There are many definitions of 'evidence'. Evidence continues to be described as 'inherently uncertain, dynamic, complex, contestable, and rarely complete' (Lomas et al. 2005). However, definitions such as this help only to repeatedly state the obvious. Moving beyond these definitions to a state of comfort about what evidence or information should be taken more seriously and which should be viewed with more caution, requires a good understanding of the limitations associated with how evidence is collected and what this is based on. Of the many views on evidence, the debates can become polarised with those who align with the belief that scientific (rigorous and replicable) research alone identifies whether an intervention can work versus those who believe evidence can comprise a range of sources, including that derived from personal experience and personal beliefs (Davies 2005; Lomas et al. 2005). In practice, high-quality health promotion has always drawn from both these positions to create programs. The challenge now is to document these types of evidence and how they are used in decision-making processes. It is also important to be mindful of these issues when working in a multisector environment. Some sectors may use scientific, context-free evidence while others may rely on colloquial, context-sensitive evidence. Understanding the advantages and limitations of these types of evidence is important for interpreting the findings and using them in making a decision.

There is an emerging discussion about the differences between 'evidence-informed' and 'evidence-based' practice and policy. While 'evidence-informed health promotion' is a term used conversationally by academics, researchers, and practitioners, it is only just starting to be explored in published literature (e.g. Bowen & Zwi 2005; Lomas et al. 2005; Mulgan 2005). Using the term 'evidence-informed' recognises that decision-making in health promotion policy and practice is *informed* by evidence (i.e. not directed solely by it) given the absence of an evidence base of well-researched comparable interventions (due to differences in contexts and the stronger approach to community development approaches, or community-consulted intervention designs). Further, at the point of integrating evidence into the decision-making process, as with more established areas of evidence-based research, such as clinical medicine, many additional factors influence the decision-making process including organisational capacity, availability of resources, political climate, and stakeholder obligations.

HOW DOES THE HEALTH SECTOR WORK WITH OTHER SECTORS TO CREATE AND USE GOOD QUALITY EVIDENCE?

We argue that working with sectors outside health is crucial to effective health promotion practice. In health there is a strong imperative to gather information to justify our approach (to assist with decision-making) and to contribute to knowledge (de Leeuw & Skovgaard 2005). The use of multisectoral interventions in health promotion raises the issue of what should count as evidence across sectors and what part it plays in the decision-making process.

In preparation for writing this chapter, the authors sought to review the 'evidence' (broadly defined) that other sectors use in decision-making. A brief search of the relevant literature within each sector was undertaken to examine whether this field of interest was established or emerging in other sectors and then to consider how multisector evidence could be generated and/or used. This resulted in very little new information, and sector-specific or cross-sectoral information about 'evidence-informed practice' was difficult to ascertain without sector-specific knowledge.

What information was found confirmed expectations: when working across sectors it makes professional sense to consider how your partners define evidence, how they generate evidence, what types of evidence or research they put most emphasis on, and for what purposes they use evidence. These factors will influence how that partner in turn responds to evidence presented by, and to requests for evidence from, the health sector.

However, given that a large proportion of the sectors with whom health promoters would join to collaborate towards improved health outcomes are based in government, at least in many countries of the global community, it makes sense to consider the types of knowledge that matter to modern governments. Therefore, understanding what knowledge is required is likely to stimulate the development of evidence to further inform debate. Different types of knowledge include:

- statistical knowledge
- policy knowledge
- scientific knowledge
- professional knowledge
- practitioner views[†]
- public opinion[‡]
- political knowledge
- economic knowledge
- classic intelligence (e.g. terrorist networks) (Mulgan 2005).

The types of knowledge required by governments and other decision-makers need to be considered within a sectoral context. While public health and health promotion compete with clinical medicine for a portion of the health budget, similar conflicts occur in other sectors. This is likely to impact on the type of evidence required for decision-making. The path from research to policy development and implementation is rarely linear and inherently complex and, therefore, the current activity within a policy field is likely to impact on knowledge needs. Accordingly policy fields have been categorised into 'stable policy fields', 'policy fields in flux', and the 'inherently novel policy fields' (Mulgan 2005).

[†], [‡] This list is taken directly from Mulgan 2005. The authors' believe that public opinion and practitioner views should also be considered genuine forms of knowledge.

- *Stable policy field*—where knowledge is reasonably settled (e.g. some areas of curative medicine, some labour market policy)
- *Policy fields in flux*—contested knowledge base and lack of agreement about theoretical approaches (e.g. health promotion, some areas of traffic management, some areas of education)
- *Inherently novel policy fields*—genuinely new areas of interest with unknown outcomes (e.g. biotechnology, Internet-related technologies).

These categories provide a basis for considering the types of knowledge needed by different sectors and need to be extended by the types of knowledge or information needed to make decisions within these categories. In health, the type of evidence needed is not only focused on effectiveness but also on ensuring interventions do no harm (Macintyre & Petticrew 2000). This is similar in other sectors. For example, in transport, decisions concerning the building of a new freeway need to consider the effectiveness of increasing traffic flow and also the need to reduce both pedestrian and vehicle accidents. The balance between different types of knowledge is likely to be affected by external influences; for example, political influence in some sectors and the need to work with community in others. In the health care sector, emphasis is often placed on 'levels of evidence', with the randomised controlled trial widely considered to be the highest quality design to establish evidence of effectiveness. Additional information derived from qualitative designs are called on to establish the appropriateness and applicability of the evidence. This chapter seeks to explore whether similar expectations and/or hierarchies are applied to evidence in other sectors. Ideally, a mutual commitment to inform the evidence base across sectors could be a catalyst for initiating more multisectoral initiatives with both sector-specific and mutually defined outcomes.

CROSS-SECTORAL VIEWS ON EVIDENCE

In order to seek information that extends beyond the available literature, the authors sought to examine views on the generation, collection, and use of evidence from across sectors relevant to multisectoral health promotion. A purposive sample of sector-specific contacts familiar with decision-making processes were selected from individuals referred to the authors through academic, government, and non-government networks, inclusive of social welfare, transport, primary industries/ agriculture, local government/planning, and education. These individuals were interviewed by one of the authors using a set of five broad questions. The views provided are limited to the findings of this relatively small sample of interviewed individuals, and future research will need to be undertaken to provide a more extensive study. However, they do provide an initial insight into evidence-related decision-making paradigms and begin to highlight some potential issues in common with the health sector, as well as differences. The views are summarised below under the five pre-set question areas. They have not been aligned to the sector from which they derived but presented as a collective summary across sectors.

Box 7.1: Summary of responses from sectors to specific questions about evidence

What does the word 'evidence' mean to you/your sector?

Most respondents replied that it meant research. Other associations included 'what the situation is', 'examples of what works', 'data', 'evaluating the performance of projects'. Gathering evidence is often seen as a task beyond the core function of ground-level practitioners. A member of a peak non-profit body representing professions involved in planning cities, towns, regions, and places commented that 'evaluation is a real luxury, particularly for those in local government who struggle to simply keep up with their day-to-day work'. 'They report back on some performance measures like numbers of people but anything more than that is a luxury.'

What do you base practice and policy decisions on in your sector?

Responses to this question included the use of internal and external research, models of good practice, regulations (though open to interpretation), what is popular (political factors), outcomes of pilot projects, data collection, and/or reviews (generally narrative) of the national and international literature. Many relied on information gathered during the course of their own projects or research conducted in-house, including qualitative and quantitative research (Randomised Controlled Trials (RCTs), before and after surveys, and focus group methodologies were mentioned). A representative from a peak independent coordinating body of social and community services said their organisation relies on volunteers to help them conduct their own research as funding for paid research is limited.

Where do you go to find/source information/evidence?

- Sources of information to inform decision-making included: relevant databases, conferences, membership on listservs, population data collection (from national statistics bureau, health departments, and own department research section), universities, networking channels, and conference proceedings.
- Some felt that their sector databases were often not comprehensive and intervention research was often more descriptive of the interventions rather than evaluations of whether the intervention actually worked. Some respondents commented that their own funded projects were evidence-generating and used to inform decision-making thereafter.

- Access to PhD supervisors through sector-funded scholarships.
- A respondent from the agriculture sector contended that her department rarely goes outside their own sector to source evidence. However, she did comment that in determining why farmers do or don't adopt a promoted idea they look to other sectors such as business, management, environmental campaigns, and traffic campaigns, 'but not health specifically'.
- A representative from a statutory body with responsibility for management of parks, reserves, and other public land stated that those in health and academia have acted as knowledge brokers to illuminate the health benefits of nature. So where previously there was an emphasis on scientific evidence—on the health of the environment itself—in more recent years they have started to collect impact and satisfaction information about visitors—who comes, why, and what do they do. Further research has been commissioned to consolidate the evidence linking increased contact with nature to health and well-being outcomes in order to support their new marketing focus.

Why and how do you use evidence?

Evidence was used by some for advocacy purposes (to write submissions in response to government policy—offering government workable solutions to identified problems). Responses also included: 'To put us in a better light with political masters; to develop funding/project proposals; to model or determine future needs; to report on performance measures; and to show whether interventions work in order to get funding'.

Small-scale pilot projects were conducted and results used to develop methods for future initiatives and/or to lobby for more funding to increase the scale of the project.

Evidence was also used to inform and develop partnerships. One organisation noted that they had been looking 'from the inside out' but are now recognising the need to also look 'from the outside in' (i.e. from others' perspective), in order to compete with other interests.

How does evidence filter down to ground-level practitioners? Does it filter back up (i.e. is practice knowledge used to inform the evidence)

Information was presented at conferences, through newsletters, industry journals, industry and government awards, and through specific forums. Some thought that working collaboratively with peak bodies and networks helps information to filter 'down and back up'.

A lot of the evidence is derived from ground-level projects, i.e. action research (do it, review it). One sector representative also mentioned that internal information-sharing was starting to be practised, rather than top-down approaches.

One individual from the planning sector contended that the perception was that peer review journals were for academics and that ground-level workers don't read them. From the transport sector it was thought that evidence filtered up through the data collection process.

FINDINGS FROM CROSS-SECTORAL INTERVIEWS

The sector interviews highlighted that non-health sectors were struggling with similar issues to those in health promotion, such as identifying what kinds of evidence they need for decision-making, and also identifying factors that indicate that progress is being made (intermediate indicators), as opposed to being able to monitor longer-term outcomes. A few interviewees reported the need to link evidence about 'how well something is being done as planned' (process evaluation) with project results (impact evaluation) to show progress towards broader goals (outcome evaluation). The ethical implications of intervention implementation was also a concern for some interviewees with reports of not being able to conduct RCTs due to the reported 'ethics' of withholding interventions to the control group by government departments.

An interviewee from the agricultural sector commented that while many of their initiatives were multisectoral in their effects, there is minimal sharing of evidence across sectors to inform program content. However, she acknowledged that useful information had been gleaned from pooling of data from a number of sectors, including health and human services, which allowed each sector to use and interpret the data as appropriate to their own evidence needs. Sponsored evaluations of farming cooperatives, for example, have called for evaluations of the effect not only on the triple bottom line but on the environmental, social, and health effects of the initiative. Data made available from outside the agricultural sector, from health, justice, and education for example, would obviously prove invaluable in illustrating such multifaceted effects.

Further, interviewees reported that some sectors were collecting information similar to other sectors (especially demographic data) that could be shared across sectors. However, barriers to more effective collaboration for producing mutually beneficial evidence can originate at the data gathering stage. A representative from the transport sector commented that they try to use schools in research projects but it is sometimes difficult to get them to participate. There was some suggestion that information was being brought together via whole-of-government initiatives and working groups. There is often a conscious approach not to put interpretations on the collective data so that each department or sector could use it for their own purposes.

Not unlike the health sector, the degree of emphasis on using evidence was reported to depend on the preferences of key strategic people (e.g. CEOs) within an organisation. It also may depend on where senior staff have come from. It was reported by one interviewee that 'those who come from academia' tended to value research and evaluation more so than those who did not. There were reports that it might be possible to get public servants to use evidence, although encouraging and enabling its use higher up the hierarchy (as political involvement increases) is more difficult.

So, how do health promoters engage in an evidence debate with sectors that may perceive evidence differently? Does the health sector place more emphasis on evidence in making decisions or is it just that the discussions about evidence, per se, are more prevalent? Our preliminary consultations have initiated an essential broader research and practice agenda to strengthen the mechanisms for the development and evaluation of interventions that are more likely to produce beneficial than harmful outcomes, and to contribute to reducing health and social inequalities. Focusing on the separate and shared information needs appears to be an 'evidence-informed' position to start with!

TOWARDS AN EVIDENCE BASE THAT USES KNOWLEDGE FROM, AND IS USEFUL TO, OTHER SECTORS

The development of good quality evidence is somewhat dependent on the conduct of good quality research. Given that one of the strongest policy-oriented reasons for research is to develop and implement interventions, the predominant focus of the evidence orientation has been to determine the effectiveness of interventions. Several reasons have been identified that limit the capacity of intervention-oriented research: complexity, methodology, timescale and return structure, and theory (Millward et al. 2003). If health promotion practitioners are to work successfully across sectors to contribute to a sound evidence base for interventions, these issues need to be considered. Table 7.1 provides some strategies for addressing these issues.

In order to work from an evidence-based perspective across sectors, it is essential that there is discussion and a shared understanding and agreement on what level of evidence is desirable, is acceptable to funders, is needed to inform decision-making, as well as discussion about the trade-offs in relation to bias and utility (Thomson et al. 2004). Case Study 7.1 is a brief illustration, based on an intervention involving the health and welfare sectors.

Table 7.1 Strategies for improving intervention-oriented research

ISSUE	STRATEGY
Complexity	Develop understanding across sectors about the determinants of public health issues. Clearly identify with partners the levels at which interventions should be targeted.
Methodology	Work towards developing a consensus for intervention research techniques and levels. Without a consensus it will be difficult to engage with partners.
Timescale and return	Need to understand the role of politics in funding health promotion initiatives. Use this knowledge to advocate for the prioritisation of long-term health gains. This also highlights the importance of using the existing evidence, with agreed consensus about what constitutes evidence.
Structure	Develop structures to support the conduct of intervention research. This includes working with university and governments to prioritise health promotion research that provides equitable solutions across the population.
Theory	Develop shared understanding of the theoretical frameworks and paradigms that influence how each sector does their business, and therefore how they make decisions and what evidence will be required.

Case Study 7.1: Income supplementation and health

A pilot study conducted by researchers in the UK identified substantial health gains when elderly people received an 'attendance allowance'.§ As a result, the researchers decided to pursue a larger study that would explore the health effects of income supplementation. While the researchers initially considered conducting a RCT, they encountered several problems. These related to the ethics of either withholding or delaying the receipt of the allowance for people deemed to be in need. When the researchers proposed a less rigorous study (before and after study of benefit recipients) they were unable to secure funding. They assumed that the funders deemed that because there was no control group, no useful information would be provided. This raises an important question, 'what sort of evidence is acceptable in such situations?' (This case study is described in more detail in Thomson et al. 2004.)

USING SYSTEMATIC REVIEWS TO IDENTIFY EFFECTIVE INTERVENTIONS

Systematic approaches to synthesising the available evidence to inform health policy, management, and practice has been increasingly supported. The Mexico Statement on Health Research, produced at the conclusion of the recent global

---

§ An attendance allowance is payable to people aged 65 plus who need frequent help or supervision and whose need has existed for at least 6 months.

Ministerial Summit on health research, identified the need to promote access to reliable, relevant, up-to-date evidence on the effects of interventions, *based on systematic reviews of the totality of available research findings* (Ministerial Summit on Health Research 2004: 2). Such calls are in recognition that 'reviews of research are a better basis for informing policy than a single study or expert opinion' (Sheldon 2005: S1: 1). Relying on the latter carries risks associated with low statistical power, researcher/expert bias, contextual variability, methodological and theoretical incompleteness, and policy irrelevance (Sheldon 2005).

Lavis et al. (2005) present a clear definition of systematic reviews as:

> Reviews of the research literature with five components: an explicit question; an explicit description of the search strategy; an explicit statement about what types of research evidence were included and excluded; a critical examination of the quality of the studies included in the review; and a critical and transparent process for interpretation of the findings included in the review.

Research evidence for inclusion in a systematic review can be derived from a range of sources and certainly should not be restricted by sectoral boundaries. Case Study 7.2 illustrates the need to step outside traditional health sources to identify relevant studies to inform a review on the effectiveness of housing initiatives to improve health outcomes.

As Case Study 7.2 illustrates, systematic reviews are increasingly common-place among tools to inform health promotion practice and policy. However, while essential to decision-making processes, systematic reviews alone are insufficient in informing policy and practice, and 'the effects of policies and practice will always remain a matter of judgement' (Chalmers 2005: 235). While debate still continues about the most appropriate syntheses and review methodology for health promotion intervention effectiveness (e.g. Mays, Pope & Popay 2005), examples can be found across the spectrum; from those using the most rigorous methodology to the more unstructured forms. The Cochrane Collaboration is an international conglomerate of registered entities, focused on the production of high-quality systematic reviews of trials evaluating health care interventions. Cochrane reviews are subject to rigorous peer review, updated periodically, and disseminated electronically through the Cochrane Library (Bero & Rennie 1995; Dickerson & Manheimer 1998). While originally focused on medical interventions, Cochrane reviews now cover diverse topics such as: area-wide traffic calming in preventing traffic-related crashes, injuries, and deaths; school-based interventions for the prevention of illicit drug use; and policy interventions implemented through sporting organisations for promoting healthy behaviour change. These examples illustrate the acceptance by the Cochrane Collaboration of the multisectoral approaches to health promotion and public health. This trend is promoted and supported by the Health Promotion and Public Health Field of the Cochrane Collaboration (www.vichealth.vic. gov.au/cochrane). There are several other organisations conducting high-quality systematic reviews of the effects of health promotion interventions and website links are provided at the end of this chapter.

Case Study 7.2: Housing improvement and health gain: a summary and systematic review

The authors of this review asked the question, 'Can poor health be improved by improving housing?' To answer this question they examined all housing research that had assessed the health of residents whose houses had been improved, searching a wide range of databases from a number of sectors. They searched for studies from anywhere in the world that had been carried out in the past 100 years, and utilised health databases such as Medline, the Cochrane Controlled Trials Database and HealthSTAR, but also social science databases (e.g. ASSIA—Applied Social Sciences Index and Abstracts, Social Science Citation Index, IBSS—International Bibliography of the Social Sciences and PAIS International, (the database of the Public Affairs Information Services, covering the full range of the social sciences), the Campbell Collaboration's Social, Psychological, Educational and Criminological Trials Register, Urbadisc/Acompline (covering urban and regional planning and policy issues), PSYCHINFO, and the SIGLE (System of Information for Grey Literature in Europe)).

This was combined with other sources of evidence including: bibliographies of all sourced reports, papers, and textbooks; emails sent to subscribers to the Housing Studies Association newsletter and the Health Action Zone discussion group requesting relevant information. Project managers at the Joseph Rowntree Foundation were asked to provide any information on ongoing projects and delegates at a major international housing conference were asked for any information on relevant studies. An Internet search of the following sites was also conducted: Scottish Poverty Information Unit; Housing Corporation Innovation and Good Practice and Research Database; The Joseph Rowntree Foundation; projects funded by the joint DH/DETR/MRC research programs on air pollution; UK National Research Register; United States Department of Housing and Urban Development; Office of Policy Development and Research (US); National Database on Social Science Research (UK); National centre for Social Research (UK); OHN in Practice Current Controlled Trials. Interestingly, the reviewers found that housing improvements can improve residents' health, in particular their mental health; housing improvements can result in rent increases, which in turn can actually make people's health worse; the original residents may move to another area and not benefit from the housing improvements; and housing improvements can have negative as well as positive effects on health.

Source: Thomson, Petticrew & Morrison 2002

Systematic reviews can be used by health promotion practitioners and decision-makers to highlight gaps in the research, the poor quality of existing studies, or indeed to illuminate quality evidence to support the uptake or rejection of a health promotion initiative. Identification of evidence of effectiveness will be affected by the *degree* to which evaluation is undertaken, and its usefulness dependent on the *quality* of the evaluation undertaken. Therefore, the findings of systematic reviews can only reflect the quality and the breadth of the primary studies that exist in the area under review. Health promotion practitioners, researchers, and funders have a role in advocating for good quality research/ evaluations that can produce reliable and useful information to add to the evidence base. There is also a need for those in health promotion to engage in the debates about what types of study designs are appropriate in different situations and to work to develop methodologies that will produce findings that are reliable, valid, and useful to decision-makers.

It is also worth noting that while the evidence debate continues in the resource-richer countries there is increasing concern about how evidence is developed and used in developing countries (McQueen 2001). To date much of the published evidence focuses on interventions conducted in more richly resourced countries with a predominantly English-speaking population. Therefore, it is essential that contextual information (such as political factors, the physical environment, and cultural values and norms) are highlighted in syntheses of the available research so that findings of research conducted in one part of the world can be interpreted and examined for wider generalisability in a global context. This is especially important for work conducted across sectors.

The Cochrane Health Promotion and Public Health Field's 'Guidelines on Conducting Systematic Reviews of Health Promotion and Public Health Interventions' (Jackson & Waters 2005) suggests that caution should be taken when making generalisations from one context to another. To order to assist with generalisability, context-related information, such as characteristics of the target population (e.g. socio-economic, cultural, literacy levels, place of residence) should be extracted from intervention studies for inclusion in systematic reviews. Researchers are increasingly extending their investigation of context to include inter-organisational networks within which the host organisation operates (Hawe 2004). While examples are at this stage limited, it is anticipated that more work will be conducted in this area over the coming years.

GAPS IN EVIDENCE FOR CROSS AND INTERSECTORAL HEALTH PROMOTION PRACTICE

The Ottawa and Bangkok Charters for Health Promotion highlight the need for those promoting health to work across sectors (WHO 2005), although there is limited evidence to show the effectiveness of multisector partnerships to address health concerns (Federal, Provincial and Territorial Advisory Committee on Population Health 1999). This is not intended to argue that these partnerships have not been effective; however, it does identify the need for multisectoral partnerships to become more active in assessing and reporting on their effectiveness. This will provide useful information about partnership processes (partnership development, the implementation of interventions using a partnership approach, and effective strategies for evaluating multisector interventions) and the impact of partnerships on health outcomes. A Partnerships Analysis Tool has been developed by a non-government health promotion agency that may assist in further developing this evidence base (VicHealth 2005c).

Combining evidence from multisectoral interventions can also produce challenges (though these can also be found in within-sector evidence summaries). For example, in their systematic review on promoting walking and cycling (see Case Study 7.3), Ogilvie et al. (2004) identified that studies had used a range of metrics for describing the primary outcome measure (shift from cars to walking or cycling). They were therefore unable to synthesise results based on a single measure but needed to undertake a summary of the effects of overall distribution of transport choices by calculating and comparing absolute change.

Case Study 7.3: Promoting walking and cycling as an alternative to using cars: a systematic review

A systematic review was conducted by UK researchers to identify interventions that have been effective in promoting a population shift from using cars to walking and cycling to identify the related health impacts of these interventions. Twenty-two studies that met the inclusion criteria were identified. The authors categorised studies into: targeted behaviour change programs (n=4), agents of change and publicity campaigns (n=4), engineering studies (n=6), financial incentives (n=2), providing alternative services (n=3), effects on health (n=6) and social distribution of effects (n=11). The authors identified that agents of change, publicity campaigns, engineering measures, and charging road users have not been effective 'in our terms' (Ogilvie et al. 2004: 3). In addition, car-share clubs and telecommuting were not only found to be ineffective but may also be associated with negative effects. The authors acknowledge that 'evaluation studies are often not designed to assess effects on important population health determinants such as physical activity'. Further they suggest 'many transport policy interventions constitute natural experiments in which effects on population health could and should be evaluated using well designed prospective (and, where appropriate, controlled) studies' (Ogilvie et al. 2004:4). The authors of this review conclude by highlighting that their findings echo those of the Wanless report (2004), 'that we know relatively little about the likely impact on health of interventions to influence the wider determinants of population health'.

Ogilvie et al. 2004

SEARCHING FOR THE EVIDENCE
Practical, easily accessible electronic information

It is difficult to determine accessibility of access to electronic databases. Even where access is available, little is known about the uptake of these databases by those seeking to promote health. As highlighted in Case Study 7.3, accessing databases relevant to other sectors complicates the process of identifying effectiveness of interventions across sectors. Context is likely to play an important role; those working in smaller organisations or in poorer countries may be less likely to have good Internet access (Petticrew et al. 2004). Librarians and universities may play a crucial role supporting skill development in this area and the Cochrane Health Promotion and Public Health Field incorporates a study-searching component in their systematic review training. This material is available online (www.vichealth.vic.gov.au/cochrane/training).

A practical but underutilised method of identifying and accessing relevant information is to establish a cross-sectoral advisory committee. This committee may be useful in identifying relevant databases and/or unpublished literature (Jackson & Waters 2005). It may also be worth considering conducting a deliberative session where stakeholders bring along lists of sources and forms of evidence (articles, books, reports, etc.) (Lomas et al. 2005). For example, if a health department wanted to encourage multisectoral partnerships for infrastructure to support physical activity it would be worthwhile running a deliberative process to identify the range of evidence available. This could also be conducted at a local level by inviting partners to attend.

Cross-sectoral research methods

One of the main problems with the lack of comparable methods and utilities is the challenge of building the evidence base for the successes in health promotion. Widely lauded initiatives, such as the Healthy Cities project, are largely absent of an evidence base on effectiveness (de Leeuw & Skovgaard 2005). How and why this has happened is worth considering. It may be in part due to the lack of evaluation. It may be because of the methodology on which the intervention or program is based or it may be a result of multisector involvement where data have been collected but not adequately utilised.

As a result there is an emerging call for the use and acceptance of a range of evidence. Ogilvie et al., for example, contend that 'it is preferable to reach conclusions, however tentative, that are based on the best available evidence rather than simply stating that no evidence is available' (2005: 891). Health promotion practitioners and decision-makers have a practical and strategic role to play in filling these gaps.

USING KNOWLEDGE TRANSFER STRATEGIES TO ENSURE DISSEMINATION OF RESEARCH TO DECISION-MAKERS

Knowledge transfer, as previously discussed, refers to the use of evidence or research findings to inform policy and practice. This is an important area as 'there is unfortunately no correlation between the quality of science and the policy derived from it. Good science does not always guarantee good policy [and] bad or even no science does not necessarily lead to bad policy' (Choi et al. 2005: 634).

While basing policy on evidence might seem like a logical process, health promotion practitioners should be aware of the challenges and the different decision-making imperatives of those involved (Choi et al. 2005; Petticrew et al. 2004). These issues highlight the need for the development of systems that allow the identification, synthesis, and appropriate dissemination of research evidence that, in many countries, appear to be not well developed (Petticrew et al. 2004). 'Researchers who want to influence have to understand the game; how it's played, who to approach, and how the political apparatus is structured' (Petticrew et al. 2004), and Canadian research findings suggest that knowledge transfer requires:

- Time
- Credibility and reliability
- Information quality and timing
- Applicability and customisability
- Mode of delivery
- Opportunities for training and education (including systematic reviews (definition, significance and appraisal), purpose and methodology of the registry of systematic reviews, information management and credibility of online information sources) (Dobbins et al. 2004).

Table 7.2 Facilitators and barriers to policy-makers using the evidence derived from research

FACILITATORS	BARRIERS
Personal contact between scientists and policy-makers	Absence of personal contact between scientists and policy-makers
Timeliness and relevance of research	Lack of timeliness and relevance of research
Research that includes a summary with clear recommendations	Mutual mistrust between scientists and policy-makers
Research that confirms current policy or endorses self-interest	Power and budget struggles
Good quality research	Poor quality of research
Community pressure or client demand for research	Political instability or high turnover of policy-making staff
Inclusion of effectiveness data	

Source: Innvaer et al. 2002 as cited in Choi et al. 2005

Further, Lavis et al. (2005) also found that factors such as the interaction between researchers and health care policy-makers, and timeliness of the presentation of research findings increased the prospects for research use among policy-makers in health. They also contended that health care managers and policy-makers would benefit from researchers highlighting information that could be adapted to their local situation (including contextual factors and harms and risks as well as potential benefits of interventions). It is not unreasonable to assume that these are issues that would be applicable to managers and policy-makers in sectors outside health, where pressures of time and local conditions also play a significant role in decision-making.

SUMMARY

This chapter highlights the need for health promotion practitioners to consider the types of evidence used by their partners to inform decision-making. Understanding these types of evidence and their level of influence will help facilitate decision-making that is multisectoral and inclusive of health outcomes. In order to do this, health promotion practitioners need to ensure that their work is rigorously evaluated and contributes actively to the evidence base.

USEFUL WEBSITES

The Campbell Collaboration (covering interventions in education, social work and welfare, and criminal justice): <www.CampbellCollaboration.org>

The Cochrane Library: <www.thecochranelibrary.org>

The Cochrane Collaboration: <www.cochrane.org>

The Cochrane Health Promotion and Public Health Field lists relevant Cochrane protocols and reviews at: <www.vichealth.vic.gov.au/cochrane/activities/reviews.htm>

Evidence for Policy and Practice Information Centre (EPPI-Centre):

Health Evidence: <www.health-evidence.ca>

NHS Centre for Reviews and Dissemination: <www.york.ac.uk/inst/crd/>

Health Evidence Bulletins—Wales:

Effective Health Practice Project: <www.myhamilton.ca/myhamilton/CityandGovernment/HealthandSocialServices/Research/EPHPP/>

National Institute for Health and Clinical Excellence:

Evidence base reviews available at: <www.publichealth.nice.org.uk/page.aspx?o=508295>

Medical Research Council Social & Public Health Sciences Unit:

The Community Guide—Guide to Community Preventive Services—Systematic Reviews and Evidence-Based Recommendations: <www.thecommunityguide.org>

Informed Health Online: <www.informedhealthonline.org/item.aspx>

Nerida Joss

NAME	ORGANISATION	WHAT DOES THIS RESOURCE OFFER?	WHERE TO FIND IT
1978 **Alma Ata Declaration for Primary Health Care**	World Health Organization	This declaration brought health promotion ideas and concepts into the global area and therefore is known as the origin of health promotion to many people. Held in Alma Ata in the former USSR, the declaration changed the way many countries responded to health issues by introducing key health promotion philosophies.	<www.who.int/hpr/NPH/docs/declaration_almaata.pdf>
1981 *Global Strategy for Health for all by the Year 2000*	World Health Organization	As a result of the success of Alma Ata, WHO responded with a series of measurable targets and goals in health. This further fostered the idea of health promotion globally.	<whqlibdoc.who.int/publications/9241800038.pdf>
1986 **Ottawa Charter for Health Promotion**	World Health Organization	The first international conference on health promotion was held in Ottawa and produced the Ottawa Charter. The now famous charter acknowledged health promotion work of the past and provided a strong, directive framework to foster further action. It is considered one of the most important documents in health promotion today and provides a framework under which health professionals everywhere, can work.	<www.who.int/hpr/NPH/docs/ottawa_charter_hp.pdf>
1986 **Australian Better Health Commission**	Commonwealth Government of Australia	The Commission produced review of the nation's health from a social perspective published in three volumes making recommendations on national health problems.	Available in libraries but not available online

(Continued)

(Continued)

NAME	ORGANISATION	WHAT DOES THIS RESOURCE OFFER?	WHERE TO FIND IT
1988 **2nd International Conference on Health Promotion**	World Health Organization	Held in Adelaide, Australia, recommendations from this conference drew attention to the need to build healthy public policy to strengthen the action areas listed in the Ottawa Charter.	<www.who.int/hpr/ NPH/docs/adelaide_ recommendations. pdf>
1991 **3rd International Conference on Health Promotion**	World Health Organization	This conference, held in Sundsvall, Sweden, called upon people to actively engage in creating supportive environments to promote health.	<www.who.int/ hpr/NPH/docs/ sundsvall_statement. pdf>
1994 **International Union of Health Promotion and Education**	IUHPE	The International Union of Health Education added health promotion to its name, to become the *IUHPE*.	<www.iuhpe.org/>
1997 **4th International Conference on Health Promotion**	World Health Organization	Held in Jakarta, Indonesia, the focus of this conference was on the inclusion of the private sector in decision-making. As a result the Jakarta declaration listed five priority areas for future commitment.	<www.who.int/hpr/ NPH/docs/jakarta_ declaration_en.pdf>
1999 **5th Global Conference on Health Promotion**	World Health Organization Pan American Health Organization	Held in Mexico, the focus of this conference was on equity and inequities within and between countries, and future actions, particularly through health promotion.	<www.who.int/hpr/ NPH/docs/mxconf_ report_en.pdf>
2005 **6th International Conference on Health Promotion**	World Health Organization	Held in Bangkok, the focus of this conference was on the determinants of health in the context of the globalised world. The Bangkok Charter calls for strengthening of commitment from a wide range of stakeholders towards achieving health for all.	<www.who.int/ healthpromotion/ conferences/6gchp/ hpr_050829_ %20BCHP.pdf>

NAME	ORGANISATION	WHAT DOES THIS RESOURCE OFFER?	WHERE TO FIND IT
UN Millennium Development Goals	United Nations	The 8 Millennium Development Goals (MDGs)—which range from halving extreme poverty to halting the spread of HIV/AIDS and providing universal primary education, by 2015—form a blueprint agreed to by all the world's countries and all the world's leading development institutions to meet the needs of the world's poorest.	<www.un.org/ millenniumgoals/>

GUIDEBOOK

GUIDEBOOK 2:
HEALTH PROMOTION ASSOCIATIONS, ALLIANCES AND ADVOCACY ORGANISATIONS

Nerida Joss & Helen Keleher

NAME	WHAT DOES THIS ORGANISATION OFFER?	WHERE TO FIND IT
Australian Health Promotion Association (AHPA)	National Committee; annual conference State Branch Committees; local programs including workforce development, mentoring, and seminars Auspice for *Health Promotion Journal of Australia* Membership is open by subscription Members receive the AHPA e-list, which includes regular postings of job advertisements, and advice about conferences and seminars.	\<www.healthpromotion.org.au\>
Public Health Association of Australia (PHAA)	National Committee; annual conference State Branch Committees; local programs including workforce development, mentoring, and seminars Auspice for *Australian and New Zealand Journal of Public Health* Membership is open by subscription Members receive the PHAA e-list, which includes regular postings of job advertisements and advice about conferences and seminars.	\<www.phaa.net.au\>
CLICK4HP	E-list open to subscribers at no cost The list has an international membership that ensures a rich flow of information. Good source of program information.	click4hp@yorku.ca
SDOH e-list	E-list open to subscribers at no cost The list has an international membership that ensures a rich flow of information. Good source of advocacy and activist information.	
International Society of Equity in Health	ISEqH promotes equality in health and health services internationally. It has a list serve and newsletters.	\<www.iseqh.org\>
People's Health Movement	The PHM advocates for Health For All Now. Membership is open to all. They run a moderated mailing list called PHM exchange.	\<www.phmovement.org\>

GUIDEBOOK 3:
KEY RESOURCES ABOUT THE SOCIO-ECONOMIC DETERMINANTS OF HEALTH

Helen Keleher

NAME	ORGANISATION/ AUTHORS	WHAT DOES THIS RESOURCE OFFER?	WHERE TO FIND IT
Commission on Social Determinants of Health	World Health Organization	Website that reports on the work of the Commission, newsletters and updates, and reports of meetings of the Commission and its Areas of Work: Country Action, Knowledge Networks, Global Initiatives; Civil Society Organisations; and WHO Action to integrate the work of the Commission with WHO programs.	<www.who.int/ social_determi- nants/about/en/>
Commission on Social Determinants of Health: Imperatives and Opportunities for Change	World Health Organization	This is the background paper to the work of the Commission.	<www.who.int/ social_determi- nants/strategy/ stratdoc18Feb05/ en/index.html>
Social determi- nants of health: the Solid Facts, 2nd edition	Richard Wilkinson and Michael Marmot (eds)	This document was published by the WHO following the UK Acheson Inquiry in Health Inequalities. It con- tains information about 10 deter- minants but significantly does not include gender or culture.	<www.who.dk/ document/e81384. pdf>
Understanding health: a determinants approach	Helen Keleher and Berni Murphy (eds)	This contributed volume provides an introduction to the determinants of health.	Oxford University Press, Melbourne
Social determi- nants of health: Canadian perspectives	Dennis Raphael (ed)	Uniting top academics and high- profile experts from across the coun- try, this contributed volume is the first of its kind published in Canada. It summarises how socio-economic	Canadian Scholars Press Inc <www.cspi.org/ books/s/socialdeter. htm>

(Continued)

(Continued)

NAME	ORGANISATION/ AUTHORS	WHAT DOES THIS RESOURCE OFFER?	WHERE TO FIND IT
		factors affect the health of Canadians, surveys the current state of eleven social determinants of health across Canada, provides an analysis of how these determinants affect Canadians' health, and explores what policy options would contribute to better health outcomes.	
What determines health?	Population Health, Health Canada—the Public Health Agency of Canada	This site provides good overviews of what determines health, explanations of twelve key determinants of health and the research and evidence base, as well as health status indicators.	<www.phacaspc. gc.ca/phsp/phdd/ determinants/ index.html>
Swedish National Public Health Strategy	Swedish National Government	The Swedish Public Health Strategy explicitly uses a determinants of health framework.	<www.fhi.se>

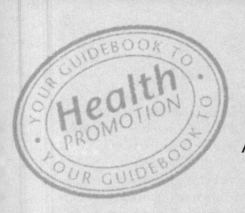

GUIDEBOOK 4:
HEALTH PROMOTION AS
A GENDERING PRACTICE

Catherine Mackenzie

Applying feminist principles and research methods can enable health promoters and policy-makers to reveal otherwise hidden mechanisms of power and privilege that maintain the oppression of particular groups of people based on sex, class, race, ethnicity, age, and disability (Travis & Compton 2001).

A first step in traversing this terrain is to be alert to the ways in which health promoters, researchers, epidemiologists, and policy-makers attach meaning to the terms 'sex' and 'gender'. While sex and gender are not interchangeable, they are connected (Doyal 2003). The terms are still being debated, but nevertheless there is general agreement that 'sex' refers to the biological sex of a person (usually either 'female' or 'male') whereas 'gender' is a principle of social organisation that is based on biological sex but is not a characteristic of a person. In other words, women and men are ascribed a socially constructed gender because of their biological sex (Office for Women and University of Adelaide 2006).

Policy-makers, researchers, and health promoters commonly treat the terms 'sex' and 'gender' as though they are the same. This is evident in the various forms, surveys, and demographic collections for citizens to fill out in their daily lives. Commonly these offer two 'gender' tick boxes marked: 'male' and 'female'. Here, 'gender' is read as an adjective (Eveline & Bacchi 2005). If one is describing a person as *being* male or *being* female, one is really saying that their biological sex (rather than their gender) is male or female. If by contrast we use 'gender' as a verb, we 'do' gender rather than 'be' gender (Eveline & Bacchi 2005: 506; Office for Women and University of Adelaide 2005: 10).

Gender varies according to time and place and intersects with other social determinants: for example, ethnicity, class, culture, (dis)ability, race, and age (Eveline & Bacchi 2005; Council of Europe 1998). In most societies, gender is a process by which hierarchical relations between women and men are created and reproduced so that women are disadvantaged and men are advantaged (Office for Women and University of Adelaide 2006).

Production of public policy is one of the sites where gender roles and responsibilities are allocated and reproduced as 'the norm'. Health promotion workers and policy-makers need to be alert to ways in which they may be unintentionally contributing to the gendering process. For example, physical activity policies and programs that aim to address women's role as unpaid carers by child care provision could instead (or in addition) advocate for the redistribution of caring responsibilities between women and men. Thus, it is useful to attend to gender relations within sites such as policy production where gendering processes occur (Eveline & Bacchi 2005).

Researchers need to explore how best to gather evidence that examines the everyday lives of women and men. While there are often sex-disaggregated data available, these data identify differences and similarities between women's and men's various activities, but do not tell us underlying reasons why they exist.

Health promoters, researchers, and policy-makers need to ensure that policies are informed by gender-based data, which examine how social structures influence different groups of women's and men's experiences of and activities in everyday life. Through this exercise, power imbalances that exist between groups of people can be revealed and addressed by policy.

TRAVEL TIPS FOR HEALTH PROMOTERS

- In research and program planning use sex to mean biological distinctions (for example statistical differences) and gender to discuss social constructions and resultant power imbalances.
- When travelling through the field of policy-making, be mindful of the ways in which you may be gendering the people who will be affected by the policies you produce.

Table G4.1   Gender and development: concepts and definitions

Culture	The distinctive patterns of ideas, beliefs, and norms that characterise the way of life and relations of a society or group within a society
Gender Analysis	The systematic gathering and examination of information on gender differences and social relations in order to identify, understand, and redress inequities based on sex
Gender Discrimination	The systematic, unfavourable treatment of individuals on the basis of their sex, which denies them rights, opportunities, or resources
Gender Division of Labour	The socially determined ideas and practices that define what roles and activities are deemed appropriate for women and men
Gender Equality and Equity	Gender equality denotes women having the same opportunities in life as men, including the ability to participate in the public sphere Gender equity denotes the equivalence in life outcomes for women and men, recognising their different needs and interests, and requiring a redistribution of power and resources
Gender Mainstreaming	An organisational strategy to bring a gender perspective to all aspects of an institution's policy and activities, through building gender capacity and accountability

Gender Needs	Shared and prioritised needs identified by women that arise from their common experiences as a gender
Gender Planning	The technical and political processes and procedures necessary to implement gender-sensitive policy
Gender Relations	Hierarchical relations of power between women and men that tend to disadvantage women
Gender Training	A facilitated process of developing awareness and capacity on gender issues, to bring about personal or organisational change for gender equality
Gender Violence	Any act or threat by men or male-dominated institutions that inflicts physical, sexual, or psychological harm on a woman or girl because of their sex
Intra-household Resource Distribution	The dynamics of how different resources that are generated within or that come into the household are accessed and controlled by its members
National Machineries for Women	Agencies with a mandate for the advancement of women established within and by governments for integrating gender concerns in development policy and planning
Patriarchy	Systemic societal structures that institutionalise men's physical, social, and economic power over women
Sex and Gender	Sex refers to the biological characteristics that categorise someone as either female or male; whereas gender refers to the socially determined ideas and practices of what it is to be female or male
Social Justice	Fairness and equity as a right for all in the outcomes of development, through processes of social transformation
WID/GAD	The WID (or Women in Development) approach calls for greater attention to women in development policy and practice, and emphasises the need to integrate them into the development process. In contrast, the GAD (or Gender and Development) approach focuses on the socially constructed basis of differences between men and women and emphasises the need to challenge existing gender roles and relations
Women's Empowerment	A 'bottom-up' process of transforming gender power relations, through individuals or groups developing awareness of women's subordination and building their capacity to challenge it
Women's Human Rights	The recognition that women's rights are human rights and that women experience injustices solely because of their sex

Table adapted from Reeves & Baden 2000

GUIDEBOOK

WHERE TO FIND FURTHER INFORMATION

Development Gateway—gender
<www.topics.developmentgateway.org/mdg/rc/BrowseContent.do~source=RC
ContentUser~folderId=2800?source=RCContentUser&folderId=2800>

Institute of Development Studies
<www.ids.ac.uk/ids/>

Institute of Development Studies—Gender Group (if you click on BRIDGE you will find excellent reports and gender analysis material)
<www.ids.ac.uk/ids/GenderWG/index.html>

Office for Women—Gender Analysis
<www.osw.sa.gov.au/site/page.cfm?nav_id=634>

Status of Women Canada

Sustainable Development Department—Gender Sensitive Indicators: A key tool for gender mainstreaming
<www.fao.org/sd/2001/PE0602_en.htm>

Women's Health Victoria—Gender Impact Assessment
<www.whv.org.au/health_policy/gia.htm>

World Health Organization—gender and health
<www.who.int/reproductive-health/publications/WHD_98_16_gender_and_
health_technical_paper/WHD_98_16_table_of_contents_en.html>

PART 2
HEALTH PROMOTION PRACTICE

All health promoters need an array of technical skills for effective health promotion practice so these are the focus of Part 2. Chapter 8 begins Part 2 with an overview of program planning and evaluation, arguing the need for strategic thinking as the foundation of planning. This chapter presents a new planning model that reframes health promotion in order to actively address the social determinants of health and inequities. In order to do this, health promotion program planning needs to begin from a determinants perspective, and remain solidly connected to the issues as they are defined by those affected by the issues. Chapter 9 takes up this theme in its critique of community participation and engagement. Chapter 10 is concerned with empowerment in health education, arguing that health education needs careful rethinking and reframing to ensure that it is equity-focused, and not causing harm by its approaches and the values on which those approaches are developed. Chapter 11 discusses communication strategies in terms of building capacity. The theme of capacity-building follows through to Chapter 12 and its arguments for building organisational capacity for health promotion. The next three chapters (13–15) address the policy skills and knowledge necessary for effective health promotion practice. Chapter 16 is a short chapter that sets out core health promotion competencies that guide health promotion. Two different sets of competencies are put forward, from Australia and New Zealand. Part 2 finishes with a chapter on reflective practice, arguing the need for a career-long approach to reflection and principles of empowerment.

Part 2 is supported by seven guidebooks:

- Guidebook 5: Health Promotion Program Planning and Evaluation Resources
- Guidebook 6: Resources on Health Equity
- Guidebook 7: Capacity-building Resources
- Guidebook 8: Preparing for a Media Interview—Ten-point Checklist
- Guidebook 9: Developing Training, Facilitating, and Presenting Skills
- Guidebook 10: Preparing a Press Release—Ten-point Checklist
- Guidebook 11: Cross-cultural Communication

HEALTH PROMOTION PLANNING AND THE SOCIAL DETERMINANTS OF HEALTH

Helen Keleher

Key concepts

- Addressing the social determinants of health is core to health promotion program planning.
- Health promotion planning requires a determinants perspective from which to think and act strategically.
- A conceptual framework and a program plan with specific steps to address equity will increase effectiveness.
- Intersectoral action is needed because the drivers for health and well-being arise from many sectors.
- Multilevel interventions and multilevel outcomes are necessary for effectiveness.
- Addressing more than one outcome level ensures that the focus of the program is beyond that of individuals towards more upstream levels of action.
- Program + context = outcomes. But the context may be more important than the program in delivering outcomes.

Key terms

- Strategic planning
- Health promotion planning
- Equity-focused health promotion planning model
- Health promotion evaluation

OVERVIEW

Health promotion is about making a difference to people's health and the conditions that support health. Basic principles characterise health promotion initiatives, which are that they are:

- Empowering: enabling individuals and communities to assume more power over the personal, socio-economic, and environmental factors that affect their health.
- Participatory: including all concerned at all stages of the process.
- Holistic: fostering physical, mental, social, and spiritual health.
- Intersectoral: involving the collaboration of agencies from relevant sectors.
- Equitable: guided by a concern for equity and social justice.
- Sustainable: bringing about changes that individuals and communities can maintain once initial funding has ceased.
- Multistrategy: using a variety of approaches—including policy development, organisational change, community development, legislation, advocacy, education, and communication—in combination (Rootman et al. 2001: 4–5).

Planning for health promotion is both an art and a science—the science of high-quality planning, and the art of strategic thinking. Planning and evaluation are core functions for health promotion work. Building on the foundations laid in Part 1, this chapter explains the steps involved in planning and evaluation for health promotion. The 'Two-Tier Health Promotion Plan' is set out with essential steps for integrating the determinants of the problem on which the plan is focused, and steps to build in an equity focus. The two tiers are 1) a *conceptual framework for health promotion program planning* and 2) a *technical program plan*. Both integrate steps for equity.

Tier 1, the conceptual framework, is essential to ensure that the program is able to work from a determinants of health perspective. Tier 2, the technical program plan, has six stages, based on program logic, from partnership development through to evaluation and dissemination.

This chapter is supported by Guidebook 5, Health Promotion Program Planning and Evaluation Resources. There is a huge literature available on health promotion program planning and evaluation—Guidebook 5 highlights some of the useful websites that have more detailed information about 'how to' undertake these aspects of health promotion work that cannot be covered in this chapter.

Capacity for strategic thinking is a critical aspect of high-quality planning for health promotion that should pervade every aspect of work that is intended to address the determinants of health, so let's begin this discussion with strategic thinking and planning.

STRATEGIC THINKING AND PLANNING

Strategic thinking and strategic planning are tools of organisational development that come from the management and business literature but have been adopted by many sectors. For organisations that are serious about making an impact on the determinants of health and thus making a difference to the health of people and their communities, the capacity to develop alliances and to work intersectorally is essential. This organisational capacity requires both strategic planning and strategic thinking.

Strategic thinking is about reinventing traditional ways of working, envisioning potential futures that are significantly different from the past, breaking away from doing 'business as usual'. Strategic thinkers advocate imaginative approaches to thinking about outcomes. In health promotion, that means tackling the fundamental causes of poor health and well-being—the determinants of health. For the health sector, this may mean reorienting from risk factor approaches; for other sectors, it may mean a more explicit incorporation of mental, physical, economic, and social health and well-being goals into outcome measures. For the sectors of community arts, recreation, and leisure, all levels of government, or education (for example) it means understanding the effects of policy and programs on the health and well-being of citizens and the incorporation of health and well-being outcomes in planning and evaluation. In many communities and regions, the changes required to re-establish good health and well-being may be substantial. Only substantial changes to the way organisations work, and to policies and programs, can overcome entrenched factors of health, social, and economic degeneration.

Strategic planning is a systematic programming of strategies from which action plans are developed. Planning tools are usually models that set out the flow of tasks to be followed, implementation and evaluation plans, and budgets. Plans are essential to clearly define the vision, goals, objectives, and actions to be taken, although planning may be as much about the process that partners have gone through than about the end result (Senge et al. 2002: 521).

The difference between strategic planning and strategic thinking is that the latter is a synthesising process utilising intuition and creativity that integrates a vision for intermediate and longer-term outcomes. Traditional planning approaches are usually focused on a particular health condition or narrowed to a risk factor. Such a planning focus may undermine rather than allow strategic thinking that has a more integrated approach to working on problems at different levels and with a longer vision. So to reduce the risk factors associated with smoking, the approach should tackle those factors in the environment that contribute to young people taking up smoking, and may begin with a project to engage with what it is about young people's environments that encourages them to start smoking. The experiences of Len Syme (2003) are illustrative of how health promotion needs to change its focus. He and his high-level team of health promoters/researchers discovered the need to have a longer-range view after the failure of traditional risk factor programs in disadvantaged communities in the USA. They engaged in strategic thinking to work out why their risk factor programs were not achieving the results they wanted, and they realised that what the community wanted was not what the researchers thought the community wanted. And they realised that they needed to invest in hope before, or alongside, smoking reduction programs.

I will return to strategic thinking and planning later in the chapter—let's turn now to the details of the Two-Tier Health Promotion Program Plan. This has two planning instruments: the conceptual framework and the technical program plan. They are both critical because one without the other is lacking in necessary detail.

BUILDING IN STEPS TO ADDRESS EQUITY

Steps to ensure that health promotion addresses inequities fit at several levels of the conceptual framework and then need to be embedded into the program plan (NSW Health 2001):

1   Take a population health approach using actions strategies such as:
    a   Community engagement and capacity 'releasing' work
    b   Community development
    c   Advocacy
    d   Organisational change to develop the organisation's capacity to influence the health of disadvantaged communities including:
        i   Management support for equity and collaborative working to be embedded into policies and programs
        ii   Staff in-service to develop knowledge and skills about equity-working
        iii Demonstrated commitment to respectful, fair, and equitable work practices, including recruitment and retention of staff
    e   Partnership work and interagency coordination
2   Include consideration and review of the incorporation of equity strategies into both tier 1, the conceptual framework, and tier 2, the technical program plan.

PROGRAM LOGIC

Program logic is a term used to describe program plans that ensure all conceptual and technical elements of the program are linked through logical connections—the determinants drive the goals that are connected to objectives from which strategies/interventions are derived. Program plans that follow a logic design include a plan for evaluation, which in turn is useless without a good quality program plan to guide the measurement of program effects. These principles apply to both large-scale and small-scale programs and evaluations.

Figure 8.1, *Program Logic* (based on a version included in VicHealth 2005b) illustrates the links between all elements of a program. Note the relationship between the determinants and goals, and then between goals, objectives, and strategies, and where the levels of evaluation fit into the logic schema.

To ensure change is both deep and enduring, health promotion outcomes need to be measured at more than one level. Four main levels for action are identified (Health Education Authority 2001; NSW Health 2001; VicHealth 2005a):

1   Strengthening individuals and families: this means increasing social connection through sustained involvement in group activities; access to supportive relationships, to education and income support; and increasing health literacy (including emotional literacy).
2   Strengthening communities: providing environments that are safe, supportive and sustainable, with healthy environments, evidence of social cohesion and social inclusion. The community could be a township, local area, or school community.
3   Strengthening organisations: for example, bringing about change in health-promoting organisations with explicitly stated values in relation to equity; developing capacity for working in partnerships and collaborations; ensuring that health promotion is included at all levels of planning and reporting, and that health promotion is managed and implemented by a core staff of skilled practitioners; that internal and external partnerships are supported; and that quality frameworks are in place for health promotion.
4   Strengthening sectors or whole societies: addressing social and structural barriers to good health that involve a wide range of sectors including, for example, education, employment, housing, environment, justice or protecting human rights, or tackling discrimination through legislation.

Figure 8.1   Program logic

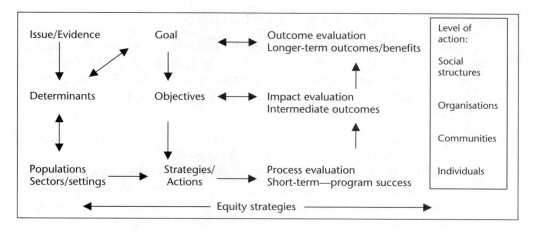

It is critical that outcomes should be planned at more than one level for effective and sustainable change. A decrease in the level of teenage pregnancies, for example, requires more than a change in knowledge about use of condoms. Schools need to change their approaches to sex education. Or to support young mothers, education systems need to establish programs that allow young mothers to return to study, and communities need to provide stronger social and economic support to single-parent families. Working at only one level of health promotion action will minimise the degree of change and effectiveness that is possible with a program.

An effective health promotion program will seek to affect one or more determinants of health at one of more of these levels of action. It may be necessary to develop sub-plans for say, the work conducted with individuals and the work conducted for organisational change, with visions/goals, objectives, and actions that relate to intermediate and longer-term outcomes. Or another way to capture the different levels of action could be to ensure that your overall program goal takes account of more than one level of change, and that you have objectives for each level of action.

Box 8.1: Projects or programs?

The language of projects and programs is frequently interchanged, so be sure to have a common understanding of what different stakeholders mean when they use these terms. As a guide, the term *project* is used here to refer to something done on a small scale, perhaps with partners with a quite defined topic and a short timescale; while the term *program* is used to refer to more layered and longer-term health promotion. A health promotion program is a course of action operating at multiple levels and with a number of stakeholders, and more likely to be over a longer period of time than a project.

SUCCESS AND EFFECTIVENESS

The principle of logical design extends to the inclusion of the program evaluation in program plans. Health promotion program evaluations should be designed to demonstrate *effectiveness* (change in intermediate and longer-term outcomes) as well as *success* (the implementation of the program elements).

Success is about the following:

- Quality principles—were program materials, the communication strategy, document management, and so on of good quality?
- Reach and engagement—did the program reach those most vulnerable or disadvantaged and particularly those experiencing compound social disadvantages, and were/are they engaged in the processes that were developed?

- Appropriateness—was the program appropriate in terms of culture, gender, language, and technical approaches?
- Satisfaction—to what extent were the program participants satisfied with the program?

Effectiveness is about whether or not the program was successful in creating change, or making a difference, in terms of outcomes, at both intermediate and long-term levels.

GOALS AND OBJECTIVES

The development of goals and objectives is a technical process that all health promotion practitioners need to master. They are essential steps in program logic:

- *Goals* (or aims) are statements about long-term benefits or changes the program seeks to influence, change in terms of one or more determinants of health. Goals are measured by outcome evaluation.
- *Objectives* are statements of change designed to achieve the goals—they are more direct and specific than goals/aims. Objectives are linked to intermediate outcomes and are measured by impact evaluation.
- *Strategies/interventions* are methods that are used or actions that will be taken to achieve the objectives and are measured by process evaluation.

You will find different uses in different sectors of the terms actions, interventions, strategies, and frameworks. One sector's strategy is another sector's intervention—and a framework could be a policy strategy or an outline plan for interventions. When working outside your own sector, check the language used, and clarify terms so you have a common understanding of the hierarchies used in planning.

At this stage, it would be a useful exercise for you to visit Guidebook 5, and find resources on how to develop goals and objectives. The online tools provided by the Planning and Evaluation Wizard of the South Australian Community Health Research Unit (SACHRU), The Bush Book and The Health Communication Unit are all practical and clearly written, and include templates for practice.

MULTILEVEL INTEGRATED HEALTH PROMOTION

Integrated health promotion is a term in common use, as is the term multilevel health promotion, but are they the same thing? Integrated health promotion is described as a program design that uses a mix of health promotion interventions and capacity-building strategies to address priority health and well-being issues (DHS 2003). Multilevel health promotion is used to describe work conducted across sectors and levels of action. We actually need both integration and multilevel working so the term 'multilevel integrated health promotion' seems useful to support the conceptual framework and technical plans. Multilevel integrated health promotion involves collaborative work between organisations across sectors, using a mix of health promotion action at distinct levels of action.

Tier 1: conceptual framework

Tier 1, the conceptual framework for health promotion program planning, is about getting the building blocks right so that the program plan is evidence-based and designed to create effective and sustainable change. These are parallel processes that are consistent with a socio-ecological approach to health promotion. Constructing a conceptual framework begins with evidence that indicates the nature and scope of a problem or issue, and/or points towards the existence of an inequity. It could be thought of as moving through specific layers of planning: Table 8.1 demonstrates these layers, drawing on elements of the VicHealth Framework for Mental Health and Wellbeing (VicHealth 2005b):

In summary, the steps for developing the conceptual framework are:

- identify the evidence that establishes the problem
- establish the determinants of the problem or issue that your program seeks to influence—the size of the program will be related to the number of determinants on which the program is focused
- identify the population group(s) or community of interest where health advancement is desired
- work out the health promotion action areas that will create change in the determinants of health identified in Step 1—refer to the Framework for Health Promotion Action in Chapter 3 and Figures 3.1 and 3.2 for a range of possibilities
- establish the settings for those actions that will promote effectiveness
- determine the levels for action, selecting more than one—individual/family, community, organisational, societal
- make decisions about the desired outcome levels at the intermediate level and then the longer-term benefits that will result from the program.

This conceptual framework will then inform the development of your technical program plan which is discussed a little further on.

Tier 2: technical program plans for health promotion

Tier 2 is the technical program plan, which comprises the planning steps that may be more familiar to health promotion practitioners because there have been many other program plans developed (see for example Naidoo & Wills 2000; Tones & Green 2004). Some planning models are straightforward and some are very complex (for example, Green & Kreuter 1999). As a general rule, more

Table 8.1 Tier 1: conceptual framework for health promotion planning

EVIDENCE OF ISSUES/PROBLEMS/INEQUITIES			
DETERMINANTS OF HEALTH (1–3) (E.g. Social Inclusion)			
POPULATION GROUPS OR COMMUNITY OF INTEREST (by age, sex, life-stage etc)			
HEALTH PROMOTION ACTION AREAS (REFER TO CHAPTER 3, FIGURES 3.1 AND 3.2)			
SETTINGS FOR ACTION E.g. Education, Health, Justice, Politics, Sport, Community, Housing			
LEVELS FOR ACTION			
INDIVIDUAL/FAMILY	COMMUNITY	ORGANISATIONAL	SOCIETAL
INTERMEDIATE OUTCOMES (Foreign Social Inclusion)			
INDIVIDUAL/FAMILY	COMMUNITY	ORGANISATIONAL	SOCIETAL
Programs that enhance: Social support and social inclusion Empowerment Knowledge Literacy Self-esteem and self-efficacy Skills	Programs that enhance: Environments Inclusion Social support and connectedness Acceptance of diversity Community development	Programs that enhance: Research that respects lay knowledge Equity approaches Community engagement Respect for culture Partnerships and collaborative working	Programs that enhance: Healthy public policy Social stability Income support and wealth redistribution Appropriate resource allocation
LONGER-TERM OUTCOMES			
Individuals and families who have access to the resources they need, healthy food, affordable education and health care	Communities that are cohesive, stable, and prosperous	Organisations with the capacity for integrated multilevel health promotion	A society with greater equity and reduced health and social inequalities

complex models require a higher level of resourcing, and can be perplexing for practitioners who are pressed for time and with multiple responsibilities.

The steps in tier 2 are based on program logic, which is necessary for quality, transparency, and effectiveness. The difference with models provided elsewhere is that the Two-Tier Health Promotion Plan is built by first developing the conceptual framework, to guide the integration of the determinants approach, and additional stages that ensure a focus on both equity and outcomes, and then the technical plan. Tier 2 (the technical plan) then, has six stages, each of which will be explained further on.

Figure 8.2 Tier 2: the technical plan

```
1   Partnership development
2   Vision setting
3   Goals and objectives
4   Action mapping
5   Implementation
6   Evaluation and dissemination.
```

Health promotion planning models may look linear on paper but in reality the phases overlap, and they are more cyclic than linear because of the plan—evaluate—reflect—plan cycle. They also need to have some flexibility built into them. Cyclic processes are important because of the need for continuous learning about the program design, implementation, and outcomes to inform future health promotion work. Flexibility is important to enable programs to be responsive to emerging needs and issues, consistent with community development principles. For example, there seems little point in continuing to expend program resources (two staff, room hire, catering) on a peer-led parent education program if, after several weeks, only three parents, all with post-secondary levels of education and good incomes, have ever turned up to the program. Resources would be better spent on research to better understand the needs and priorities of a wider range of parents so that the program can be redesigned to meet needs of those not currently making use of the program. An equity approach would require a refocusing on the original population of interest to the program, which the funding body was told would be vulnerable parents with limited access to resources.

Six stages of tier 2

Stage 1: Partnership development and rationale

Partnership development is critical at the outset. The development of partnerships should be deliberate—it is also an equity strategy (NSW Health 2001). Partnerships lead to collaborative working, which strengthens all aspects of your program processes. Every program benefits from the input of a number of stakeholders, so from your networks, develop a stakeholder group that represents at least one other sector in addition to your own and, of course, include local community folk. The partnership, whether internal at first, or internal and external, is when the evidence is reviewed, and the social determinants defined. Perhaps your group will decide on one determinant of health but because determinants are inter-related, it may be more effective to select two or three. However, any more than three determinants/factors may be beyond the capacity of the group and available resources.

The available evidence to support your plan needs to be gathered and summarised to make your case for organisational support—this is your rationale, and is a critical early step in the planning process. Draw together and summarise the evidence from a range of sources: research, local reports, local knowledge, related interventions/programs, evaluations, and practitioner wisdom. Ensure that in summarising the evidence, you make the connections between the evidence and the determinants of health you wish to influence, and that you make related inequities transparent.

Discuss and agree on the nature of the partnership (see Chapter 3)—explore expectations, assess level of commitment of potential partners, talk about available time for the work that is to be planned, and what other resources might be available. Partnerships preferably build on established relationships but, of course, all partnerships have to start somewhere! Nevertheless, partnerships work best if there is an intermediate or longer-term commitment. Refer to Chapter 3 for discussion about partnership working and collaborative practice, including the preconditions and processes of effective partnerships set out by Labonte (2003) in Table 3.3.

Table 8.2 Partnership development checklist

PARTNERSHIP DEVELOPMENT CHECKLIST	√
± The partnership has allowed time for exploration of expectations, level of commitment, available resources	
± The partnership includes genuine participation from community members	
± Key social and economic determinants to drive the program have been identified	
± Evidence summary completed, drawing links with determinants of health and making inequities transparent	
± Identification of the range of possible issues and agreement reached on the paramount issues that need to be addressed	
± In-principle support gained from relevant managers within partner organisations	

Stage 2: Vision setting

Following Senge et al. (1999), evoke strategic thinking among your planning group to develop a shared vision to inform your goals:

■   Assess the landscape: get a feel for the larger landscape; ask searching questions about the relationships between issues and problems; keep asking 'what are the real problems lying beneath the surface issues/risk factors' to get to the underlying factors that are social, economic, and environmental.

■ Discover the core questions with an equity focus: once you have posed most of the relevant questions, look for patterns in the responses and define the core problems that, if resolved, would make the most difference to health equity among the people that are of interest to your planning group.

■ There are many population groups that could be of interest to your work. You may decide to take a whole-of-community approach or focus on specific groups or populations.

Table 8.3 Vision setting checklist

VISION SETTING CHECKLIST	√
± Revisit group membership to ensure it is becoming a coalition of partners from relevant sectors—revise if necessary	
± Reaffirm commitment of partners and their level of involvement	
± Identify population groups or community of interest—whether targeted universal approaches are indicated	
± Assess the landscape, and go through a process of asking searching questions to get beneath surface issues	
± Revisit your strategy for involving community members; identify enablers and barriers to their involvement, and solutions to the barriers	
± Use group processes to discover core questions: look for patterns; define core problems; clarify factors that contribute to health inequity	
± Revisit discussions about the determinants (from the Development Phase) and unpack what they mean for the population groups of interest to this program—these will become your program themes	
± Affirm that the focus population is involved in all aspects of the program/work	

Stage 3: Goals and objectives

Goals (or aims) are statements of intent that act as a compass or reference point for the program. While they are often thought of as broad statements, the stakeholders should feel that the goal is achievable so it needs to be closer to the program than perhaps the vision articulated in the previous step. A program being designed at multilevels will need different goals for different levels, for example:

■ **Individual**: Increase social support for elderly isolated men in Pleasantville

■ **Community**: Develop a Community Advocates Program to facilitate access to services of elderly isolated men

■ **Organisational**: Build the capacity of the Board of Management to resource social approaches to health promotion by providing training to all Board members

■ **Societal**: Reduce the invisibility of older people in Pleasantville

- **Disease**: Reduce the number of night-time emergency callouts from isolated elderly people with breathing difficulties
- **Environment**: Instigate a campaign for Council to develop a walking strategy with facilities suitable for older people.

Each goal needs a set of objectives—and perhaps sub-objectives—that show how the goal will be operationalised. Objectives give structure to the program, and should not just be doable, but SMART:

Specific
Measurable
Achievable
Realistic
Time-limited

With some practice, you will see that the main difference between goals and objectives is their focus.

- **Goals** are more focused on *long-term outcomes*, so they are measured by *outcome evaluation*
- **Objectives** are focused on *intermediate outcomes*, so they are measured by *impact evaluation*
- **Actions** (or strategies or interventions) are focused on what the program is meant to achieve *immediately after its completion*, and they are measured by *process evaluation.*

By ensuring goals and objectives are written for more than one level, your program will make clear its intentions to influence change in a more sustainable way than it would by just working at one level. This is about working upstream through a multilevel, integrated program design.

Table 8.4 Goals and objectives checklist

GOALS AND OBJECTIVES CHECKLIST	√
± There is a clear link between program goals and one or more of the identified determinants of health	
± There are clear links between the program goals and objectives	
± Develop and agree goals for the partnership as well as goals for each individual agency involved in the program and the partnership	
± Objectives are written for each outcome level and not just at the level of individuals	
± Develop a draft evaluation plan linking process, impact, and outcome levels to strategies, objectives, and goals	
± Confirm that the resources and time frame are appropriate to the goals and objectives	

Stage 4: Action mapping

All too often, programs are established without a good evidence base, with the selection of interventions ad hoc and unsystematic. This may be because there isn't good evidence readily available to guide practitioners in their decision-making.

However, as the evidence base for health promotion strengthens (see Chapter 7), there are opportunities to strengthen program design, making it more robust. Mapping of evidence and intermediate and long-term outcomes is critical to prevent the diluting of impact by poorly targeted program design. Ideally, this will be a blend of evaluative evidence from previous programs or from reviews of evidence and practitioner wisdom about 'best bets' or promising work that others are undertaking.

Developing a review summary from the literature on approaches can be a useful resource for your organisation and for your partnership. Table 8.5 is an illustrative summary—the headings can be varied to suit your purposes. For example, a column can be added for references.

Table 8.5 Sample review of health promotion program approaches conducted for the *Strengthening Communities and Healthy Environments* program

INTERVENTIONS AND STRATEGIES	CONTENT	POPULATION GROUPS/ SETTINGS	EVIDENCE SUPPORT	IMPLEMENTATION ISSUES
Heart health and diabetes education	Programs that enable people to play active roles in achieving, protecting, and sustaining health should be based on thorough understanding of social and economic determinants of health	Individuals, families, groups, organisations, or communities	Poor evidence that individual health counselling is effective for more than the short term Promising evidence that community-level health education through multifaceted intervention strategies is effective	Most people likely to be preoccupied with day-to-day survival issues than concerns with possibility of developing a longer term chronic disease, particularly those in low-income groups, so focus on changing capacity, social support, and control over decision-making and resources at the individual, network, organisation, community, and political level

INTERVENTIONS AND STRATEGIES	CONTENT	POPULATION GROUPS/ SETTINGS	EVIDENCE SUPPORT	IMPLEMENTATION ISSUES
Workplace heart health programs	Low-income workplaces should be examined to gain an understanding of the particular contextual social, environmental, and economic determinants of health	Factories and other industrial workplaces	Good evidence that healthy workplaces impact on a range of health conditions	Programs should seek to increase local democracy and be evaluated for a wide range of outcomes, including changing capacity, social support, and control over decision-making and resources at the individual, network, organisation, and community levels
Organisationally based health programs	Target low-income workers and ensure that programs are based on sound understanding of determinants of health	Settings approaches	Good evidence that workplace settings are effective for health programs that increase understanding of health issues with a more holistic view than just focusing on behavioural risk factors	Work-based programs are more effective if top-down support of management is negotiated and bottom-up inclusion of staff in decision-making and goals and objectives are targeted to reach low-income workers
Income equity	Advocacy for minimum wages and secure jobs	Employment programs	Good evidence that low income over time is predictor of stress and poor access to health services and that a living wage through life prevents CVD in the longer term. Employment programs that put people into low-income jobs show little evidence of positive improvement on health	Work collaboratively with local employment programs to ensure they are health-promoting and not health-damaging

(Continued)

Table 8.5 *(Continued)*

INTERVENTIONS AND STRATEGIES	CONTENT	POPULATION GROUPS/ SETTINGS	EVIDENCE SUPPORT	IMPLEMENTATION ISSUES
Social support	One to one or group interventions including counselling	Groups at risk of CVD or diabetes	One-to-one interventions lack good evidence in relation to health outcomes More promising approaches to the provision of social support for low-income groups when they are combined with problem-solving skill building	Use settings approaches and combine with multilevel, integrated health promotion interventions Avoid top-down ownership of group processes and foster local governance and empowerment
Community mobilisation programs	Community-wide, multilevel and intersectoral	Communities particularly low income and disadvantaged by geography, lack of public transport, cultural diversity, low levels of employment	Good evidence that with high degree of diffusion of information, there is potential for community mobilisation to influence health via environmental, regulatory, and institutional policies	Ensure goals and objectives define populations of interest and evaluate for reach and engagement
High-quality centre-based preschool/ early childhood centres	Target low-income families with insecure housing and/ or who rely on public transport	Communities particularly low income and disadvantaged by geography, lack of public transport, cultural diversity, low levels of employment	Strong evidence that early childhood centres improve mental health while providing education, social support and social connectedness for mothers and children	Collaborate with early childhood programs to value add

Source: Garrard et al. 2004

The partnership needs to agree on what health promotion action areas it will focus on, such as community engagement, and/or organisational development, community strengthening, communication and marketing, advocacy, and so on.

To do this, refer to the health promotion approaches and the Framework for Health Promotion Action in Chapter 3 (p. 31).

Table 8.6 Action mapping checklist

ACTION MAPPING CHECKLIST	√
± The proposed interventions have been assessed for their capacity to address the nominated determinants	
± The types and range of health promotion action areas that the partnership can manage have been identified, and allocated to agencies that have the requisite skills and expertise	
± The actions to be evaluated have been identified	
± Intended/predicted short-term, intermediate and longer-term outcomes of the program and the connections between them have been mapped	
± The program is acceptable to key stakeholders: communities, local decision-makers, organisations	
± Mechanisms are established for monitoring and feedback by lead organisations to the partnership and agreed actions if agencies unable to comply	
± Agree timelines with start and end dates for all stages, activities, and tasks	

Stage 5: Implementation

By the time you reach this phase, your partnership should have a robust and structured program plan. Such a plan is absolutely necessary so everyone is 'on the same page' about what will be done, and with what intentions (Keleher & Armstrong 2006: 95). It is likely that you will need to develop an overall plan with sub-plans because a single plan for a multilevel program is too unwieldy to manage.

It is essential that resources issues are sorted out across the partnership so that all available resources can be identified and the limitations of those resources are understood. At this stage, it may be necessary to revisit the goals, objectives, and strategies of the program plan to ensure a better fit with the available resources.

Ensure the schema for your program plan includes the levels of outcomes that your partnership has decided to focus on—horizontally at individual, organisational, community, societal levels—and vertically, at intermediate and longer-term levels.

Implementation relies on quality management principles, including whether good standards are being met, budgets and staff are being effectively monitored, and process measures are being collected. Quality management is about ensuring performance meets agreed standards that are consistent in health promotion terms with the principles of the Ottawa Charter.

Key aspects of implementation include (Keleher & Armstrong 2006: 102):

■ communication within the project, among organisations involved and externally

■ project monitoring that includes the collection of good quality data about the project and time for reflection and analysis of that data

■ sustaining of the partnership: checking that decision-making structures are clear and functioning well, emerging problems are being resolved, and that successes are celebrated along the way

■ managing contingencies: looking out for new opportunities to augment the project, monitoring resources regularly, looking out for feedback about the project, including unforeseen issues

■ leadership and innovation: providing appropriate leadership; sharing

■ reviewing problems

■ keep political antennae working.

Table 8.7   Implementation checklist

IMPLEMENTATION CHECKLIST	√
± Identify required resources for interventions, which organisations will have lead roles on each intervention (or set of interventions)—this can serve as a reality check!	
± Ensure everyone knows who will do what and that it fits with the time frame	
± Check that the agencies involved have the necessary resources, including time, infrastructure, personnel for the program	
± Agree what process measures will be used and when, and reporting expectations	
± Ensure reports are received in a timely manner to enable reflection and quality improvement if necessary	
± Check that mechanisms are working for monitoring and feedback by lead organisations to the partnership	

Stage 6: Evaluation and dissemination

Evaluation of health promotion programs should be at least episodic through the life of the program. Evaluation plans need to include timelines and at what stages process evaluations should be collected, when impact evaluation data will be collected, by whom, how, and with what resources.

The language of outcomes in terms of program success is commonly called *process* evaluation. The effectiveness of health promotion work also needs to be evaluated (or measured) in terms of what happened as a result of the program, at both the intermediate (impact evaluation) and over the longer term (outcome evaluation). These three levels of evaluation—process, impact, and outcome—are linked to program design through the aims, objectives, and strategies/interventions.

Evaluation is regarded as requiring seven key steps (Rootman et al. 2001: 28–29):

1 describe the proposed program or initiative
2 identify the issues and questions of concern
3 design the process for obtaining the required information
4 collect the data by following the agreed-on data collection methods and procedures, ensuring information is collected from all credible sources
5 analyse and evaluate the data
6 make recommendations developed with stakeholder involvement in interpretation of the results
7 disseminate the findings to funding agencies and other stakeholders in a meaningful way.

Essentially, health promotion evaluation uses established research methods (Patton 2002; Round, Marshall & Horton 2005). Very good resources are available to assist with the development and construction of evaluation plans. Guidebook 5 introduces many of the most well-known websites that contain proformas and tools, as well as comprehensive 'how-to' guides on conducting evaluations.

Essential competencies for health promoters in conducting evaluation are included in Chapter 16, in Tables 16.2 and 16.3. They include:

■ the selection and application of evaluation instruments
■ applying and interpreting statistical and qualitative data
■ the application of appropriate methods to measure goals, objectives, and actions/strategies
■ understanding of ethical issues in research.

Within their own organisations or partnerships, health promotion practitioners are most likely to be involved with process and impact evaluations. Outcome evaluations are usually undertaken at a regional or statewide level and outsourced.

Evaluation plans need their goals and objectives matched to data collection methods. A sample evaluation plan that matches objectives to data collection methods is provided in Table 8.8.

HEALTH PROMOTION PROGRAM PLANNING TOOLS

Guidebook 5 includes a number of websites with useful tools for writing program plans that are amenable to adaptation to suit your particular purposes. Organisations with a health promotion mandate will have their own preferred formats for program and evaluation plans. Browse through the websites in Guidebook 5 and practise writing up the steps so that you become familiar with the processes involved.

Table 8.8 Evaluation planning

GOAL: TO CONDUCT AN IMPACT EVALUATION OF THE REGION-WIDE STRENGTHENING COMMUNITIES AND HEALTHY ENVIRONMENTS PROGRAM	
OBJECTIVE	STRATEGIES / DATA COLLECTION METHODS
Identify the strategies used by individual agencies funded under each individual scheme, to identify and reach the population(s) of interest	Documentary analysis: ■ Agency policies ■ Newsletters ■ Evidence of needs assessments ■ Annual (and other) reports Interviews with key personnel Analyse prioritisation processes Identify expenditure of resources
Identify to what extent community engagement can be monitored and identify most effective and feasible monitoring mechanisms for participation in community life	Survey to gather data about number and type of strategies Analyse available data of participation statistics and types of participants
Identify factors within and outside the Neighbourhood Renewal Program that facilitate or inhibit its effective implementation and the achievement of individual schemes' goals and objectives	Key stakeholder interviews
Identify examples of good practice models for increasing participation in organised community events and implementation of sustainable healthy environment practices in the venues	Case studies to highlight good practice
Examine the relationship between the Neighbourhood Renewal and other community building programs	Interviews (face-to-face or telephone) and focus group discussions Surveys to provide opportunities for feedback
Examine the link between development of healthy environment policies and their impact on practices	Organisational policy analysis Examination of 'fit' between policy and reality Questions in interviews about capacity of agency to deliver

Source: Garrard et al. 2004

HEALTH PROMOTION RESEARCH

It is impossible to optimise outcomes for communities without an organisational strategy to support health promotion or with good research evidence. Evidence informs strategic planning and articulates the fit between government policies, organisational policies, and outcomes for people. There is substantial potential for ineffective health promotion work, even though it may be undertaken by well-intentioned staff but without strategic intent, strong evidence, or quality planning.

Most local organisations are not funded to conduct research and their capacity to do so may be quite limited. Yet all organisations need to base their work on best evidence, which can be categorised into three types:

- Pre-program evidence: primary and secondary data from studies such as Burden of Disease, community profiles, and needs assessment
- Implementation evidence: best evidence about what works to inform the selection of actions/strategies
- Evaluation evidence: analysis of data from process and impact evaluations of programs conducted by your own or other organisations that have implemented a similar program.

Coalitions or partnerships (such as the Victorian Primary Care Partnerships) are responsible for the development of comprehensive data collections of local population areas for pre-program planning. Community profiles, needs assessments, and population studies are all used to inform the development of area or catchment plans with priorities for health promotion and service development.

Implementation evidence is increasingly being developed by agencies established for the gathering and review of health promotion program evidence (see Chapter 7) and it is increasingly being provided in practitioner-friendly formats that provide clear guidelines and are quick to navigate (see for example Garrard et al. 2004 and Keleher & Round 2006). Partnerships with universities and other research organisations are another strategy to get health promotion research evidence to inform health promotion program work. Finally, evaluation evidence can be found in reports for organisations, journals, and conference papers.

SUMMARY

This chapter has put forward a planning process consistent with the key message of this book—that health promotion is a social and political process of implementing and managing change. The model put forward is integrated with equity approaches and a sound understanding of the determinants of the problem or issue, the nature of the expected outcomes, and processes and actions involved in health promotion for change. What distinguishes the Two-Tier Health Promotion Plan is that it begins with a determinants perspective and a population health approach, developed through a strong conceptual framework. That framework has inherent understandings about its purpose, which is to inform the processes and actions and expected outcomes of the program plan. The Two-Tier Health Promotion Plan with its conceptual framework and technical program plan helps to explain what an upstream, multilevel, and multistrategy health promotion approach looks like. More importantly, by following through the two tiers and the stages, your approach will be both strategic and logical, and more able to produce effective outcomes and sustainable change.

9 ENGAGING COMMUNITIES

Jennie Popay

In October 2005 Jennie Popay visited South Australia as a guest of the Australian Health Inequities Project (AHIP), supported by the South Australian government. AHIP is an initiative of Flinders University and Melbourne University, funded by the National Health and Medical Research Council under a scheme to increase the capacity of the Australian workforce. While in South Australia she spoke to an AHIP function and a Department of Health function. This chapter is an edited version of her talk on community engagement.

Key concepts

- Community engagement can improve the delivery of services, help to develop good policy and effective interventions, and assist with the democratic project.
- Local and central governments have a long history of initiating, then changing or abolishing processes to foster community engagement in decisions.
- Many individual agencies and local governments try to foster engagement, but are thwarted by national governments or powerful forces. This breaks a psychological contract between communities and government.
- Lay and professional people can be harmed by inappropriate approaches to engagement.
- Communities have memories of community engagement processes that have been underfunded, abolished, or not taken seriously. These memories inform realistic assessments of the limited value of community engagement and this can lead to barriers to current and future attempts at engagement.
- We need to reframe the debate that engagement fails because the community does not have the capacity, to one that seeks to unlock capacity in community and professional structures, deal with the transfer of power, and have long-term processes that preserve engagement and meaning. Despite the problems of engagement, it is worth doing.

Key terms

- Community engagement
- Psychological contract with communities
- Policy and service improvement
- Community memory
- Capacity for engagement
- Power

OVERVIEW

I discuss community engagement in issues around health and equalities and improving the environment. What does patient and public involvement or community engagement mean and why has it become so popular in the United Kingdom (UK) in the last ten years? Is it making a difference? I am giving my answer away when I say we must ask, why not?

MYRIAD WAYS TO ENGAGE

In the UK there is a very long history of trying to involve users of services and the public in public sector services. Since the beginning of the National Health Service (NHS) we have had non-executive members of boards who are 'lay people'—they do tend to be mostly white, middle-class, older retired men but that's slowly changing. Then during the (Conservative) Thatcher years, we had *Listening to Local People* where every public agency had to listen to what local people had to say. They may or may not have taken any notice of them. We had a really interesting experiment in the 1970s of community development projects abolished after about four years, which in the UK is a sign that something is effective! *Community Health Councils* were established in the 1970s as boards of lay people. They were abolished in 2003 and replaced by a new England-wide system of patient and public involvement forums with statutory power to inspect every health trust in the UK and a *National Commission for Patient and Public Involvement* in 2003, which is shortly to be abolished. Community development is now well embedded within local government and Community Development Officers are now employed by all local authorities.

And now under New Labour we have *A Thousand Blossoms Blooming* and being abolished regularly. We have *People Banks*, which is a really interesting notion and represents the economisation of our language. We have *Scottish Social Inclusion Forums*, which seem to be having a real impact on regional planning. And we have community-run services. So community engagement has a long history and is a very diverse landscape with lots of different things happening and a lot of dedication on the part of both lay people and professionals.

But in the UK at least, community engagement and public involvement can mean just about whatever the agency wants it to mean, for example:

- 'Empowering citizens to express views on how needs are to be met'
- 'Working with local people to strengthen accountability',
- 'Bringing local people into the service delivery systems'
- 'Putting active citizens at the heart of tackling social problems'
- 'Increasingly building people's skills, knowledge, abilities and confidence to take action and play leading roles in improving services and developing communities.'

Why has it become so popular? Over the last decade there has been a shift in gear in the way the UK government is thinking, reflecting a long-term social movement where lay people have increasingly been challenging the right of professional experts to define problems and solutions. There is also, in Europe and North America, voluntary voting and as a consequence the proportion of people voting has been dropping dramatically. As a result there is real concern about what that means for the legitimate right of the state, nationally and locally, to make decisions. So the belief is that this engagement agenda will re-engage people in the democratic process.

And then there is undoubtedly an element of learning from the past, that attempts to improve services, attempts to regenerate areas have failed. Salford, a city near Manchester for example, has been regenerated many times and they've failed every time to produce a significant improvement in the quality of life of the people involved. They've got wonderful housing stock now but as a place to live it's still not succeeding. And similarly central government reorganises the health service frequently and they're not getting the improvements they're expecting. And so there is a belief that there must be a way in which we can enlist lay knowledge, lay wisdom, to do these things better. For many individual practitioners I think that belief is genuine.

THE GOOD, THE BAD, AND THE UGLY

My account of the engagement agenda is taken from the spaghetti western starring Clint Eastwood, *The Good, The Bad and The Ugly*.

The *good*: people genuinely believe that lay and public involvement is opening space within publicly funded services for transformation rather than fiddling around the margins. There is potential for 'working both sides', or developing community capacity and organisational and professional capacity at the same time.

The *bad*: the concern that engagement and involvement is really an agenda around the state withdrawing from service provision, the hollowing out of the state, the commercialisation of citizenship, and a privatisation of provision.

The *ugly:* the challenge that lay knowledge represents to professional knowledge and the experience that wherever engagement is genuine, it will be a struggle for power. Here we have to accept that if there isn't a sense of struggle for power then there isn't a transfer of power going on. People don't give power away, you have to take it. And that struggle is undoubtedly leading to casualties in terms of lay people who are getting burnt out and damaged by the process and the front-line workers who are expected to deliver an engagement agenda without the right support from organisations and local and national governments.

DOES ENGAGEMENT MAKE A DIFFERENCE?

Despite these problems the current UK Government seems to be taking engagement and involvement seriously because there are important policy drivers in place now. For example Section 11 in the *Health and Social Care Act 2001* has placed a mandatory duty on all public agencies to consult local people on all major decisions. All National Health Service (NHS) organisations have to produce a baseline assessment and strategic plan for patient and public involvement. There is a Patient and Public Involvement Forum linked to every NHS organisation: trust, acute, specialist, primary. These lay bodies have the statutory power to go in and inspect the trust. They cannot be refused. They can negotiate other timing but they can't be refused and they have the statutory power to push their results up to the inspection agency. All the inspection agencies are now required to involve lay people in inspection and audit.

Is it making a difference? There's some evidence that patient and public involvement and community engagement is leading to better outcomes and control of disease. We are getting some evidence of more appropriate and sustainable services. In some areas community engagement is leading to improved material and social conditions. There are some people, individuals and some communities, who have become more assertive as a result of their experience of being engaged. So there is a lot of evidence at an individual level but the lack of a collective voice is where the really serious problem lies.

THE PSYCHOLOGICAL CONTRACT

One way of thinking about this lack of progress is that a psychological contract is being broken. Consider a public agency charged with delivering a new deal for community involving a multimillion (English) pound regeneration initiative. The agency tells communities *you're going to lead this initiative, it's your initiative.* But within a very short space of time, a year even, the central government demands early wins. So the delivery of those early wins bypasses the community engagement structures and processes and as a result these communities are feeling severely let down, frustrated, angry. Here, there is a psychological contract between the local state and local people, which is being broken with severe long-term implications for that relationship. This damages lay and professional people and relegates most good practice to the margin. It's not changing the mainstream of the way health-related decision-making specifically or public sector decision-making is being done, so it's ticking boxes.

BARRIERS TO SYSTEMATIC COMMUNITY ENGAGEMENT

So what's getting in the way? As part of a project funded by the UK Department of Health, which aimed to develop ways to support public sector organisations to 'do' community engagement better, we developed a barrier model and a resource pack. The resource pack based on this work is available as a free download from <www.nccce.lancs.ac.uk>. Figure 9.1 shows that the model is necessarily messy as it highlights barriers in the public sector at a local level and nationally.

Figure 9.1   Barriers constraining capacity for partnership working with lay people

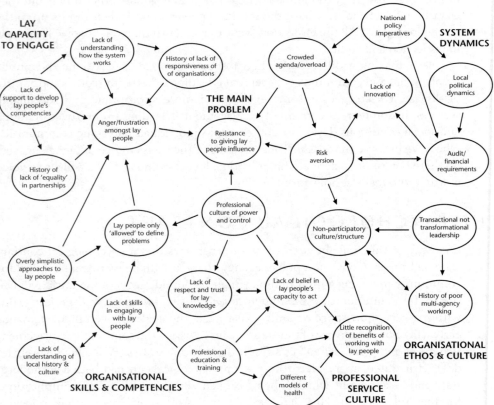

The barriers in the public sector that are highlighted in this model are the result of many things but the most important are:

■ Lack of appropriate skills and competencies among individual practitioners: this gets most of the attention because it is the easiest thing to 'fix'. If you are really imaginative you can get local people in to do some of the training!

■ Entrenched professional and organisational cultures. Focusing attention on the need for organisational culture change is still pretty rare in the UK—although the SAFEC project did just this. This has a lot of potential to change things in terms of community engagement but it requires more commitment from senior managers than they may be willing to give.

■ Wider system dynamics, including demand for the quick wins! Even if a local authority or a local health trust wants to do engagement properly, they are faced with central governments using the rhetoric that they want it done but then demanding results too quickly. This undermines any authentic attempt to engage and results in a negative reaction from the community, making it more difficult to engage in the future. In many UK communities this experience of the psychological contract being broken goes back to the 1950s. Individuals and communities have memories, so past actions of the national state to undermine what the local state might be trying to do have cast long shadows for today's engagement agenda.

■ Lack of clarity of purpose: overlaying all of these barriers, and in part resulting from them, is a lack of clarity about the purpose of community engagement. Or maybe it isn't that policy-makers lack clarity but that they do indeed have a very restricted role for community engagement—that is as a mechanism to delivery services or policy initiatives rather than an end in itself. And while policy-makers may have this perspective—the community might really believe that more fundamental change is in the air—the scope for profound disillusionment increases when the penny drops as drop it will.

REFRAMING CAPACITY FOR ENGAGEMENT

Finally, let's reframe capacity. Research with local people and service users has shown barriers among patients, users, and the public. These barriers are not primarily about a lack of capacity to engage or a lack of knowledge. That means the notion of community capacity-building and community development is really problematic because of the paternal, professional assumption that lay people have to learn to participate. We have to reframe the debate because there is rarely an assumption that professionals and organisations have to learn to participate. It's usually the professional experts who teach about how to participate and they have what we sociologists would refer to as positional power.

I will conclude by referring back to some research we did as part of the Salford Social Action Research Project, exploring people's experience of engagement. We found that people have high levels of attachment to the places as they had been, and as they could be, but low levels of attachment to the places as they are.

Paradoxically, while there was a lot reciprocity between neighbours, there was very little collective community engagement or action. People said they would act collectively if they thought there were issues that were important and if they could make a difference, but very few people were engaged in the process that the local authority was trying to get going.

In our work we constructed three groups from our interviews. There was a small group of *engagers* for whom getting engaged in decision-making with the local government or the health authority had transformed their lives. So they got educated and got jobs. A slightly larger group had been *damaged* by the process, finding themselves in the middle between the authority and the local people and leaving everybody frustrated. And then the largest group, the *reluctant*, had never been engaged in the public sphere, and could see no evidence why they should get engaged because they believed that it wouldn't change anything. And these are people who have seen peers trying and not having an effect over three or four decades past, of things that have happened in the place—a community memory.

So the central paradox in the UK is that the genuine commitment in the public sector to engage lay people more equally in decision-making is counterbalanced by people in disadvantaged communities who are learning from experience that it's not worth getting engaged.

SUMMARY

So what's to be done? Involvement in engagement is not a silver bullet but although it can be iatrogenic, there are many reasons why we should continue to do it better. Let's try and reframe it as *releasing capacity* not building it within organisations, user groups, and communities. That gives us a focus on reducing barriers on all sides rather than building capacity with lay people only. If you only build capacity on the lay side without reducing barriers on the professional side then you'll get more forces against community engagement. And, crucially, lay people need to experience power being redistributed and engagement having real impact if they're going to not just engage but sustain and spread engagement.

So the key to engagement is to be clear about the purpose and recognise that it is more than involving people in decisions about what treatment they should receive, how services should be organised, how their money gets spent. The most important public health purpose is to come right back to lay knowledge and create enduring processes to allow people to have a real say in how life is to be lived. That's the meaning issue and one of the reasons why consultation exercises can be so hollow. You can only get at that if you have long-term conversations of possibility between agencies and the people that they're there to serve.

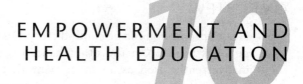

EMPOWERMENT AND HEALTH EDUCATION

Helen Keleher

Key concepts

- Empowering approaches to health are the new generation of health promotion, seeking to impact on social change, power relations, and inequity.
- Empowerment works at individual, organisational, and community/ political levels.
- Health teaching for well-being is a more empowering approach than traditional individualised health education approaches.
- Structural health determinants are effective entry points for organisational and community capacity-building and development.

Key terms

- Empowerment
- Health education
- Health teaching for well-being

OVERVIEW

Health promotion can be contradictory. On the one hand, it is intended to improve people's health. On the other hand, it can be disempowering and alienating, inadvertently used as an instrument that maintains the status quo of power relations between professionals and their health promotion audience. Jennie Popay has explained in Chapter 9, the potential for engagement to be iatrogenic, and how damage to people can occur if the engagement is not authentic and followed through.

Health education is another strategy that can put people at risk by attempting to domesticate people, reinforcing and perpetuating inequalities, 'serving the interests of the powerful to the detriment of the powerless' (Patterson 2006: 218). Should such programs be allowed to call themselves health promotion? Too often, programs are delivered under the banner of health promotion but are not designed on empowerment or equity principles that are at the heart of health promotion. When health promotion is not designed for empowerment and equity, people with income and other resources will gain more advantage than those who have fewer resources (Victora et al. 2003), thereby increasing inequities.

This chapter reviews the concepts of empowerment, health education, health teaching for well-being, community capacity, and development. This chapter is supported by Guidebook 7, Capacity-building Resources.

EMPOWERMENT

Empowerment is a term much used, abused, and misunderstood; but used appropriately in health promotion, empowerment approaches are a key to reframing practice. This section reviews the concept of empowerment at three outcome levels: psychological, organisational, and community/political levels. Psychological levels are discussed in terms of a critique of health education and the introduction of the concept of learning for health and well-being. Organisational empowerment and community/political empowerment are discussed in terms of the concepts of community capacity-building and development.

Empowerment strategies are not new. They were the basis of the Alma Ata Declaration for Primary Health Care (1978), which discussed community participation and equity. Community participation became a buzz word during the 1980s. Then the Ottawa and Jakarta Charters for Health Promotion (WHO 1986, 1997) provided empowering principles for health promotion, which are discussed in Chapter 2. Despite its popularity, participation, whether at individual or community levels, has been shown to be insufficient to promote better health or impact on inequity. More multifaceted processes and approaches are necessary if people and communities are to gain control over their own affairs and their lives and to change social environments. Empowerment strategies are a means towards better health with the potential to impact on health status, but sometimes empowerment is a sufficient end in itself because the skills and capacities developed are prerequisites for healthy people and healthy communities.

Empowerment is a complex concept that encompasses various levels of working with people. At the level of individuals or within the context of families, empowerment draws on psychological theories including locus of control theory and concepts of self-efficacy derived from social learning theory. Empowerment also has roots in adult education theory, which draws heavily on the work of the Brazilian Paulo Freire (1970), whose radical adult literacy method was based on the idea of conscientisation—a dynamic cyclical process of critical understanding, reflection, action, and learning from action (praxis).

However, empowerment is not just used in psychological theory, as empowerment has multidisciplinary associations. Social-structural and socio-ecological theories from political science and sociology also inform our understanding of empowerment, drawing in concepts of power relations, social exclusion, and inequity, as Wallerstein (2006) explains:

> Empowerment is an action-oriented concept with a focus on removal of formal and informal barriers, and on transforming power relations between communities and institutions and government. It is based on an assumption of community cultural assets that can be strengthened through dialogue and action … and focuses on power relations and intervention strategies.
>
> Empowerment includes both processes and outcomes with empowerment of marginalized people an important outcome in its own right, and also an intermediate outcome in the pathway to reducing health disparities and social exclusion (Wallerstein 2006: 18).

For empowerment to be used effectively in health promotion, specific attention to both process and outcomes is required. The processes used are as important as the overall context in which the work takes places (Wallerstein 2006)—both process and context are necessary for effective outcomes.

Empowerment outcomes can be achieved at multiple levels:

- Psychological empowerment of individuals is one level
- Organisational empowerment outcomes is the second level, and
- Community/political outcomes are a third level (Wallerstein 2006).

Change can be affected at all levels. Wallerstein (2006) provides a useful table of empowerment program components or strategies in relation to the action areas of the Ottawa Charter:

Table 10.1 Empowerment program components/strategies

PERSONAL SKILLS	SUPPORTIVE ENVIRONMENTS	COMMUNITY ACTION/ PARTICIPATION	HEALTHY PUBLIC POLICY	REORIENTING HEALTH CARE
Planning/actions Access to information	Supportive groups Dialogic approach Indigenous knowledge	Meaningful decision-making Use of lay leaders Leadership Advocacy Organisation capacity	Collective actions Effective organisation structures Transfer power Promote transparency	Involve constituents

Source: Wallerstein 2006

In straightforward terms, power is about the capacity to create or resist change (Kuyek & Labonte 1995 in Labonte 1997: 31). Labonte (1997) discusses the power used by health workers:

- Power-over: the person exercising power attempts to have others behave according to his or her desires such as:
  - □ domination, exploitation, and hegemony (the way professional powers are sometimes used to control how others come to see themselves as powerful or powerless), but also seen in public health legislation over quarantine or smoking laws for example
  - □ economic exploitation, where 'the neutral language of the market ... is blind to distributive justice' (Labonte 1997: 31)
- Power-with: based on the principles of respect, generosity, and service to others from an ethic of caring and justice.

HEALTH EDUCATION

Health education one of the most common strategies used in health promotion but also one of the most problematic. Health education is very commonly designed as an intervention for people with complex health challenges, and is seen as a prerequisite for self-management of chronic conditions such as diabetes, asthma, renal disease, and arthritic conditions. Indeed, health education for self-management is regarded as the cornerstone of care for people with diabetes (Steed et al. 2005). Diabetes health education (for which there is a huge literature) has an overwhelming emphasis on symptom control via lifestyle self-management interventions (see for example Clark, Hampson et al. 2004) through programs directed at improving health behaviours and glycemic (blood sugar) control.

Health education is usually delivered by health professionals in either a brief intervention of say, 10–15 minutes, or in a series of sessions that vary a great deal in contact time, format of delivery, and approach. An evidence-based health education program covers those things which clinicians and health educators regard as important. The health educator will usually have been trained to deliver the program, and indeed, may have delivered the program many times over. Typically, health education programs are evaluated against a narrow range of outcomes about knowledge—attitudes—behaviours.

Freire (1970) refers to domesticating models of health education that are designed to reinforce a kind of certainty about people's social reality. Australia's Aboriginal people call this 'health education through white man's eyes' where professionals name the problems, identify what they see as a person's learning needs, and see compliance as the goal based on a belief that behaviour change is externally motivated (Patterson 2006: 219).

The problem is that behaviours are shaped by the social and economic environments in which people live (Raphael et al. 2003), the stress from which produces health-compromising practices such as tobacco, alcohol and drug use, and poor nutrition. Health education programs make many assumptions about people's capacity to understand the content of health education programs, their capacity to make changes in their lives including their level of resources, and the availability of enabling social circumstances for any change to occur.

Broadly, there are two main models of health education—the *traditional medico-centred model*, and a *client-centred model*. The traditional medical/ professional–patient model is concerned with compliance and planning for people, and relies on passivity and dependence (see Chapter 2, Table 2.1). This model is not concerned with the effects of social exclusion and marginality, power relations, or inequities.

Client-centred health education is frequently described as an empowerment model, using terms such as patient autonomy, active participation (which may just mean giving a person opportunity for discussion), the development of individualised written management plans or tailoring of self-management plans. People are assessed for their readiness to participate in such programs, and perhaps an assessment is done of a person's perceptions of the barriers or benefits of their participation in a health education program. To a degree, client-centred health education could be regarded as having concerns with a person's agency in decision-making but it is through a psycho-social lens at the midstream, drawing on psychological theories of behaviour change, motivation, counselling, and self-efficacy. Theories of behaviour are not concerned with the effects of social exclusion and marginality, power relations, or inequities. The focus on behaviours can lead to victim blaming, an over-emphasis on the ways, however unhealthy, in which people cope with their lives, and fails to address underlying reasons why vulnerable and disadvantaged people adopt such behaviours (Raphael et al. 2003).

Client-centred health education developed because of the lack of effectiveness of the traditional medico-centric model but the long-term effects of client-centred health education are not well proven and studies show variable results (Goudswaard et al. 2004). Those most likely to benefit are people with good education and literacy, social support, personal and economic resources, and a good sense of control over the determinants of their health. Health education, both traditional and more client-centred models, is likely to actually increase health inequalities because these models are not effective for many groups who are marginalised by poverty, culture, discrimination because of race, disabilities, illness or social stereotyping, and difference. It is necessary therefore, for health promoters to understand the role of powerlessness in people's lives and the power relations involved in health education, and to develop new approaches that are effective in reaching socially excluded populations in order to overcome health disparities (Labonte 1997; Wallerstein 2006). This is powerful evidence that health education must move beyond the advice-giving—knowledge-transfer—symptom-control model to one of empowerment.

HEALTH TEACHING FOR WELL-BEING

If we are to understand the purposes of empowerment as incorporating practices of enabling, mediating, and advocating, and if we also understand that empowerment may work at the level of social or political impacts before having a health impact, then a reframing of health education is to understand it in terms of health teaching for well-being. Necessarily, health teaching for well-being incorporates principles of empowerment. In other words when programs are designed for empowerment, learning for health and well-being becomes a process that also facilitates or enables people to gain control over the determinants of their health to improve their quality of life (Wallerstein 2006). Health teaching is intended to be liberating education, which sits in contrast to the domesticating model of education—'it invites people to believe in themselves and to believe that they have knowledge' (Patterson 2006: 218). Health teaching does not begin from the perspective of a professional culture of 'teaching' someone what professionals think that lay people need to know. If that latter approach is taken, then it is still a health education model. Empowerment through health teaching for well-being is a form of psychological empowerment because it relates to people's self-efficacy and control in their lives but power relations are also addressed, so there is an equal relationship between clients and professionals that is based on respect.

Empowerment is not a stand-alone strategy—it is increasingly effective when part of a comprehensive approach. For example, to address empowerment for Indigenous people with diabetes in a local community, there will need to be individual and group health teaching as well as organisational change, community engagement, and policy change. The intervention program components of Table 10.1, based on the Ottawa Charter, set out the program components for empowerment and the elements of a comprehensive approach.

Use of an empowerment model with people who have Type II diabetes, for example, requires different starting points than symptom management and glycemic control. Type II diabetes is more likely to affect people experiencing social and material deprivation, with a greater burden on vulnerable populations (Raphael et al. 2003), graphically illustrated by the burden of Type II diabetes on Aboriginal people. The burden of diabetes is felt not just on the individual but on the health and well-being of families and the whole community.

There is a great deal written about health education principles (Ewles & Simnett 1999; Patterson 2006). However, understanding what comprises an empowerment model is critical, albeit under-researched. Drawing on Raphael et al. (2003) and Wallerstein (2006), Table 10.2 provides insights into the principles of empowerment-based learning for health and well-being that should be the foundations of any health teaching:

Table 10.2 Principles of empowerment-based health teaching for well-being

PRINCIPLES OF EMPOWERMENT FOR HEALTH TEACHING	CHECKLIST FOR YOUR PROGRAM. DOES IT INCLUDE:
Sensitivity to health care needs defined by people themselves	
Respect for culture: a necessary prerequisite for all people involved in learning for health and well-being	
Cultural and local sensitivity of programs	
Educational materials and opportunities examined for their underlying assumptions about race and culture	
Autonomy in decision-making	
A sense of community and local bonding	
Use of small groups to build supportive environments and a deeper sense of community	
Family and individual empowerment strategies to increase patient's abilities, use health services more effectively, and increase care-giver coping skills and efficacy	
Reinforcement of authentic participation	
Increase people's skills and control over resources	
Increase access to relevant information	
Use of lay leaders and helpers (see Case Study 10.1)	
Fostering of advocacy and leadership development	
Time and space to identify structural barriers and facilitators to empowerment interventions	
Mechanisms to overcome structural barriers and facilitators to empowerment interventions	
People will be provided with full knowledge of what options are available to thems in setting their goals and managing their personal behaviours	
Understanding of the role of material and social forces that underpin constraints to good health conditions or personal health skills	

Keeping in mind that a central purpose of health promotion is social change, it is very likely that programs designed to enable health teaching for well-being will not begin with the presenting problem that the health professional may see as the most important. Sensitivity to health care needs defined by people themselves means that professionals need to engage with people and listen to their concerns before jointly deciding on the processes and content of learning for health and well-being programs. Such participation must be understood as a 'complex and iterative process ... not predictable in its outcomes and happens with or without professionals. Therefore, professionals' roles should shift from dominant to supportive or facilitative' (Wallerstein 2006: 8).

Health teaching for well-being requires the integration of initiatives that are much more far-reaching than short-term interventions. The transfer of health knowledge remains an important program element of health teaching but it must be integrated with processes and strategies that build trust as a precondition for joint decision-making about what are very often complex issues. Participation, client autonomy, and psychological empowerment will be constrained by the unwillingness of professionals to acknowledge power and change power relations, unwillingness to extend their engagement beyond a superficial level of knowledge transfer, lack of respect for culture, and professional's lack of knowledge about empowerment processes and the need for long-term engagement. These are classic problems in communities who are experiencing social, cultural, and political disempowerment and disadvantage and whose problems are frequently 'diagnosed' from a medical model perspective rather than framed from a socio-ecological perspective.

> Even when our social situation accords us power-over other people, the intention with which we exercise that power-over can lead to its transformation into power-with ... use of power that seeks to transform the very relationship within which it is exercised ... Power-with ... is the energy and optimism we create when we act together ... pool our different abilities and learn from one another (Labonte 1997: 36).

The problematic nature of health education is when we are overly concerned about the health-behaviours of others without examining our own behaviours. Labonte (1997: 29) suggests the behaviours on which we would be better to concentrate:

Table 10.3 Empowering behaviours and attitudes

BEHAVIOURS	ATTITUDES
Process	
Active listening	Non-judgmental
Eye contact: open body language	Non-threatening

BEHAVIOURS	ATTITUDES
Validating, positively reinforcing, trusting, identifying inner strengths	Belief in person's capacity ability
Calming	Caring, valuing the importance of 'being in the moment'
Sensitive, slow in advising	Respectful
Self-talking, open, sharing, negotiating, abandoning expert jargon	Empathic, reflective
Assertiveness	Willing to challenge
Affirming, motivating talk	Optimistic
Forgiving	Caring, permitting human mistakes
Hearing our voice	Willing to learn with others
Content	
Materially: emotionally, supporting, persisting	Committed to person
Linking self to others, to resources	Creating change through larger mutual support networks
Risk-taking, reaching out, accepting power inequalities as part of problem's roots	Willing to give up power, wishing to create equity (fairness)
Sharing ideas and strategies	Analytical, critical
Providing perspective	Having a wider view
Focusing on problem/solution	Creating positive change in the short term
Affirming spiritual connection	Action from spiritual base, beliefs
Solution-seeking, modelling	Solution-oriented

Source: Labonte 1997: 29.

COMMUNITY CAPACITY AND ORGANISATIONAL EMPOWERMENT

NSW Health suggest that the language of capacity-building is widely understood by leaders in the health system. Nonetheless, the language of capacity-building risks being seen as paternalistic, jargonistic, and 'top-down' (Labonte & Laverack 2001a,b; NSW Health 2001). Building of capacity is not a program in its own right—indeed, health promotion may only play one part of the overall process. Various methods are developing about how to develop community capacity. Guidebook 7, Capacity-building Resources, will assist you to access some key resources.

For those considering programs in community capacity-building, critical thinking is necessary on many aspects of programs. These include the values and assumptions of all stakeholders involved in capacity-building: who has program control, who controls resources, how leadership is developed and devolved, and the effectiveness of participation and engagement (Labonte & Laverack 2001a).

Whether or not participation is empowering can be examined through key characteristics (Wallerstein 2006):

■ People's access to information on public health issues
■ Their inclusion in decision-making
■ Local organisational capacity to make demands on institutions
■ Governing structures and accountability of institutions to the public, and
■ Human rights (Rifkin 2003).

Local community organisations are necessary for partnerships to find solutions that may (for example) replenish communities that have been distressed or depleted, whether through employment or education or health development strategies. Land Councils, Health Councils, neighbourhood houses, domestic violence shelters, local learning and employment networks, and community housing associations are examples of community-based organisations being formed to address local problems. Organisational empowerment is linked to democratic freedoms, which in turn are builders of people's capacity to act, and work together—and of enabling people to find the capabilities within them to lead the kind of lives they value (Sen 2001). The language of community building or regeneration is frequently used to describe the processes of rebuilding and sustaining community life and well-being.

Increased participation by people in local organisations can have many benefits both for individuals, the organisation, and the community. The WHO Charters for Health Promotion (1986, 1997) and the Alma Ata Charter for Primary Health Care (1978) establish the foundations of participatory strategies. They suggest worldwide support for empowerment interventions that include 'group dialogue, collective action, advocacy and leadership training, organizational development, and transfer of power to participants' (Wallerstein 2006: 9). Such interventions need to be linked to outcomes that are steps towards, and prerequisites of, health and well-being, such as:

> Collective efficacy, the belief that people together can make a difference, outcome efficacy, the belief that one's actions can produce results, political efficacy, the belief that one can influence the political process, organisations and communities, critical thinking ability and participatory behaviour' (Wallerstein 2006: 9).

Community capacity and development are core skills for health promotion where action is needed to address the social–structural determinants of health such as poverty, unemployment, gender inequity, or discrimination. Empowerment

Case Study 10.1: Community Health Advocate Programs

The Community Health Advocate (CHA) program trains community members to assist and advocate for other members of the community regarding health and other community issues. The Center for Healthy Communities at the University of Wisconsin reports on its program to develop and sustain community—academic partnerships with a public housing community. Principles followed to develop the partnership included the building of trust over many, many weeks or even months, open communication, respect, shared goals, sharing of credit for outcomes, a focus on strengths and assets, and sharing of resources. Based on a philosophy of community capacity-building, the staff work with underserved communities who have a high prevalence of health issues such as low health status, drug and alcohol issues, mental health concerns, safety issues, and poorly managed chronic illnesses. Community strengths such as active resident organisations were identified and a program was developed in partnership. One part of the program was an identified need for the development of a core group of resident leaders so training was provided to strengthen leadership skills. Recruitment of natural leaders and building of their skills were core strategies. It was thought they would function as opinion leaders and disseminate health promotion strategies and mobilise the community to improve the quality of life of residents. Many activities, such as community festivals and the provision of health-care information in culturally appropriate languages and linking of residents to health workers, have resulted. CHAs have successfully improved access to and the quality of health services, have empowered communities to implement change, and have improved collaboration among community members and health care providers in order to identify and resolve health care issues and improve quality of life (Wolff, Young, Beck et al. 2004).

processes and strategies are critical in addressing inequities arising from these determinants.

The wider social benefits of organisational, community, and political empowerment such as enhanced civil society, governance (transparency and accountability), and human rights are at the heart of health and human development (Labonte & Laverack 2001a,b; Wallerstein 2006).

SUMMARY

We can improve the ways in which we theorise, research, and practise health education by consciously reflecting on our assumptions about how health promotion works and how people with whom we seek to work actually learn, grow, and become empowered. We must interrogate our understanding of how people generate their own knowledge, and strive to overcome professional tendencies for top-down strategies that can be disempowering and alienating. Through critical reflective evaluation we can uncover and understand how our implicit and explicit theoretical orientations affect our day-to-day practice. Only then can we begin the otherwise daunting task of changing the health promotion world as we know it—a world where professional knowledge, power, and action dominates local knowledge, power, and action. In the powerful world where professionals dominate, downstream activity will also predominate. In the health promotion world, power must be shared, as well as resources and knowledge. Only then will our actions be empowering for health and well-being.

STRATEGIC COMMUNICATION

11

Berni Murphy

Key concepts

- In order to enable, inform, educate, mediate, negotiate, persuade, facilitate, and advocate, health promoters need a broad range of functional communication skills in their professional toolkit.
- Functional communication skill sets tend to be anchored in the here and now, while strategic communication is more future focused.
- High-level forms of health activism can be effective in instigating action to address the determinants of health at multisectoral levels, bringing in players from a range of social, economic, and political arenas.
- As we seek to strengthen links within and beyond the health sector, health promoters must develop and practise ways to strategically communicate our ideas in a language that the intended audience can understand and embrace.

Key terms

- Health communication
- Functional communication skills
- Strategic communication
- Enabling, mediating and advocating
- Health activism
- Health promotion 'speak'

OVERVIEW

This chapter explores the communication skills and strategies that underpin health promotion action. The Ottawa Charter recognises that improvements in health will be gained when we *enable*, *advocate*, and *mediate* (WHO 1986). Each of these strategies typically utilise specific communication skill sets, together with a tactical approach designed to generate change. Google-search the term 'health communication' and you are likely to be overwhelmed by hundreds of thousands of websites about social marketing campaigns, health education exemplars from around the globe, or issues pertaining to one-to-one communication in clinical settings between health professionals and patients. Unsurprisingly, health communication is therefore often conceptually limited to notions of awareness-raising and education about risk and protective factors linked to chronic conditions such as diabetes and cardiovascular disease. This chapter seeks to stretch the boundaries beyond this narrow focus to consider the meaning of strategic communication in a contemporary health promotion landscape. This chapter is supported by the following guidebooks:

- Guidebook 8: Preparing for a Media Interview—Ten-point Checklist
- Guidebook 9: Developing Training, Facilitating, and Presenting skills
- Guidebook 10: Preparing a Press Release—Ten-point Checklist
- Guidebook 11: Cross-cultural Communication

THE ROLE OF COMMUNICATION IN HEALTH PROMOTION WORK

A quick scan of job advertisements provides a useful insight into the nature and scope of the communication skills implicit in the day-to-day work of a health promoter. Box 11.1 provides an example of a recent advertisement for a health promotion position in regional Australia.

As an exercise, create a mind map of the communication skills that you think are required in order to fulfil the demands of these selection criteria. Some of the following skills should appear on your mind map: ability to present to a range of audiences; ability to facilitate groups and meetings; ability to mediate and negotiate using recognised strategies; ability to develop and lead workshops; ability to work effectively with the media; ability to contribute to health debates in a persuasive manner; ability to lobby effectively; and ability to write reports/submissions for internal and external audiences. Guidebooks have been included following this chapter to assist you in developing some of these skills.

The importance of communication skills in the health promotion field are also manifest in the following account by a recent graduate who is now working

Box 11.1: Job description for a health promotion professional

Position Description: Integrated Health Promotion Professional

Qualifications

Degree in health promotion or public health preferred

Knowledge and attitudes

1   Understanding of the social model of health
2   Understanding of the determinants of health and their impact on populations
3   Knowledge and understanding of strategies for effective organisational capacity building
4   Knowledge and understanding of strategies for effective community capacity building based on an empowerment model
5   Knowledge and understanding of a range of evidence-based planning and evaluation approaches
6   Commitment to working respectfully with culturally diverse groups and communities

Skills

1   Proficiency in community engagement and consultation
2   Ability to engage and work collaboratively with a range of stakeholders both within and beyond the health sector
3   Ability to develop and facilitate integrated health promotion training as required
4   Ability to communicate integrated health promotion principles and initiate appropriate action within the networks and partnerships in a timely manner
5   Capacity to strengthen existing partnerships and to foster new ones
6   Demonstrated skills and experience in planning, implementation, and evaluation
7   High-level written communication skills as required for operational plans, reports, and funding applications
8   Experience in effectively managing programs and teams
9   Ability to write media releases and to conduct media interviews as required
10 High-level interpersonal communication skills to conduct meetings, and to speak at conferences and other public forums
11 Capacity to represent the organisation in negotiations with external stakeholders
12 Demonstrated computer proficiency as required to carry out duties

in regional Australia. Box 11.2 provides an excerpt from an interview with this graduate about her experiences as a health promotion worker.

Box 11.2: Communication skills in day-to-day health promotion work: Experiences of a new graduate

When I left university, I had a strong theoretical understanding of health promotion frameworks and models, underpinned by knowledge of the determinants of health. I felt very well prepared to contribute to program planning, evaluation, and policy development. Since graduating, I have been working in a rural community with a population of about 2000 people spread over a huge geographical area. I have found that while the theoretical knowledge provides scaffolding for the work that I do, my day-to-day activities are all about creating networks, building partnerships, mediating between stakeholders, and engaging groups in the community. I negotiate with other sectors such as sport, recreation, education, local government, and transport to link them into a health agenda. At university we were taught about the importance of partnerships and collaboration. I wish I had been taught more about *how to* engage community members and other stakeholders, how to contact them, how to persuade them, how to link them together, how to lobby, how to work with them to access and utilise resources. Creating systems and structures for effective, evidence-based health promotion action means considering different ways of working ... It means building relationships, being inclusive and respectful, building trust, establishing guidelines for operating. I need a range of communication skills to be at ease in all of these situations. And I need to use these skills effectively if I am going to make a difference. Strategies to address a local health priority might typically be conceptualised at a formal Primary Care Partnership meeting, but it can also be sparked by an informal chat with key stakeholders at the local netball or football game. Opportunistic and informal approaches are quite important in small communities like mine. I could sit in my office and write a brilliant health promotion program plan for this community but in the end nothing much would change. In truth the real work happens when I walk out of the office door and start talking to people.

(Verbal report to Berni Murphy by Lou-anne Mooney, a new graduate recently employed as a health promotion worker at Omeo District Health in regional Victoria)

FROM FUNCTIONAL TO STRATEGIC COMMUNICATION

Mittelmark (2004) argues that 'public health professionals are notorious for their failure to communicate with decision-makers in ways that have the intended impact. Health professionals are trained to communicate on a professional level with colleagues. At the highest form this takes place in the pages of professional journals (p. 35). Hoffman (2003) asserts that the use of technical language by health professionals can also result in failure to capture the imagination of the target audience (e.g. the public, interest groups, decision-makers). In reality then, not all forms of communication utilised in health promotion action are in fact strategic. Consider the following scenarios:

1   A health promotion worker consults with a group of new arrivals about health issues of concern to them. The consultation process breaks down due to cultural insensitivity on the part of the worker. For some time after this experience, this community group is reluctant to engage with other health workers.

2   An academic is interviewed on television about a health issue that has shot to prominence in the public arena. This academic is excited about the opportunity to raise awareness about the issue, inform the debate, and to potentially influence decision-makers. During a two-minute interview the academic manages to use all of the following terms: *intersectoral collaboration, target group, settings for health, sustainable integrated health promotion, silo interventions, downstream, midstream and upstream approaches, socio-ecological determinants, proximal and distal factors influencing health outcomes, social constructions of health, key stakeholders, capacity building, empowerment models, infrastructure, and health inequities.* Predictably, the general public did *not* connect with this academic and interest in the issue subsequently waned.

3   A prominent researcher publishes important findings in a reputable peer-reviewed journal but fails to take any other steps to get his message across to the field and decision-makers.

4   A health promotion worker writes an excellent media release about an innovative program currently happening in her community. Several journalists from around the country try to follow up but are unable to contact her. The story eventually only runs in the local paper.

5   A report is commissioned by a health promotion network to explore opportunities for improving the health of the community. While the 96-page report is described as *cutting edge*, a plain language summary of the report is never distributed as originally intended, beyond the eight-member network.

In each of these scenarios, particular written and verbal communication skill sets are required to conduct the community consultation and media interview, and to produce the journal article, media release, and in-depth report. However, in each instance the opportunity to influence interest groups and instigate change at perception, policy, and practice levels has been lost by a strictly *functional* rather than *strategic* approach to communication.

Fundamental to notions of strategic communication are the following key issues:

■   WHAT is the message and how can it best be packaged? Finding a shared language is essential.

- WHO should the message be delivered to? The adage 'speak truth to power' is relevant here.
- WHO should be the messenger? As Labonte (2005) says, ' ... not everybody needs to be the advocate but we can all support the advocate'.
- WHEN should the message be delivered? Timing is important. Sometimes the process will need to be carefully planned and iterative, while at other times it will of necessity be opportunistic and seemingly chaotic.
- WHY? Being clear about the purpose and knowing the machinations of political processes and current trends is also critical to strategic communication. Assuming that simply presenting evidence to decision-makers will result in funding or policy changes ignores the realities of the political process.

Functional communication operates in the immediacy of the here and now. It's about having the skills to write a press release, to speak at a conference, to publish an article, to engage a group, to facilitate training. Strategic communication on the other hand is future focused. It is about understanding the purpose, conceptualising the vision, and predicting the short-term impacts and longer-term outcomes. As health promoters we are expected to have a range of functional communication skills in our professional toolkit, but we also need to learn and practise the skills of strategic communication.

ENABLING, MEDIATING, AND ADVOCATING THROUGH A COMMUNICATION LENS

Health promotion is often described as a process of enabling people to increase control over and improve their own health. The Ottawa Charter recognises that improvements in health will be gained when we *advocate, enable,* and *mediate* (WHO 1986). Each of these strategies use specific or *functional* communication skills sets, together with a tactical or *strategic* approach designed to generate change.

Enabling: Just how strategic are we?

Over the past thirty-plus years, health promotion action to *enable* has largely focused on informing and educating individuals and groups, usually by raising awareness about health risk and protective factors, and by increasing knowledge and skills through education to prevent or manage chronic conditions. The vast majority of the literature informing this work tends to fall into two main categories. In the first instance, health communication literature explores theories about the communication mechanisms required to ensure that our message reaches the target audience, is relevant to them, and resonates in ways that will influence health behaviour. In the second instance, the literature documents findings from evaluation studies of awareness campaigns and education programs, often utilising narrow criteria as markers for success or failure (e.g. recall of the key message from a social marketing campaign; increased knowledge following an education program). More recently an emerging body of health communication literature questions the merits of traditional awareness raising and education, suggesting that the evidence about the impact of behaviourist approaches is at best patchy.

Behaviour change programs that are delivered in a cultural vacuum, while ignoring the social determinants, are unlikely to generate any lasting positive impact. Tilmouth (2006) laments that while we ignore the issues that impact on Indigenous communities such as employment, housing, systemic discrimination, and loss of identity, and we continue to deliver health education programs devoid of a cultural context, 'we are in fact not promoting health for all but health for some'. Reid (2006) argues that traditional models of informing and educating can serve to amplify rather than reduce health inequalities, with discourses of blame, shame, and undeservedness typifying the values and attitudes enshrined in such programs. Further, she challenges health promoters to move away from focusing on the lifestyles of disadvantaged groups with poor literacy, low locus of control, and little hope of sustaining change, to instead 'changing our own behaviours and the ways that we do business' with those groups.

It would appear that efforts to inform and educate the workforce can also be problematic if organisational cultures and contexts are not deliberately factored into the change process. In 2001, the Victorian Department of Human Services (DHS) developed a five-day Health Promotion Short Course (HPSC) as part of its workforce capacity-building strategy. One of the key objectives of this initiative was to increase knowledge and understanding about health promotion among traditional and non-traditional health sectors. The evidence suggests that the course has indeed achieved this objective. Course participants are now better informed and more knowledgable. Heward (2006) contends however that 'such courses can run the risk of being to workforce development what the much maligned health information pamphlet is to individual behaviour change'. HPSC participants reported returning to their organisations with new knowledge, understanding, skills, and enthusiasm to embrace different ways of working. However, unless a change process was conceptualised and overtly managed back in the work context, in the end nothing much changed (Heward 2006). Clearly the lessons we have learnt from our attempts to *enable individuals* and expect them to change their behaviour in unsupportive environments must now be applied to *enabling in organisational development contexts*.

This chapter does not seek to replicate the work of existing texts and resources in providing templates for developing social marketing and health education programs, or explanations of the functional communication skills required to deliver such programs. Instead, the purpose here is to encourage the reader to consider what a strategic approach to enabling might look like in their own work setting. At the very least a more *strategic communication approach to enabling* should overlay functional communication skills ordinarily utilised to inform and educate with notions of culture, context, determinants, values, power relationships, and impacts, whether intended or inadvertent. If, however, we are willing to rethink the construct of 'enabling' and expand its parameters, increased awareness, knowledge, understanding, and skills no longer become the end point of the process, but instead can be conceptualised as an important part of a bigger process. In this milieu, empowering and unlocking capacity then become pivotal strategies in effecting change.

Mediating: Strategic opportunities

- Throughout this text, building capacity and fostering intrasectoral and intersectoral collaborative partnerships has been emphasised as being critical to improving health outcomes. Further, it is often argued that health gains in the future will mostly come from outside the health sector. With this in mind, Catford (2005) contends that the domain of *mediating* provides untapped opportunities for health promoters.
- By definition, a mediator brings parties together, finds and connects the links, and intervenes to seek resolutions when the parties are in dispute. A health promoter can therefore act as a mediator when fostering and strengthening partnerships and when working to build capacity or unlock existing capacity in organisations and communities.

Functional communication skills in the mediator's toolkit typically include:

- understanding *how to* network and build trust
- capacity to recognise and capitalise on synergies
- capacity to recognise and cope with competing interests
- ability to negotiate and persuade
- ability to manage conflict with integrity.

While high-level communication skills are clearly fundamental to *mediating*, capitalising on strategic opportunities requires a sophisticated synthesis of these skills together with a capacity to avoid potential barriers that might occur along the way. When mediating for health breaks down or is ineffective, one or more of the following elements are usually evident:

- The mediator fails to identify and/or engage the key players.
- The mediator is positioned as being central to the process rather than a facilitator of the process.
- The health promotion mediator insists that it's all about health, i.e. demands that other sectors reframe their goals and core business to reflect a health agenda and health outcomes.
- The mediator alienates potential partners by using jargon and non-inclusive language.
- The mediator fails to understand the complexities of the group's dynamics.
- The mediator fails to show initiative or to provide leadership when it is required.
- The mediator is unwilling to fade into a supporting role as the partnership strengthens.
- The mediator is unwilling to challenge and confront.
- The mediator asks 'why' in ways that alienate and enrage rather than engage.

Case Study 11.1 illustrates the potential of mediation as a strategic communication initiative when engaging other sectors, such as transport, in a health agenda. In this narrative, the health sector mediates with transport in order to improve access to essential health care for disadvantaged groups. In this regard, the health sector has acknowledged transport as a significant social determinant of health for these groups, and has therefore deliberately engaged with key players from the transport sector to create a solution. In this partnership, the transport sector is not expected to restate its core business as being about health outcomes. Instead, opportunities to overcome the problem are considered, and the logistics

---

Case Study 11.1: Let's Get Connected Project

Anecdotal reports from community health services and other health providers in rural Victoria indicated that patients in urgent need of specialist treatment available only in Melbourne were missing appointments simply because they could not get there. During 2003 project officers were appointed by the Department of Human Services (DHS) in Victoria to help overcome this problem. The project workers initially conducted a transport audit of each of their regions. They then identified key stakeholders and commenced a consultation process with the aim of creating easier access to Melbourne for people without the means and support networks to make their own way there. In most cases these patients were disadvantaged, elderly, isolated, or a combination of these factors. The project workers liaised closely with several stakeholders including V-Line train and bus operators, taxi companies, the Red Cross, and Traveller's Aid to negotiate a satisfactory arrangement. A typical illustration of how the system operates is as follows: A community volunteer picks up a patient from their home at a designated time and drives them to the bus or train, then assists them in getting onto the transport and comfortably seated. Red Cross meets the patient on arrival in Melbourne and liaises with Traveller's Aid to deliver them to their appointment or to overnight accommodation if required. Taxis and any other assistance required are coordinated in advance to minimise the stresses often associated with getting around a big city. An online booking system coordinates all transport and other arrangements, and also provides opportunities for others needing to travel to Melbourne at the same time to be linked into the system and accommodated. The project workers need excellent interpersonal communication skills to make this project happen, together with negotiation skills, flexibility, a calm demeanour, knowledge of legislative change processes, and, of course, persistence. They keep in close contact with each other to share and learn from their experiences. This project is all about being strategic in order to improve access opportunities for disadvantaged people who might otherwise miss out on essential care. The system is not yet perfect and is described by those involved as a work in progress. It is clear however that much has been achieved since the project was initiated. Mediation and coordination work will undoubtedly continue into the future to fine-tune the Let's Get Connected Project.

(Verbal report to Berni Murphy by Lesley Murray, Manager of Home Based Care and Hostel Services, Orbost Regional Health, 2006)

negotiated in terms of roles, responsibilities, and outcomes. It is important to realise that partners can work together very effectively for mutually beneficial goals even though they might attribute quite different meanings to the work of the partnership. While one partner might describe the partnership's work as being about addressing health inequities, another partner might describe the same work through a cost-effectiveness and efficiency lens. The skilled mediator will recognise and work with the synergies rather than insist that all partners must adopt a shared vision and common goals.

Advocating: Skills and strategies

> Effective communication strategies are not meant to manipulate and tell the public what to think, but what to think about (Ratzan 2001: 211).

Health promotion advocacy can take many forms. We might issue a press release, disseminate our evidence at conferences, or lobby influential people whether informally or formally. Too often though we use our research and technical skills to document the evidence in a language that is understood by those in our own field, but fail to then communicate in jargon-free language the significance and logical implications of that evidence to those in positions to take action on it. We must learn to speak plain truth to power, and to construct a pathway for change that makes sense based not only on the evidence, but also on what is politically and economically savvy at that time. The nexus between evidence and health promotion action invariably requires targeted and strategic communication. When should we consider rolling out a media campaign to raise awareness, generate debate, and ultimately influence decision-makers, policy, and funding arrangements? And how do we actually do this? Do we in fact all need to be advocates? How can we best support the advocate? When should the communication campaign adopt a softly softly approach, perhaps utilising some of Cialdini's influence strategies (1984), or when should we rage against injustice (Labonte 2005). These are some of the challenges for the field as we seek new ways to effect change.

Some of the approaches available to the health promotion *advocate* include:

- Advocating through the media
  - □ write a letter to the editor of a newspaper
  - □ speak on talkback radio
  - □ issue a press release (refer to Guidebook 10)
  - □ conduct a media interview (refer to Guidebook 8)
  - □ write an opinion piece

- Advocating within and beyond the field
  - □ publish in journals, newsletters, reports, online
  - □ advocate through professional associations
  - □ present at conferences (e.g. oral presentations, posters)
  - □ present at meetings, networks, and forums
  - □ facilitate seminars and workshops (refer to Guidebook 9)

    ☐   contribute to community networks and alliances in culturally sensitive ways (refer to Guidebook 11)
    ☐   contribute to health promotion course curricula

- Lobbying those in positions of power
  - ☐ influence policy at legislative levels
  - ☐ build relationships and provide evidence to those with influence
  - ☐ make feasible recommendations
  - ☐ act as a conduit for public reactions to the issue

MEDIA ADVOCACY

In this section we will look specifically at the role that the media can play in generating debate, raising awareness, and informing the public and decision-makers about health issues. We will also consider strategies that you, as a health promotion practitioner, can employ to effectively utilise media advocacy. The media can be utilised in relation to public health issues by:

- raising awareness about a health issue or an emerging trend
- informing and influencing public perception
- shifting the focus of a debate
- persuading key policy- or decision-makers
- raising the profile of an organisation and its work.

The Office of Health Economics in Britain estimates that over 80 per cent of the population identify mass media as their key source of information when it comes to health (Naidoo & Wills 2000). Other studies have found that senior policy-makers also mention news as their major source of health and medical information (Lupton 1994). Case Study 11.2 illustrates the planning and processes involved in deliberately engaging with the media in order to raise awareness of a health issue with a view to instigating change.

Case Study 11.2: Working with the media to raise awareness and shift an agenda

During August 2002, Professor John Catford, Dean of Health and Behavioural Sciences (HBS), invited mainstream media (TV, radio, print) to a Deakin University HBS roundtable. Several journalists attended this event to hear about emerging health issues that the university's prominent researchers were addressing. The purpose here was threefold:

1   To increase awareness of these issues among the journalists, and through them, the general public.
2   To utilise media advocacy as a tool for persuading decision-makers to take action.
3   To raise the profile of Deakin University's research into these issues.

The Faculty's Public Relations (PR) officer organised this media event. The Dean invited five highly respected researchers to talk for a few minutes each about their areas of interest and to then respond to questions from the journalists. Professor Catford raised concerns about a number of health issues, including the escalation in childhood obesity in Australia. He was particularly strong on arguing the case for banning sugary drinks in schools. The following day an article entitled 'Experts fear children's health at risk' by Jen Kelly was published in the *Herald Sun* (27 August 2002). This article specifically focused on Professor Catford's call to ban soft drinks from sale in schools.

The next day (28 August) two things happened. The *Herald Sun* Editorial refuted Professor Catford's push for a soft drink ban, instead arguing for schools and parents to better *inform and educate* children about obesity and the dangers of drinking soft drinks.

Rather than consider this a blow to the cause, Professor Catford's PR officer was thrilled that the issue was firmly in the public arena for debate. Talkback radio raged about the issue, its underlying causes and possible solutions. While much of this debate was not necessarily well informed, the fact was that the issue was now firmly on the agenda.

Later that same day the (then) Minister for Health, John Thwaites, announced that the Victorian Government was very concerned about childhood obesity. He declared that a two-day summit would be held in October 2002 so that prominent experts and other stakeholders could debate the issue and make recommendations to redress it. He announced that Professor Catford would chair this summit. The Dean's PR officer reported that in the weeks immediately after the roundtable, Professor Catford fielded up to thirty media enquiries about health issues per day, mostly about childhood obesity. This roundtable was therefore deemed to be very successful in raising awareness about the issue, engaging the media, politicians, and other stakeholders, as well as raising the profile of Deakin University.

These events did not happen in a vacuum—peak bodies such as the Public Health Association of Australia (PHAA), and nutrition groups have been advocating and lobbying for many years for these changes to be made in government policy. Their policy development paved the way and provided important evidence-based information to be used in advocacy by others.

So what was the outcome of this media advocacy? On 24 April 2006 an article by Natasha Robinson entitled 'Schools to expel sugary drinks' was published in the *Australian* newspaper. This article reported that the Victorian Education Minister Lynne Kosky had declared a ban on selling sugary soft drinks in schools from 2007. Minister Kosky had further announced that fatty foods and lollies were also likely to be restricted. The lesson here is that well-planned media advocacy can be a very effective strategy in raising awareness about a health issue. However, the political processes required to effect change might not happen immediately, and persistence is required to keep the issue prominent in the public arena.

ADVOCACY: PITCHING, LEADING, AND FADING

In seeking to engage decision-makers to take action, the advocate must be prepared to *pitch and lead, then fade*. This usually involves *initiating* the campaign then *driving* the agenda. Once decision-makers or those in power engage with the process, the advocate might need to assume a less prominent supporting role. The skilled advocate must be prepared for each of these phases. The following key questions are useful in helping to plan an advocacy campaign:

■ Is the message 'pitch' likely to capture the attention of the intended audience (i.e. those involved in formulating policy, decision-makers, funding bodies)?
■ Will they understand the nature and scope of the problem?
■ Will it resonate with them?
■ Will they understand the options for tackling the problem and the potential consequences of any action taken?
■ Will they understand the merits of getting involved (i.e. for themselves as well as for those affected by the problem)?
■ Will they recognise the role that they or their team can play in addressing the issue?
■ Can they be persuaded and supported to take the lead in the change process?

SHIFTING HEALTH PROMOTION ADVOCACY INTO A HIGHER GEAR: HEALTH ACTIVISM

Right now health promotion's version of advocacy is too often so politically correct. Our organisations vet the letters we write to ensure that they won't cause offence or portray the organisation in a negative light. We don't attend rallies. We don't challenge the status quo with any passion. We don't rage against injustice. Instead we quietly advocate to each other in our own field where it's safe. Maybe it's time for health promotion advocacy to get messy (Serena Everill, Delegate at the AHPA Conference Alice Springs 2006).

Health activism is defined by Zoller (2005) as a 'challenge to existing orders and power relationships that are perceived to influence negatively some aspects of health or impede health promotion. Activism involves attempts to change the status quo, including social norms, embedded practices, and power relationships'(p. 360). Brown et al. (2004) contrast health activism with health advocacy, with health advocacy described as focusing on education and working within the existing system. In this regard, advocates tend to rely on *expert knowledge* rather than inserting lay knowledge into expert systems. *Reformative focused activism* typically seeks increased funding and policy changes, while *transformative focused activism* seeks broader changes in social norms or economic practices. Zoller (2005) observes that elite-based, reform-oriented activists often have greater access to political decision-makers. Hoffman (2003) cautions, however, that technical language, so often the currency of the elite, can quickly disengage those in positions to influence change, including the public.

Top-down approaches to advocacy can be very effective, but they can also quickly become disconnected from the communities they seek to help, and in some ways mirror the silo interventions that have characterised much of health promotion's early work. With this in mind, advocacy campaigns must overtly avoid being silo activities. Instead they need to be organised, coordinated, cohesive, and conceptualised as being part of a bigger health promotion agenda. Zoller (2005) argues that high-level health activism needs to address the determinants of health (e.g. poverty, race, gender, health care access, quality of life, environment, work) at a multisectoral level, bringing in players from a range of social, economic, and political arenas (p. 358). She cautions, however, that forming alliances to advocate for better health is not always straightforward. While government departments and powerful organisations can undoubtedly contribute greater access to resources, they can also hamstring the alliance's capacity for activism, particularly if bound by traditional or conservative modes of operating.

THE LANGUAGE OF HEALTH PROMOTION— ARE YOU TALKING TO ME?

In reality, the language that health promoters use to describe ideas can be interpreted by others as alienating and controlling. Health promoters seeking to engage with other sectors or the public through media campaigns need to be wary of *health promotion speak*, as it is not necessarily a language that is well understood or valued beyond academic and bureaucratic health promotion circles. Table 11.1 presents a snapshot of data from a study into the meanings that people attribute to common health promotion terms. Representatives from a range of sectors including education, sport and recreation, local government, and community development, together with members of the general public, were asked to explain the meaning of several health promotion terms such as *upstream determinants of health*, *silo interventions*, and *health inequities*. The findings presented in this table highlight the level of misunderstanding that can occur when we fail to articulate our ideas in plain language.

Clearly, some terms such as 'intersectoral collaboration' were reasonably well understood by study participants, while other terms such as 'silo interventions' were completely misinterpreted. The negative impact that such misunderstandings could have on building and strengthening partnerships for health are obvious. It would appear then that health promoters need to tune into a jargon alert if we are to ensure that the language we use to get our message across connects with the intended audience. In the pursuit of strategic communicating, *health promotion speak* must therefore be tempered with a dose of plain language and common sense!

Table 11.1 The meanings that others attribute to common health promotion terms

COMMON HEALTH PROMOTION LANGUAGE	WHAT HEALTH PROMOTERS MEAN BY THIS TERM	HOW EDUCATION INTERPRETS IT	HOW COMMUNITY DEVELOPMENT INTERPRETS IT	HOW LOCAL GOVERNMENT INTERPRETS IT	HOW SPORT AND RECREATION INTERPRETS IT	HOW A MEMBER OF THE PUBLIC INTERPRETS IT	HOW ANOTHER MEMBER OF THE PUBLIC INTERPRETS IT
Intersectoral collaboration	Sectors like health and education working together to improve the health of a community or a population	People from different sectors talking to each other and working together	Health, government departments, welfare, and others working together	Collaboration, e.g. between sections of an organisation	Sectors working together	Sectors working together to share resources and skills	People cooperating with each other
Upstream determinants of health	Factors at the macro level that influence health (e.g. access to transport, housing, and education)	Working against the usual patterns	I have no idea	Factors beyond our control that impact on health	No idea—is this about pushing shit uphill?	No idea— is it about swimming or fishing?	Causes of health and wellbeing
Infrastructures for health	Systems and support mechanisms that impact on health, such as policies, funding, and resources	Systems to deliver health care	Building better hospitals	Technology and systems that support health	Systems, procedures, and resources for health	Services for health treatment	Services for health, such as allied health

(Continued)

Table 11.1 (Continued)

COMMON HEALTH PROMOTION LANGUAGE	WHAT HEALTH PROMOTERS MEAN BY THIS TERM	HOW EDUCATION INTERPRETS IT	HOW COMMUNITY DEVELOPMENT INTERPRETS IT	HOW LOCAL GOVERNMENT INTERPRETS IT	HOW SPORT AND RECREATION INTERPRETS IT	HOW A MEMBER OF THE PUBLIC INTERPRETS IT	HOW ANOTHER MEMBER OF THE PUBLIC INTERPRETS IT
Health inequities	Unequal access to resources for health	Unequal distribution of resources for health	Some people are healthier and have better access to health care than others	Not sure—is this about the stock market?	Health deficiencies	Comparing one person's well-being to another	People having different levels of access to health care
Silo interventions	Stand-alone interventions that isolate health issues, groups, or risk factors and in so doing fail to recognise the wider context	Intervening in food storage	Government departments working alone	Interfering with wheat containers	Preventing building silos	Something to do with the wheat industry	This is about accumulating health care processes and information
Socio-ecological approaches to promoting health	Takes into account the complex inter-relationship between multiple factors that influence health outcomes	Combination of social and environmental influences on health	This is about social and environmental factors	Taking into account ecosystems and society	No idea	I don't know	People's backgrounds influence their access to health and health care

(Adapted from a current study—as yet unpublished—into the meanings and interpretations of health promotion language, conducted by Berni Murphy during 2006.)

SUMMARY

Communication underpins virtually all health promotion action. With this in mind, a broad range of functional communication skills need to be developed and practised by those seeking to work in the health promotion field. Good communicators have the ability to convey complex concepts in a language that speaks to the intended audience. They use metaphors and analogies to make sense of the ideas. As health promotion seeks to strengthen its links within and beyond the health sector, we must develop and practise ways to *strategically communicate* our ideas in a language our audience understands and embraces. The role of strategic communication will become even more important as we move towards more sophisticated and effective models of health promotion and, in so doing, promote health for all.

USEFUL WEBSITES

How to run a workshop: <www.eldis.org/static/DOC16284.htm>

Toolbox for Trainers, Canadian Child Care Federation: <www.cccf-fcsge.ca/sub-sites/familytp/english/toolbox_en.htm>

Strengthening Personal Presentations, The Health Communication Unit: <www.thcu.ca/infoandresources/Step8MessageDevelopment.htm>

Count me in!:

WHN (the Count Us In! project):

Producing information materials through participatory writeshops: <www.mamud.com/writeshop.htm/>

Conducting a workshop, Community Tool Box: <ctb.ku.edu/tools/en/sub_section_main_1113.htm>

12 ORGANISATIONAL CAPACITY

Paul Laris & Colin MacDougall

Key concepts

- Healthy public policy is ecological in perspective, multisectoral in scope, and participatory in strategy, and is neither made, nor implemented, in a calm, rational way. Nor is it made in the health or public health sector. Rather, it is a messy enterprise, involving many agencies, interests, and competing power structures.
- Advocacy for healthy public policy faces major hurdles in the form of distinctly unhealthy policy positions advocated by powerful interests. Without adopting an effective model of advocacy, proponents of healthy public policy may find themselves playing a game they cannot win.
- The dominant paradigm for advocacy for healthy public policy within public health organisations remains problem-focused, based on strategic control by public health professionals and an adversarial approach.
- Organisations that can develop and articulate a *civic philosophy*, supported by a *custodial role* and an *externally focused organising capacity*, will have a greater capacity for advancing healthy public policy than those that accept the neoliberal agenda of problem-based, value-free strategic planning.

Key terms

- Healthy public policy
- Organisations and public health organisations

OVERVIEW

As Chapter 14 explains, healthy public policy is a complex concept, imbued with debates about values and ideology, and necessarily involving power and interest groups. Chapter 15 provides tools for health promoters to use when looking at the impact of current or proposed policy on health, well-being, and environmental sustainability. Inexorably, the roads for the policy analyst searching for healthy public policy lead to organisations. At the moment these organisations are often within the health sector but, as this book argues, we should at the very least be making stronger alliances with organisations and sectors whose policies and values determine health and well-being. And ideally we should work alongside these so-called determinants sectors, supporting their journey and working comfortably with their agendas. All this sounds fine in theory, but in practice we find that the biggest barriers to any change are located fairly and squarely in organisations.

Our thinking behind this chapter sees three possible pathways for organisations aiming to support the development of healthy public policies:

- *Value-added* pathways reflect the implicit expectation in both public and private sectors that organisations will more accurately define and measure performance and, as a consequence, continuously improve efficiency;
- *Value-free* pathways reflect the likelihood that, taken to extremes, such a reductionist approach becomes focussed entirely on doing the thing right, rather than asking what is the right thing to be doing. Values are irrelevant if accountability is only about technical efficiency;
- *Adding values* is about organisations articulating what they stand for.

In this chapter we propose that those interested in health promotion concentrate their efforts on the latter pathway as a fundamental strategy for building healthy public policy. We argue that if health promotion can engage with organisations that then more readily develop and articulate a civic philosophy, there will be a positive influence on the society in which they operate. Furthermore, a set of strategic approaches flow from these values, which enable organisations to take the initiative in promoting healthy public policy, rather than being reduced to responding to others' agendas.

We argue for the third approach, *adding values*, because our experience is that the history of health promotion has been one of struggle. Advocates for health promotion based in organisations, particularly health sector organisations, have often found themselves lonely as they confront the agendas of large and powerful interest groups such as the arms, tobacco, alcohol, sugar, and processed food industries. Notwithstanding some significant gains (such as tobacco controls in some countries), the work of health promotion is both unequal and intensely adversarial, which can lead to health promoters feeling helpless and powerless. At its worst, this leads to health promotion workers showing each other their scars and bemoaning glorious defeats. With the advent of a wider appreciation of the role of the social determinants of health, the focus has moved from behavioural and regulatory approaches towards the broader development of healthy public policy. That is, policy that promotes the health of populations across all sectors, rather than just through the health care sector. Our concern in this chapter is that advocacy for healthy public policy also faces major hurdles in the form of distinctly unhealthy policy positions advocated by powerful interests. There is a risk that, without adopting a more effective model of advocacy than we use now, proponents of healthy public policy will find themselves playing a game they cannot win.

HOW HEALTHY PUBLIC POLICY IS GENERATED

Healthy public policy has been defined by Nancy Milio as *ecological in perspective, multisectoral in scope, and participatory in strategy* (Milio 1988). Such policy is neither made, nor implemented, in a calm, rational way. Nor is it made exclusively or even primarily in the health or public health sector. Rather, it is a messy enterprise involving many agencies, interests, and competing power structures. Because it is public policy *for* health, rather than just policy of the health care or public health sectors, effective policy development and implementation must happen across a much wider public arena. This arena encompasses contested fields where political, economic, and social interests vie for influence. In many countries, the goals, outcomes, and processes of healthy public policy run counter to those of the dominant paradigms often reflected by the actions of those 'central' agencies that control the levers of power, such as Departments of Treasury and Finance and large national and multinational corporate interests.

Our experiences of teaching management and engaging in management consultancy in public health confirm a discourse in both practice and the literature of advocacy for healthy public policy as a difficult, often lonely battle against powerful odds. According to this discourse, it is essential to analyse barriers in public health organisations that inhibit the implementation of healthy public policy. Then, the activist manager draws on charisma and guile to engage in strategic planning, coalition building, persuasion etc. in order to drive organisational change. This is a technical and strategic process working within the existing power structures and processes. While the ends may be selected on the basis of civic values, the process is essentially value-free. The organisational change task is usually conducted broadly from within the public health system; often by people or units in marginalised or misunderstood positions. In South Australia, the Generational Health Review commissioned by the incoming government in 2002 had strong recommendations about reorienting the health care system to a primary health care focus. The document was based on a civic philosophy and rationale for health services reform. However by January 2006 the state Australian Medical Association was complaining that:

> Much time and effort has gone into creating health regions, changing governance structures and re-organising health administration, while the reform of the clinical services lags behind. Advice from clinicians on rationalising services for Rehabilitation and Acute Cardiac Services is simply ignored by the Regions (Cain 2006).

Overall, this sort of exercise can be a dispiriting task leading to feelings of frustration or burnout. It is an adversarial model, fighting against often overwhelming odds in a moral crusade often doomed to glorious defeat. Ironically it echoes the unhealthy public policy approaches of 'wars' against drugs or terror. By targeting the barriers we may inadvertently lead to their reinforcement, just as prohibition policies create the very markets drug dealers depend on for profitability. A more recent example has been the Commonwealth Scientific and Industrial Research Organisation's publication of a diet book promoting increased meat consumption for lowering the risk of heart disease, funded partly by the meat industry and criticised by the journal *Nature* (Cauci 2005). The adversarial debate among nutritionists distracts us from the unhealthy public policy of private business interests funding the nation's leading public science research body.

Box 12.1: Lessons for the field

When health promotion tries to move from behavioural and lifestyle interventions to the pursuit of healthy public policy, it clashes with the values and practices of powerful interests and organisations.

Health promotion workers need to analyse their stance with key organisations to avoid playing a game that they cannot win and becoming scarred by defeat after defeat.

Where possible, approach organisations and encourage them to add values by articulating what they stand for.

THE SOCIAL AND POLITICAL CONTEXT

So how has recent history shaped the values and cultures of organisations that we seek to work through to achieve healthy public policy? In the late 1970s and early 1980s, governments in South Australia and New South Wales instituted management reforms to achieve their social democratic aims. Governments hoped to create accountable management by experimenting with corporate planning and program budgeting, leading to encouragement for government agencies to work with, and raise money from, the private sector to generate profits to feed into the agencies' mainstream activities. This in turn led to what became known as *managerialism*, which, in its early days, aimed to overcome bureaucratic stifling of public accessibility, hindering of social and political reforms (e.g. equal opportunity, open government) and enabled Labor governments to seek tighter management and control to implement policy changes (Considine & Painter 1997).

The climate changed as Public Service Boards and Commissions were in decline and other forms of procedural regulation were dismantled. Managers were given room to bring about more effective and low-cost services and flexibility in the public sector, in order to scale down public employment. The language of efficiency and effectiveness replaced the language of collective action and progressive social democratic ideals (Considine & Painter 1997).

Governments came to appreciate enthusiastic technocrats who were perceived as aggressive and effective managers. Labor and Liberal Ministers alike rewarded the drive and single-minded focus on outputs, performance indicators, and a discourse of doing more with less. From the mid 1980s governments became more intent on contraction, and there was an emerging doctrine that governments had failed to provide services and should import private sector management methods and models to replace traditional bureaucratic modes of operation (Considine & Painter 1997). Both Labor and Liberal governments instituted microeconomic reform of the public service on market principles.

John Hyde, known at the time as a Liberal politician and supporter of the free market, organised a 'Crossroads Conference' of believers to discuss persuasion, action, and tactics to move Australia towards a market economy (Hyde 2002). This group, strongly influenced by the ideas of Adam Smith, Friedrich Hayek, and Milton Friedman, became known first as 'economic dries'. This led to a series of think tanks, with neutral and unremarkable names, sponsored by business and disenchanted with universities and conventional sources of policy advice: e.g. Centre for Independent Studies, Australian Institute for Public Policy. These think tanks combined bureaucracy, business, and media interests (Kelly 1992) and gained powerful support from media such as *Australian Financial Review*, calling for lower protection, microeconomic reform, and structural adjustment. New networks united a new generation of academics, business people, public servants, and journalists (Kelly 1992). Quiggin has noted the evolution of the term 'economic rationalism' in Australia from the 1970s through to the 1990s when:

> critical and sceptical thinking that characterised the first phase of economic rationalism was gradually replaced by a dogmatic, indeed, quasi-religious, faith in market forces and the private sector. More and more, economic analysis was based on deductions from supposedly self-evident truths, which were effectively immune from any form of empirical testing (Quiggin 1999).

These ideological and value shifts fell on fertile ground in the form of organisational cultures akin to a contract state that had begun in the 1980s. The public service was restructured using economic theory that sought to separate regulation from policy delivery, introduce competition, and recast government trading enterprises as businesses, often to be sold off entirely. If markets could not allocate resources, substitutes such as benchmarking were used to mirror competition (Davis 1997). This led to organisations becoming prone to an excessively introverted focus on their own aims rather than a wider focus on the public good. Single-purpose organisations overlooked government objectives and public policies that crossed agency boundaries (Trosa 1997).

Box 12.2: Key tools of economic rationalism

- Comprehensive corporate planning based on centrally determined goals
- Program budgets allocating resources to policy and management goals
- Management improvement with private sector managers as models
- Highly paid senior managers on contract
- Accountability through central audit review, and performance monitoring of individuals and organisations.

All these tools are nested within an ideology of the primacy of the free market, individual choice and responsibility, and the drive for governments to leave planning to market forces.

LIVING WITH THE LEGACY IN THE NEW MILLENNIUM

A decade or more of organisations infused with neoliberal economic theories has nurtured a paradigm of apparently value-free, problem-focused, public health advocacy based on strategic control by public health professionals and an adversarial approach. In Australia, the National Public Health Partnership's *Planning Framework for Public Health Practice* makes this approach very clear (NPHP 2000). While noting the importance of engaging with stakeholders along the way, its primary focus is on the problem:

1 define the problem and identify its causes or determinants
2 assess which of these determinants should and can be addressed
3 identify interventions and evaluate the evidence on them
4 decide, on the basis of the information gathered, the interventions that will make up the portfolio
5 turn the portfolio into action
6 evaluate the portfolio.

The NPHP approach can be read as an ideal type of a modernist mission, guided by strategic planning, implemented with resolute efficiency, with no obvious room for messy stakeholder partnerships, the need to work through complex agendas, conflicting priorities, or rapidly changing circumstances: all of which are the day-to-day realities of policy development and implementation. A predominantly rational approach assumes a sole subject for policy development that is framed as an object or problem to be acted upon. Messy partnerships or high-level policy conflicts may be assumed or subsumed, but remain hidden from first glance.

THREE KEY FEATURES FOR ORGANISATIONS ADVOCATING HEALTHY PUBLIC POLICY

Thus, the new public organisation in the neoliberal age is often narrowly focused, driven by the management style of a reductive strategic tactician: clarifying and reducing goals to 'deliverables', and achievement to what can be measured by key performance indicators. Risk aversion (avoid engaging the real issues and avoid trouble) is presented as risk management. The role model is the military officer, at war with the problems. We argue that this adversarial organisation is both too narrow and particularly inappropriate to advancing healthy public policy. We suggest that organisations that can develop and articulate a *civic philosophy*, supported by a *custodial role* and an *externally focused organising capacity* will have a greater capacity for advancing healthy public policy than those that accept the neoliberal agenda of problem-based, value-free strategic planning.

A civic philosophy

Beaglehole and Bonita's assessment of the potential for public health into the new millennium reinforces this central tenet: that it is time to shift away from a narrowly disease- or risk-factor-focused approach to one based on an appreciation of the socio-structural factors that are the foundations for health. They identify the motivating concerns for this new approach as the pressure of inequities in health, associated with extremes of health and illness, poverty and wealth, and global environmental issues. They note also that:

> public health requires a strong and clearly articulated theoretical foundation based on a clear appreciation of the history of public health in order to avoid being at the mercy of the prevailing ideology. Progress in public health will be easier when there is a more sympathetic attitude towards collective endeavour (Beaglehole & Bonita 1997).

A public health organisation that effectively promotes healthy public policy must have the capacity to envision the desired outcome and to inspire that vision in others in order to build effective alliances for change. That 'strong and clearly articulated theoretical foundation' must be congruent with the organisation's responsibilities, its capacity, and its ability to build both capacity and support. A civic philosophy is based on the rights and responsibilities of the organisation as a citizen committed to the health of the society, and links with the reframing of health as a human right in Chapter 5 of this book. The values that underpin such a foundation include:

- Equity and social responsibility: a strong commitment to social justice and a collective social responsibility for ensuring all people have access to the basic requirements for life with dignity. This in turn implies beliefs that health is a human need, health care a right of citizenship, and population health a public good.
- Autonomy and participation: the rights and responsibilities of individuals in (at least notionally) a democratic society to shape their own lives and to participate in processes to shape their society.
- Beneficence and non-malfeasance: to strive to do good (within the context of the two principles above) and, above all, to do no harm.
- Global bio-sustainability: the aim of ensuring that human organisation and activity helps to sustain not only human life and the lives of future generations, but also the diverse and intricately interdependent and dynamic life that makes up the biosphere on this planet. Good planets are hard to find.
- Change: to value and be comfortable with rapid, constant, and moderately chaotic change and to value and use the learning that comes with this. This is perhaps of a different order, being as much a personal characteristic as a philosophical belief. It is driven by the need for organisations and their managers to be prepared to embrace new ways of working, often with unfamiliar partners, in unfamiliar fields for objectives that have not previously been within the scope of public health as an endeavour.

Corporate ethics?

Postmodernism has encouraged a pragmatic, eclectic approach to organisational planning. Modernism was about grand theories and projects—such as Marxism or feminism. Postmodernism is based on a distrust of these 'meta-narratives' and an eclectic, more localised and case-specific approach, trying to articulate and understand the 'discourse' of how things work and how they might be changed. Critics of strategic planning such as Mintzberg (1994) have highlighted the value of synthesis and lateral thinking; of *strategic thinking*, rather than *linear strategic planning*, delivering plans 'set in stone'. Critics argue that the eclectic postmodern approach is extreme and in the absence of any social values may also become a tool of self-interested opportunism.

Since the demise of the USSR, the power and influence of private corporations has grown apace. Korten and others have noted with concern the capacity of global corporations in geopolitics to 'buy out democracy' (Korten 1995). Brown cites increasing evidence of corporations' roles in decisions to invade other countries, privatise human resources (including armies and police), and what he sees as an undermining of democracy. It is deeply ironical that these trends coexist with a boom in corporate discourse about ethics, governance, and legitimating the relationship between the corporation, the state, and civil society. The case of

KPMG provides a graphic example. On their website, KPMG provide an article on 'Ethical Business and Sustainable Communities', which argues that:

> With the fall of communism and the re-affirmation of capitalism as the only sustainable model of economic society, we have witnessed a transformation of business's position. It has evolved from a narrow focus on generating income and wealth to one of strategic partnering with the government and the community sectors to play an expanded role in shaping the social context of nation states (KPMG: <www.erc.org.au/busethics/kpmg_ethical_bus.pdf>).

The article goes on to argue that good ethics promote transparency, choice, and a focus on good corporate reputations—which is good for society and good for business and what is good for business is good for everyone. However, this born-again fervour should be seen in the context of KPMG's recent history. After the demise of Arthur Andersen, another of the big five major corporate accounting companies, in the wake of the ENRON collapse, KPMG faced numerous charges of tax avoidance by marketing dishonest and illegal tax shelters for six years. According to the *Washington Post*, the state handled KPMG with kid gloves on this issue because there was fear that the collapse of yet another of one of the 'final four' major accounting corporations would have serious consequences on the stability of the economy (Sloan 2005).

Thus, while private corporations may profess an ethical base and a civic philosophy, this must always be appreciated in the context of their underlying aim of returning a profit to their shareholders. Public organisations do not have the same imperative, and their approach to articulating and implementing their civic philosophy carries a greater prima facie legitimacy because of this. This fundamental weakness of private corporations as advocates for an ethical society means their inputs into healthy public policy must be taken with caution. Conversely, public and civil society organisations that have no commercial interests have an opportunity and a responsibility to use their commercially disinterested legitimacy for the public good. For all these reasons, health promotion workers have a legitimate argument for working with public sector organisations to debate civic philosophies, ethics, and healthy public policy.

The custodial role—accountability beyond numbers

The *custodian* is the responsible public administrator (or, quite possibly, the administrator of a private enterprise with public or social goals). The custodian has a responsibility to ensure the organisation delivers what its stakeholders expect. These expectations are set out in the organisation's charter or mission statement and embodied in the way it conducts its day-to-day business. They are expressed through the organisation's civic philosophy, be it implicit or explicit. Because stakeholders know what the organisation stands for, they know for what it must be held accountable. While these expectations may change over time, the custodian is accountable to ensure that the organisation maintains and builds its capacity to deliver on these expectations. This will involve planning and managing the ways in which this can be done most effectively and efficiently.

Managing the internal coherence and function of the organisation implies a number of key duties including staff management, financial management, public sector management, and cultural capacity-building. Cultural capacity-building includes the promotion of healthy public policy and building an understanding of why and how this must be so. Education and inspiration are important. So is a culture and a structure that recognises and encourages ideas and innovation from its own people, rather than punishing deviance and rewarding risk-averse conformity. The term 'learning organisation' is often used to describe organisations that can take ideas from the edge and bring them to the centre as part of a process of continual renewal. This cultural capacity means that when the organisation needs to work in a new way in a new field with new collaborators, staff, structure, and resources have the flexibility, motivation, and competence to make a difference.

The organisation as civic organiser

The neoliberal strategic planning model has the organisation retreating to a focus on core business for which it has comparative advantage in the market place. However, the core business for an organisation with a healthy public policy agenda must lead to an external focus. Influencing the wider polity is about exploring and developing partnerships with other agencies and groups and managing the relationships with funders, users, and other key stakeholders. Essentially it is about partnership and the organisation's capacity to be both a partner and a facilitator of partnerships. Both functions are important. The organisation that facilitates the development of an effective partnership may achieve most by then working as a relatively minor partner. Saul Alinsky (1972) makes a useful distinction: the difference between a leader and the organiser. Leaders go on to build power to fulfil their desires, to hold and wield the power for purposes both social and personal. They want power for themselves. Organisers find their goals in the creation of power for others to use (Alinsky 1972). The organisation that can act effectively as organiser as well as partner is likely to have most of the following features:

- A vision of the gains that might be achieved through the organisations working together. An organising organisation has the capacity to envisage and to articulate what might be possible, to inspire and motivate others. Part of facilitation is enabling a developing discussion that identifies shared, achievable objectives that none of the partners could achieve by working in isolation.
- An understanding and respect for each other's position, core business, capacity, and responsibilities. Each organisation must have structures and processes that are reasonably transparent. Their individual goals for involvement in the partnership and roles in its implementation must be 'upfront' and accepted by the other partners.

- A preparedness for change. Engaging in a partnership process is engaging in a change process. The roles of each organisation are likely to renegotiated as the process runs. All participants can expect to be changed to some degree through their involvement.
- An ability to deal with conflict: Each partner will have their own agendas. It is highly likely that at some point on some issues, partners will be in conflict. This is not a bad thing—but it must be managed. Resolution of such conflict is another generator of organisational change.
- A capacity to trust and to generate trust. Organisations as partners must trust their collaborators to a significant degree. It is even less possible to micro-manage a partnership than it is to micro-manage an organisation of any size. By demonstrating trust organisations can build trust. The corollary of this is that to build trust you must take risks—informed and hopefully minimal risks, but risks nonetheless.

A CRUCIAL COMPLEMENTARITY

The key feature of these three sets of characteristics, *civic philosophy*, *custodial role*, and *civic organising capacity*, is the way in which they interact, modify, and therefore complement each other. While the civic philosophy has primacy as both the underpinning of the approach and its key in changing the wider social and political culture, it is interdependent on the custodial and external organising roles. A strong civic philosophy enables a custodial organisation to have an ideological compass with which to navigate a rapidly changing social, economic and political environment. Its custodial management of staff and other resources is informed by a shared understanding of, and commitment to, its purpose. A coherent civic philosophy enables an organisation organising partnerships for change to articulate its position and its role in a way that minimises the risk of misunderstanding from its potential partners. A clear understanding of its custodial responsibilities enables an organisation to maintain and build its capacity to realise its philosophical aspirations and to be a competent and valued partner for change. The capacity to organise and participate in partnerships again enables the realisation of philosophical aims, but also helps build custodial capacity as those same principles and practices of effective partnership building also work within organisations to create dynamic and effective relationships among staff.

AND SO TO THE MEANING OF LIFE

It goes without saying that different mixes or emphases of the three characteristics will be appropriate for different organisations in different settings. The trick is to think through how to work on, in, through, and despite organisations, using just the right mixture for the task at hand. Some examples from this book are discussed in Box 12.3

Box 12.3: Exercises in applying knowledge about civic philosophy, custodial role, and civic organising capacity

In this box we present problems from other chapters in the book and ask you to consider how best to solve them by using the knowledge and strategies presented in this chapter.

- Christine Putland's Chapter 20 shows many ways in which the health promotion and community arts sectors share what we describe as a *civic philosophy*. Consider how organisations can increase their *externally focused organising capacity*, leading directly to consonant *custodial roles* that make working together easier.

- Chapter 19, by Iain Butterworth and Len Duhl, on healthy cities and settings, shows just how many sectors can and should be involved in creating environments that make the healthy choice the easy choice. We ask how networks of organisations can work hard on the civic philosophy of the network itself, as opposed to the individual organisations in the network. We have seen in Chapter 14 how important networks are to developing healthy public policy, so the first task here is to work on values and cultures. We ask how that knowledge can be used to underpin all other organisational change.

- Jennie Popay's Chapter 9, on community engagement, provides a salutary lesson about the consequences of organisations failing to transfer to the communities with whom they profess to engage the very power they need for that engagement. Further, she notes that the community engagement agenda can be just a code for a very different result—namely the withdrawal of the state from service provision. Popay describes these as the *bad* and *ugly* of community organisations. We ask how to remove these *bad* and *ugly* features by considering the failure of an organisation's external organising capacity, and the extent to which that failure stems from a mismatch between civic philosophy and professed policy.

SUMMARY

One thing is clear to us. We need to reverse the trend to the disorder that we have dubbed *obsessive reorganisation disorder* (ORD) towards a focus on equity, rights, and social justice. The symptoms of ORD include an unhealthy obsession with serial reorganisations, ever more fine-grained strategic planning, accompanied by little or no transfer of resources. The onset of ORD is frequently associated with the appointment of a new manager, who marks their territory by announcing

Box 12.4: Attributes of an intrepid civic philosopher

So what attributes does our intrepid civic philosopher need to change the meaning of life?

- Commitment to the values of equity, sustainability, and social justice and equitable population health outcomes.
- Passports and visas in the 'determinants sectors' such as economics, politics, and social movements that affect health through action on the big social questions.
- Knowledge and experience of the benefits of strategic thinking and the disadvantages of unfettered, uncritical strategic planning and reorganisation.
- Ability to both resolve and live with conflict and ambiguity.
- Strong communication and negotiation skills.
- Commitment to learning to navigate between sectors and translate civic philosophies into the language of core business in various sectors.
- Realism in expecting what some deem to be impossible.
- Enduring, critical, and reflective personal and professional networks to maintain hope and resilience.

a strategic planing exercise immediately after their appointment. These managers, the carriers or vectors, spread ORD by changing jobs frequently, armed with an impressive record of initiating change. The hosts of ORD are those boards and departments who seek out managers to change things, not to value things or add values.

As it spreads rapidly through the organisational system, ORD merely pays lip service to healthy public policy, while paralysing progressive action and tying up valuable skills and resources in internal reorganisation, at the expense of forging effective, external partnerships and collaborations. Instead, the quest for a civic philosophy that makes healthy public policy the easy choice requires organisations to engage with the big, bold questions of values, ideologies, rights, vision: indeed the whole human and planetary condition. The nuances of organisational structure, job titles, and nested strategic plans would be largely irrelevant in an organisation that matched a coherent civic philosophy with a transfer of resources from activities that do not improve population health to activities that seek to promote equity, rights, sustainability, and social justice, and to reduce health inequalities along the way. That means the treatment starts with marshalling the cognitive arguments against ORD, starting with the simple argument that there is little or no evidence for the effectiveness of the types of reorganisations so regularly foisted upon health promotion. Most importantly, at the first signs of the onset of ORD, the hosts (boards, departments, employers) and the vectors (managers previously exposed to ORD) should be asked to prepare a detailed study comparing the costs and benefits of reorganisation to expected population health outcomes. Failing that, they should be asked just to add up the costs in money and time and think through the opportunity costs. In other words, what else could they do with all that time?

At a time when there is such a clash between the values of health for all and the measures of neoliberalism, the best buy, we think, is for reformers to engage in debate and reflection designed to place the questions of civic philosophy on everyone's lips, at every level of the organisation. Their quest will involve at least the critical reflection on their practice that is discussed in Chapter 17 by Anne Johnson and Colin MacDougall. Then they will find the meaning of life.

13 HEALTH IMPACT ASSESSMENT AND INTERSECTORAL ACTION

Mary Mahoney & Grace Blau

Key concepts

- HIA offers a clever new way of working that encourages people operating across sectors to understand, and take account of, the potential role that their decisions will have on health both directly or indirectly through the determinants of health.
- HIA complements the social model of health, the principles of healthy public policy, and integrated planning.
- HIA requires practitioners to develop a range of skills necessary for working across disciplines within and across organisations and sectors.

Key terms

- Health impact assessment
- Intersectoral action
- Integrated policy-making
- Building sustainable partnerships

OVERVIEW

Health Impact Assessment (HIA) seeks to identify the potential, and often unanticipated, effects of a policy, project, or program on the health of a group of people before a decision is made to proceed with it. It is based on the idea that health is not only influenced by the health services people have access to, and by their own behaviour, but by a range of factors outside their control such as their neighbourhood, the quality of their housing, social networks, and physical environment, and their ability to access services through infrastructure and transport. The potential impacts that any new development or policy might have on their health may be positive, negative, or unknown and these impacts may not be spread evenly across the population. HIA is premised on intersectoral action and has been shown to be a highly effective mechanism for considering the implications of an organisation's actions on health. It has helped to build sustainable partnerships and has integrated health concerns alongside economic, social, and environmental considerations.

This chapter will examine the ways in which HIA has been used across sectors. It will explore the key lessons learnt from practitioners who have applied it, focusing specifically on the capacities needed for effective engagement and partnership working within an organisation. The challenges, threats, and opportunities of working across sectors will also be outlined. A broad range of examples will be used to support the discussion. Specific attention will be directed to the role that HIA has and can play at the local government level, where the need for intersectoral action is most obvious because decisions made are closest to the people likely to be affected by them.

INTRODUCTION

It is increasingly clear that staff in organisations are required to work outside their discipline areas to achieve their goals and the mutual goals of others. The reason for this is growing awareness that the complex problems facing society can no longer be resolved by the actions of one discipline or government department. Complex problems require complex solutions and these can only be developed through the interplay of a diverse range of professionals each offering a suite of differing perspectives and approaches. Inherent in this view is the need for mutual respect for the contribution that each discipline can make to dealing with an issue. For instance, one of the prime motivations for seeking to get health considerations onto the agendas of non-health sector decision-makers is so that they can assist in achieving the goals of improving population health and reducing inequalities and inequities in health within the population. These goals can only be achieved through a combination of approaches and the involvement of the people whose actions and decisions play a vital role in causing or contributing, either directly or indirectly, to the problems in the first place. Directing attention inwards within a disciplinary field will only ever result in partial solutions. For example, focusing on changes to the health care system or on to interventions seeking behaviour change will not succeed in addressing the broader determinants of health.

Integrated working and intersectoral action demand that practitioners possess a set of skills and a level of reflective practice that allows them to work in new ways. By its very nature, intersectoral action is not suited to all people. It requires individuals to drop traditional discipline boundaries and the arrogance that can sometimes accompany these, so that they can work to create a common 'metric' for conversations and understanding. It requires professionals to try new approaches or ways of seeing the problem or issue, developing an understanding that a 'one size fits all' approach will not work, an appreciating that other people's agendas are of equal importance to one's own, and that mutual working is advantageous to everyone. One mechanism that can support the mutual goals of the health professional as well as other decision-makers is Health Impact Assessment (HIA). HIA offers a clever new way of working that encourages people operating in other sectors to understand, and take account of, the potential role that their decisions will have on health both directly or indirectly through the determinants of health. It can also offer other tangible outcomes linked to broader organisational goals.

This chapter will describe the role that HIA can play in decision-making processes within government. By drawing on the key lessons that have been learnt by practitioners who have applied HIA in a range of sectors, it will identify the broad benefits that it can provide and then focus specifically on the role it can play in facilitating intersectoral action linked to health. The chapter will conclude by focusing specifically on the ways in which health promotion professionals can build intersectoral links to improve decision-making so that health considerations are taken into account, using local government as the backdrop for the discussions.

WHAT IS HIA?

Health Impact Assessment (HIA) seeks to identify the potential, and often unanticipated, effects of a policy, project, or program on the health of a group of people, usually the whole population, before a decision is made to proceed with it. It is based on the idea that health is not only influenced by the health services people have access to, and by their own behaviour, but by a range of factors outside their control such as their neighbourhood, the quality of their housing, social networks and physical environment, and their ability to access services or employment through infrastructure and transport. The role of the various agencies, such as the different levels of government which make decisions about these factors is, therefore, crucial. Consideration needs to be given to the ways in which policies of various government agencies might influence population health, particularly agencies who do not routinely consider health, directly or indirectly as part of their policy development process.

The potential impacts that any new development or policy might have on the health of people may be positive, negative, or unknown and these impacts may not be spread evenly across the population. HIA has traditionally been applied to development projects that involve changes to the physical environment, such as a mining development or the construction of a dam. In recent years, with the increasing awareness of the importance of understanding health from both a biomedical and social perspective and the consequential focus on the role of the social determinants of health, there has been an increasing drive within government to considering the impacts of decisions made by departments outside the health sector, such as transport, environment, and housing.

It is obvious that if one adopts a social model of health and acknowledges that health is determined by a range of factors including public policy, then the next step will be to devise mechanisms that will help to ascertain, estimate, or measure how these factors might impact on the health of the population and seek to strengthen the likely positive and ameliorate the likely negative impacts before they occur. The expanded use of HIA is, therefore, relatively new, emerging in the late 1970s, and draws on the traditions of both environmental impact assessment (EIA) and healthy public policy (Mahoney et al. 2002). It seeks to complement existing activities in health promotion and public health, such as needs assessment, equity audits, monitoring, and evaluation by adding a new step earlier in the decision-making process (Simpson et al. 2004).

To differentiate this new form from its traditional role in EIA, many practitioners have coined the term 'policy HIA'. As policies are broad, overarching ideas that translate to practices, plans, strategies, programs, and projects, it is virtually impossible to use HIA to 'assess' policies. This chapter will focus on policy HIA, the myriad activities encompassed under the umbrella term 'policy' and its use by health promotion and public health practitioners to influence decision-making. HIA focuses on five aspects: assisting with the social determinants of health agenda; identifying impacts arising from, but not exclusively, non-health sector activities; considering policy and decision-making rather than project-level applications; integrating health considerations rather than simply environmental impacts; and, reducing inequalities in health within the population. All of these ideas are derived from the principles of integrated approaches to decision-making and the consequential need to work intersectorally to achieve mutual goals.

WHY HAS POLICY HIA DEVELOPED?

One of the key drivers behind the push for the broadening of HIA from development projects to consideration of the impacts of policies has been the international health promotion movement. The Ottawa Charter (1986) made a commitment to pursuing the goal of achieving healthy public policy and the Jakarta Declaration followed this by advocating for the use of HIA. Additional high-level international drivers that have been influential in its development have included the Health for All policy approach of WHO in the 1980s, the Amsterdam Treaty of the European Union (1997), which contained a commitment to considering the impacts of the Union's policies and actions on human health, and the UK government's health policy Saving Lives: Our Healthier Nation (1999) and their commitment to reducing inequalities in health (Acheson 2001; see also Douglas 2001; Breeze & Lock 2002; Kemm 2000; and Parry & Stevens 2001). Most of these drivers make a direct connection between the health status of the population and the role of policy and they articulate the need for governments to identify likely impacts of their policies on health and inequalities.

As the origins of HIA in many countries are in environmental and scientific traditions linked to assessing potential hazards and risks of developments, there is considerable confusion about the knowledge, competencies, and conditions that are required for HIA to be applied to policies, strategies, and programs. Similarly, in countries such as Australia and New Zealand, which have a long tradition of the application of HIA within environmental management perspectives, the multiple goals of extending the use of HIA to public health, to the broader inequalities agenda, to policy-making outside the health sector, and to a range of levels of government, has caused debate about the role and efficacy of HIA (Mindell et al. 2001; Parry & Stevens 2001).

Ongoing research is being undertaken to determine the role that HIA can play within different levels of government in different countries, and the appropriate conditions needed for it to be effective in changing decision-making so that health is given equal consideration alongside economic and environmental factors. One of the major debates that has yet to be resolved internationally is deciding whether HIA is being used primarily as a *scientific tool* to identify and determine the nature of the likely health impacts and any gaps in the evidence base that is used to ascertain these impacts, or as a *decision-making tool* that can assist in providing evidence of greatest benefit to the population or sections of the population.

The first approach is of principal interest to academics and researchers and is focused on the need for scientific accuracy in the prediction of likely impacts. The latter is concerned with ensuring that policy-makers make the best decision that can be made at a given point in time, taking into account the tensions inherent in government decision-making such as confidentiality, limited consultation, and the short-term planning cycle of governments. These two perspectives draw on different paradigms and have been described as the difference between understanding the *science* versus the *art* of policy-making (Sim & Mackie 2003). One of the biggest tensions with HIA is that when it is applied prospectively (i.e. during the decision-making process), the policy, program, or project is altered because of the recommendations that arise from it. It is, therefore, impossible to compare the altered course of action with the events that have been averted (Blau & Mahoney 2005). This is extremely problematic for practitioners who are seeking to quantify the outcomes of HIA and require proof of its added value.

WHAT ARE THE GENERAL BENEFITS OF HIA?

Despite these tensions in interpretation, HIA continues to be applied around the world in a range of different decision-making contexts for a range of reasons. An analysis of reports of HIA completed to date and published papers/reports on HIA shows that it is providing the following benefits when applied at regional or local levels of government:

- *HIA has the potential to put health on the agenda where it has not traditionally been considered.* For instance, HIA has been applied systematically to all the Mayoral strategies in the new City of London. In the development of the early Mayoral strategies, which tended to focus on factors affecting the environment such as transport and air quality, HIA was clearly seen as an add-on process being used to meet a Mayoral obligation to electors. Bowen (2004) reports that later strategy development processes took health impacts into account much earlier and more comprehensively because of the success of these early applications of HIA.

- *HIA has encouraged intersectoral collaboration and is a mechanism for discussion about potential health and equity impacts.* For instance, the people involved in the development and implementation of the Bro Taf Health Authority's Health Inequalities Impact Assessment tool report that for the first time interdepartmental discussions occurred about potential health, inequalities and equity implications of planning within their local authority (Lester et al. 2001; Smith 2000).

- *HIA has encouraged those who make decisions to take into account any unanticipated effects of their decisions on population health or on different groups within the population.* For instance, the application of HIA during the redevelopment of a hospital in Salford in England showed that by consulting with a range of stakeholders early in the redevelopment process, a series of unanticipated impacts such as stress and conflict associated with traffic and parking difficulties could be avoided (Douglas 2001).

- *HIA has provided a systematic means of including evidence about potential impacts of a policy, strategy, or project during the decision-making process.* For instance, the New Zealand pilot HIA project on the potential health impacts of a proposed Integrated Transport Strategy allowed for urban transport planners and the transport funding agency to be exposed to the evidence about the consequences for human health and for the health status of different groups of the population that would arise from their decisions about transport provision (Thornley & Langford, unpublished report).

- *HIA has encouraged local ownership of decisions that have the potential to affect health by people who otherwise may never have participated in the planning process.* For instance, the HIA of Primary Care in Battersea in England allowed local residents to make recommendations about what health meant to them and how they wanted financial resource allocations prioritised during planning processes (Barnes et al. 2001).
- *HIA has enhanced the positive impacts and reduced the negative impacts of decisions.* For instance, the Feltham First Regeneration Program illustrated that there may be unintended negative impacts of a regeneration project for residents of that community if due consideration was not given to the needs of the local residents. Such regeneration schemes may improve a community so much that the cost of housing increases and local residents are forced out, thus compounding disadvantage in other poor communities (Barnes et al. 2001).
- *HIA helps identify, and make transparent, the trade-offs that are inevitable in the decision-making process.* For instance, the HIA of the City of Edinburgh Council's Urban Transport Strategy allowed for the health consequences of three different scenarios to be considered so that the trade-offs between each option, and their relative costs, could be compared (SNAP 2000).

The positioning of HIA at the different levels of government is very important as each level has a different focus or role in terms of health and the determinants of health and provides a different means of engaging with the key stakeholders who can play a role in decisions that are likely to affect health. Two very different examples include the ways in which the European Union approaches their requirements to complete HIA versus how a country such as Sweden approaches it. In the European Union, HIA is applied at a strategic whole-of-policy level with consideration being given to the ways in which the Union's policies affect health within and between each of the member states—one of which is Sweden (World Health Organisation 1999). In Sweden itself, however, HIA is applied at the local and regional levels, the county councils are responsible for health care, local transport, and public roads, and regional development and the municipal councils are responsible for schools, social services, aged care, environment, and health protection. HIA is therefore ideally positioned and is most effective at this level. The Swedish HIA tool was developed in the late 1970s by policy-makers who wanted to take health into account on a par with environmental considerations in order to facilitate policy-making that supports the objective of favourable and equitable health development for all people (Berensson 1998).

In Australia there is a mandated requirement to consider health impacts of development projects only within environmental management legislation through the use of EIA. The use of policy HIA is still under consideration at the three levels of government: federal, state, and local. As each state is responsible for health, it is logical that its application should be considered at both state and local levels.

WHAT IS THE LINK BETWEEN HIA, LOCAL GOVERNMENT, AND INTERSECTORAL ACTION?

Currently, there is an increasing understanding that local government, and the decisions that it makes, plays a crucial role in determining the health of the population and the differences in health status that can occur between the differing groups within the community. Some countries have understood this crucial role of local government and the need for intersectoral action for a long time and have developed effective ways of achieving integrated planning linked to health. Others are still in the early stages of their thinking. The WHO agendas of *Health for All*, *Agenda 21*, and *Healthy Cities* have all made, and continue to make, a crucial contribution to raising awareness of the role of local governments in influencing health and environmental outcomes (WHO 2004).

There is also an increasing willingness on the part of many council staff to both work together to achieve mutual goals and to consider the ways in which the planning and decision-making processes of local governments can impact on a range of outcomes, including health. As stated in the previous section, HIA plays an important role in facilitating intersectoral action by providing a relatively straightforward mechanism that assists local government staff to work across sectors when faced with complex policy development and planning issues. There are two main reasons why HIA is effective. First, it is a logical step-wise process that uses a range of tools to identify likely impacts. Second, as it seeks to identify impacts arising from the decisions of other sectors, it is underpinned by principles of intersectoral working. The next two sections will explore each of these reasons in detail.

All departments of government have their own perspective, responsibilities, obligations, and ways of working. In the absence of a formal imperative to work together, for one department to insist that others consider the implications of their actions on *its* outcomes is likely to be met with complacency at one extreme and challenges of territorialism at the other. For true intersectoral working, all participants need to understand the relevance of working together, derive equal or mutual benefits, be able to make an equal contribution and feel that a spirit of true partnerships is operating. This is extremely difficult to achieve because of issues of power, tradition, the capacity of staff to work intersectorally, and the capacity of bureaucratic organisations to accommodate this style of working. The challenge of getting health considerations onto the agendas of other departments is therefore exceedingly difficult and requires sensitivity on the part of the health professional.

AN EXAMPLE DRAWN FROM LOCAL GOVERNMENT

Using health and local government in Victoria as an illustration, let us consider how this plays out.

In local government, as with any policy-making organisation, there are hierarchies that have evolved over time in terms of departments, issues, and individuals who prioritise agendas. These can be based on either real or perceived power advantages within the organisation. For instance, economic considerations have traditionally been the main determinant of decision-making in local government and these control the nature, scope, and size of any initiative that is undertaken. To change the balance so that health becomes the principal factor to be considered in decision-making will require an enormous shift within the organisation. Such a shift could be driven by a formal event, such as a clear political mandate (i.e. legislation) for a change in balance, and/or from an informal event, or an increased capacity of council staff to translate the goal of considering health impacts into daily processes within council.

In Victoria, a formal event occurred in 1988 with the passing of an amendment to the *Health Act 1958*. This amendment introduced a requirement for all Victorian councils to develop and implement Municipal Public Health Plans (MPHPs) that would:

- identify and assess actual and potential public health dangers in the municipality
- outline programs and strategies that the council intends to pursue to prevent or minimise those dangers, to enable the people in the municipality to achieve maximum well-being
- provide for the periodic evaluation of those programs and strategies, as well as annually reviewing the public health plan.

However, for a range of complex reasons, this formal event did not shift the balance across the entire local government sector. It appears that some councils were not able to expand their roles and responsibilities beyond the 'core' local government services such as 'roads, rates and rubbish' for a number of reasons. Their focus was not broadened from the provision of 'hard' infrastructure to spending on public services, such as health, welfare, safety, and community amenities. It is clear that, at present, only some Victorian councils overtly consider the health and well-being of their community in their decision-making. In these councils, health considerations and economic factors are weighted equally, integrated planning is the norm, and mechanisms to support intersectoral working are common. Other councils do not appear to understand their expanded role in planning for health. Departments within these councils operate as 'silos' and opportunities for intersectoral action are limited or non-existent.

There is considerable debate about whether a driver for intersectoral working could be created by legislation (Banken 2001). Within the HIA literature there is no clear position about this, with some practitioners arguing that organisations will not adopt integrated approaches unless they are required to, whilst others argue that to force people to work together is counterproductive. In the context of this chapter, while this point is crucial and sets the backdrop for effective intersectoral working, the discussion will focus largely on institutional and personal attributes needed for intersectoral working at a staff or departmental level and the role that HIA can play in promoting this style of working.

HOW CAN HIA PROVIDE A FRAMEWORK FOR PROMOTING INTERSECTORAL ACTION?

Intersectoral action is currently not commonplace in local government in Victoria and generally requires a driver to 'force' it to occur. As each sector has its own drivers for working and its own 'language', some framework or mechanism that helps to break down the barriers that exist between sectors or departments can be very helpful.

For a number of reasons, HIA's *structured* step-wise approach to identifying and judging health impacts has been effective in promoting intersectoral action. First, a number of steps is required in HIA because impact assessment is trying to identify potential impacts and make a judgment about the necessary trade-offs of one option over another in the decision-making process. Second, impact assessment is premised on the notion that one discipline or person cannot know all the potential impacts of an action. If multiple perspectives were not required there would be no need to undertake HIA because routine decision-making processes would suffice. Third, evidence must be considered in a range of ways as non-health sectors do not routinely consider evidence of likely health impacts in their decision-making processes. Fourth, as decisions are usually made by a different group of people to those undertaking the HIA, it is important to understand that there are multiple ways and times when the decision-making process can be influenced.

Within local government some broad examples of the ways in which HIA can promote intersectoral action linked to health include:

- providing a structured way of examining how the non-health areas of council impact on the public's health
- providing an opportunity for staff across council to talk together about, or work together on, a project that is health-related either directly or indirectly through the determinants of health
- providing a local, concrete example of determinants of health rather than a theoretical discussion about the social model of health
- establishing a multidisciplinary team or committee that is not lead by a health professional, but where leadership is shared equally.

In terms of the mechanisms HIA provides for intersectoral working, the following table illustrates the role of each of the steps in it and the ways in which intersectoral working can be promoted.

Table 13.1 Using HIA to work intersectorally

STEP IN THE HIA PROCESS	FUNCTION OF THE STEP	INTERSECTORAL BENEFIT
Screening	Identifying the potential linkages between the proposal and health; determining whether an HIA should be conducted, the reasons for it and the added value that it will bring to the decision-making process	Through cross-sector discussions and use of simple evidence to encourage others to see the connection between their processes and health, e.g. the need to consider how land-use planning decisions can impact directly on health
Scoping	Once the decision for an HIA has been made, identifying the range, scope, and size of the HIA	Through the use of a steering or working group to increase buy-in by decision-makers about how non-health sector policies can impact on health, e.g. including a councillor on a working group that is completing an HIA on the ways in which an employment scheme will affect health
Impact identification	Collection of a range of evidence that identifies the ways in which a proposal will impact on health and the mapping of these impacts according to the determinants of health and to specific sections of the population	Through the use of key informant interviews or a rapid HIA workshop that includes people from the community, service sectors, and other departments in council to identify the likely impacts of the proposal on the health of the community and sections of the community, e.g. through mixing a range of people together in a group to consider the health impacts of a proposed transport strategy
Impact assessment	Synthesis of the impacts identified from the range of sources in terms of their nature (+/-/?) and likelihood (e.g. certain to happen).	Drawing evidence from a range of disciplines and working with key stakeholders to compare the differences and make judgments about interpreting it in this local context, e.g. a multidisciplinary mapping exercise
Development of recommendations	Developing a range of recommendations about the proposal based on the evidence collected and the trade-offs between different and competing options or groups	Preparation of an evidence-based set of recommendations to be presented to councillors about the impacts of a proposal they are considering e.g. adding evidence about health impacts into a decision being made on a controversial land development

STEP IN THE HIA PROCESS	FUNCTION OF THE STEP	INTERSECTORAL BENEFIT
Evaluation and monitoring	Determining both the quality of the HIA process and the extent to which it made a difference versus monitoring whether a predicted outcome occurred.	Using the evidence of impacts drawn from other studies to inform future decision-making in this council, e.g. monitoring whether the negative impacts identified by the community actually happened or not, and if they did requiring that all future planning applications address residents' concerns in the initial application process rather than during or after decision-making

The critical questions to be asked when using HIA in local government to promote intersectoral action are:

- When should HIA be used both to strengthen the council's focus on health and to facilitate the agenda items of partners?
- Who should be responsible for the application of HIA?
- What levels of support will be required by people undertaking HIA?
- How can the interplay between key stakeholders, such as other local government, local and regional service providers, state government sectors, and professional organisations that support the working of local government, be encouraged?
- How will the lessons learnt from intersectoral working using HIA be used to influence and shape better policy, planning and practice in the future (i.e. sustainability in decision-making)?
- Within all of these, what are the roles and responsibilities of the health promotion professional in facilitating intersectoral action to promote health?

HOW CAN I WORK INTERSECTORALLY WITHIN AN ORGANISATION?

HIA has been effective in both putting health on the agenda and promoting intersectoral working because its role has been to assist people in other sectors to understand why health impacts should be important in their work. As such, this success can be used to provide a basis for considering the necessary factors that practitioners need to consider when they are seeking to change the way others think about health by working intersectorally.

Based on the experiences of other HIA practitioners drawn from the published literature and from the writers' experiences of working intersectorally and in local government, this section offers two practical guides. The first is drawn from the use of HIA in local government and provides a detailed overview of all the factors that need to be taken into account by the health promotion professional when planning to work intersectorally, from three different perspectives: the organisation, the team, and the individual. The second is a generic checklist of questions that should be used to guide the first meeting of a team wishing to work together on issues of mutual concern. The examples provided are drawn from local government but can be applied to any context.

Practical Guide 1: Factors to be considered when planning to work intersectorally, specifically in local government

Organisational factors

As a bureaucratic organisation, each local government has a structure that determines the hierarchy of power, the position of key decision-makers and each work area's broad responsibilities within the context of the organisation's mission or purpose. When exploring the possibility of intersectoral work in local government, it is crucial that the health promotion professional develops a good understanding of this structure, the people in it, and their relative positions. As a health professional coming into an organisation whose primary focus is not health, you should endeavour to learn about the work that is undertaken by council's wide range of departments or divisions, as well as its recent history and its current priorities. It would also be important to know the degree of influence that both the councillors and the community have on council's decisions. A scan of the positions that are at the same level as your position in the organisational structure, will indicate the staff with whom you could make direct contact to search for 'allies' who understand the social model of health. You may be surprised to find 'allies' in such disparate departments as planning, engineering, community development, community safety, research, economic development, or the library.

When planning to work intersectorally in local government, a very good understanding of council's protocol is also essential to ensure that your actions do not waste time and do not unwittingly create tension in any part of the organisation. You will need to learn how 'things are done' and how and when people communicate, both internally and externally: via the telephone, emails, reports or briefings at formal meetings, chats over coffee, lunch-time seminars, team social events, or in the corridor.

Team factors

Whatever the title of your position, you will probably be one of a team, group, or unit comprising a range of council staff whose work responsibilities somehow relate to each other. As your team leader may not have a health background, you should learn about his/her main areas of interest and ascertain his/her understanding of the social model of health. Other members of your team may or may not be working on health-related issues, so you should not assume that they have a good understanding of the social model of health. Your goal is to understand the role and goals of others, to ensure effective team-working, and, through these, to establish areas of common ground that can be built on.

Individual factors

Although you will undoubtedly have excellent health promotion skills and a sound knowledge of the social model of health, your professional life in local government will require the development of many other equally important skills. The following list of questions can be used to prompt some private reflections about your own broader skill set and where you may need some help. It is not sufficient for you to simply possess these skills but you need to be able to use these for the achievement of intersectoral action.

- Can you explain the concept of the social determinants of health to a person from a non-health background?
- Can you recognise 'allies' who could assist your health-promoting role in the organisation, but who may be using different terminology?
- Can you network with staff in other departments, both formally and informally, to learn about their roles and responsibilities?
- What is your level of commitment to introduce the concept of the social model of health into the organisation?
  - ☐ Will you be able to persevere even though others may not congratulate you?
  - ☐ Are you able to recognise and celebrate small wins by yourself?
- Can you persuade others of the value that your work can add to council?
- Can you respect others' view of the world, even if this is very different to yours?
  - ☐ Can you tolerate working in a group that is led by someone who may not value 'health' as you do?
- Can you wait patiently while changes occur over many months or years?
- Can you keep focused on your ultimate outcome and demonstrate resilience in the face of setbacks?
- Can you accept criticism and avoid feeling personally wounded?
- Can you work to a high standard in situations where lower levels of professionalism are the norm?
- Are you willing to admit that you don't know everything and humbly concede to others?
- Can you detect when you cannot create change on your own?
- Can you ask for help when you need it?
- Are you realistic to know when to give up and/or when to try another way?
- Can you find someone/some group outside the organisation that will support you and facilitate debriefing when you are facing a difficult period?

Practical Guide 2: Checklist of questions to guide planning for intersectoral working

The following questions are designed to help you.

- What does each member/partner want to achieve through the process of working together?
- What are the main drivers for working together (e.g. formal—institutional agendas for integrated planning; informal—a history of working well with these people to better frame strategies or plans)?
- What benefits will be accrued by each member/partner?
- What organisational structures might hamper the group's ability to work together to achieve individual or joint goals (e.g. time constraints)?
- What organisational structures will support the group's ability to work together to achieve individual or joint goals and thus be used or exploited?

SUMMARY

While HIA is not perfect, like other forms of impact assessment it is premised on the notion that multidisciplinary, multiperspective understandings are essential for good decision-making. As such, it complements the social model of health, the principles of healthy public policy and integrated planning, and provides a means by which health promotion professions can work with other sectors to support the goals of other sections or departments. Others will not see either the relevance or value of considering health in their work unless health promotion professionals can translate, interpret, reflect, and recast their current approaches.

- HIA is a systematic process that provides a structured mechanism for integrated working.
- HIA has been successfully applied to a range of areas that have not traditionally considered health.
- The goal of intersectoral action is to develop sustainable partnerships so that health stays on the agenda.
- Working intersectorally is challenging and requires careful consideration of a range of obvious as well as less obvious factors.
- There is a clear set of principles for engaging other sectors around health.
- Intersectoral working involves understanding the agendas of others and facilitating mutual and non-mutual outcomes.

HEALTHY PUBLIC POLICY

14

Colin MacDougall & Evelyne de Leeuw

Key concepts

- Healthy public policy mirrors the language and intent while setting the conditions for upstream health promotion.
- Policy is a framework guiding a course of action that is both influenced by and allocates values.
- Broader policies that do not set the conditions for health promotion stand between determinants of health and health promotion action.
- Because policy expresses and opposes particular values, it is essential to draw on political science and to understand a range of theories and models for policy development.
- Healthy public policy is not a linear, technocratic concept developed in calm, evidence-based neutrality. Healthy public policy is contested, complex, and, at first sight, chaotic.
- Power, conflicting agendas, and networks combine to allocate values and determine broad courses of policy.
- Health promotion is increasingly making use of the emerging knowledge about policy implementation.
- Health promoters are in an ideal position to work with communities and networks to shape the way power is used to develop and implement policy.

Key terms

■ Policy
■ Healthy public policy
■ Policy models and frameworks
■ Agenda setting
■ Policy keepers
■ Interest groups
■ Policy networks, communities, and spaces
■ Policy implementation

OVERVIEW

At one level the definition of healthy public policy mirrors the language and approach to intersectoral and upstream health promotion. This is hardly surprising, because when Nancy Milio (1986) described public policy as ecological in perspective, multisectoral in scope, and collaborative and participatory in strategy, she was reflecting the strategies of the Ottawa Charter for Health Promotion (WHO 1986). One of the many legacies of the Ottawa Charter was to place activism, advocacy, and policy analysis—critique—development high on the agenda of health promotion. After the Ottawa Charter, no self-respecting health promoter could lock themselves away in an office writing pamphlets and self-help programs. By contrast, the Ottawa Charter, and many subsequent WHO statements, exhorted health promotion to engage in policy action to create the supportive environments that we know make the healthy choice the easy choice. Health promoters need healthy public policies to be in place so they can be ecological, multisectoral, collaborative, and participatory in their practice in communities.

After Ottawa, the policy stakes were raised again to focus squarely on the social determinants of health at the Second International Health Promotion Conference, held in Adelaide in 1988. The then Director-General of the World Health Organisation argued that healthy public policy creates preconditions for healthy living through:

■ closing the health gap between social groups and between nations
■ broadening the choices of people to make the healthier choices the easier and most possible
■ ensuring supportive social environments (Baum 1998).

Now, in the first decade of the twenty-first century, the current Director-General of the World Health Organisation has placed social determinants at the top of his agenda by establishing a Commission on the Social Determinants of Health. In March 2005, the Commission's Chair, Sir Michael Marmot said that:

People's health suffers because of the social conditions in which they live and work. The end goal of the Commission—and its follow-up—is to change this reality ... At the core of the Commission's work is the belief that a society that has organized its social conditions so that its population has better health is a better society. Health is a measure of the degree to which the society delivers a good life to its citizens. This commission is aiming to help countries to progress towards that ideal.

He said of the Commissioners:

Because they are people who have played prominent roles in various spheres, they will not only benefit the process of identifying effective means to address the social determinants of health, but they are also in positions to advocate for the uptake of these means by decision-makers. <www.who.int/social_determinants/en/>.

Here, WHO is not just identifying health problems, promising interventions, and identifying barriers. It is going much further by arguing for prominent health advocates to agitate for policy change by member states. A focus on policy, however, takes many health promoters beyond their training and experience. Consequently, in this chapter we review definitions, underlying principles, and some of the skills needed to engage with, healthy public policy.

To understand policy we need to look to the political sciences because we are mindful of an influential critique that the literature of healthy public policy can be exhortatory, proscriptive, and redundant, with the same ideas seen to be re-worked and traded back and forth (Pederson 1988). Pederson et al. claim that the literature is not theoretically grounded because it does not reference the literature of the social sciences. In this chapter, we take their advice that 'a useful research strategy would be to bring social science theory explicitly to bear on the issues of co-coordinating healthy public policy' (Pederson et al. 1988: iii). We conclude that health promotion workers are uniquely equipped to play a significant role in organising communities and social environments for policy development and implementation.

WHAT IS POLICY?

Policy is not merely a description of static, technocratic decisions, rather 'Policy is essentially a stance which, once articulated, contributes to the context within which a succession of future decisions will be made' (Ham & Hill 1993: 11). Ham and Hill (1993) summarise the following elements from a number of authors' definitions of policy, including:

- a course of action or inaction rather than specific decisions or actions
- a set of interrelated decisions concerning the selection of goals and the means of achieving them
- a stance that, once articulated, contributes to the context within which future decisions will be made.

Similarly, Blum (1974: 229) defines policy as '... a long term, continuously used, standing decision by which more specific proposals are judged for accepta-bility'. Policy, according to Blum, stipulates ends, may provide resources, and may spell out specific means to reach these ends and may be:

- a very general statement of intentions and objectives
- a past set of actions of government in a particular area
- a specific statement of future intentions
- a set of standing rules that is intended as a guide to action or inaction (Blum 1974).

The most important implication of thinking about policy as a general course is that, rather than focus narrowly on specific decisions, we should consider why judgments were made and action was taken in some circumstances and not in others. One place to look is the values associated with a policy because:

> Values explain policy and invest all its ordinary practices with meaning. From the open declarations of intent in legislation, to the unspoken preference for one means over another, and on to the measure and evaluations of the actions that result, values are titanic and ubiquitous (Considine 1994: 49).

Ham and Hill (1993) see the fundamental purpose of policy as a web of decisions and actions that allocate values. This is of particular importance when thinking through ecological and upstream health promotion, which is not only contested, but also can be out of step with the prevailing values in countries influenced by economic liberalism and its attendant ideas of rolling back the state. Lin and Gibson (2003) elaborate on the potential for a clash of values when they describe health policy as the product of three competing rationalities: cultural, political, and technical. *Cultural rationality* reflects values and ethics and what perceived societal opinion feels is right about health policy. *Political rationality* is concerned with the distribution and management of power and the creation of legitimacy. *Technical rationality* is where research evidence is used, can be helpful to the policy-maker, but is usually the weakest link in the chain. This model shows ways in which different people approach the same policy using different rationalities, and elaborates on the values question by separating cultural from political values.

Box 14.1: Competing rationalities in Australia

The Community Support Section of the Australian Government Department of Immigration and Multicultural Affairs established a Muslim Community Reference Group in late 2005. The Group works on an agenda set by the Council of Australian Governments, which initiated a national action plan at the Special Meeting on Counter-Terrorism on 27 September 2005 (<www.immi.gov.au/multicultural/mcrg/index.htm> accessed 1 March 2006).

Principles 4 and 5 of the plan appear consistent with health promotion language and the quest for evidence that underpins Lin and Gibson's (2003) notion of technical rationality. These principles are:

4 Encouraging tolerance and social cohesion through employment, public education and community activities

5 Engaging with communities including through consultations and ongoing dialogue.

Principles 2 and 3 of the plan also appear consistent with health promotion language and the quest for evidence that underpins Lin and Gibson's (2003) notion of cultural rationality. These principles are:

2 Building leadership capacity and communication skills in Australian communities

3 Supporting leaders and teachers

Principle 1, however, changes the value base for the whole plan, illustrating Lin and Gibson's (2003) notion of political rationality:

1 Improving understanding of extremism

This political dimension reframes the statements about social cohesion and community consultation, which are familiar to health promotion, into a value-laden debate about religion and extremism. The political stakes are exemplified by the following newspaper headlines from speeches made by Peter Costello, who has for a long time positioned himself as the next Prime Minister of Australia.

Costello urges migrant loyalty

Steve Lewis, chief political correspondent (*The Australian*) 24 February 2006:

> Peter Costello has called for a tougher US-style citizenship oath that demands loyalty to the Australian 'compact' as he outlined his vision for a more muscular nationalism. Lambasting the spread of 'mushy multiculturalism', the Treasurer has bluntly called for hard-line Muslims and others who don't observe Australian values to be stripped of their citizenship.

> And he said people coming to Australia should have the same respect for Australian values as visitors to a mosque who are asked to take off their shoes.

Fears of new White Australia policy

By Jewel Topsfield & Michelle Grattan (*The Age*) 25 February 2006:

> Some Liberal colleagues said the speech was about Mr Costello positioning himself to win support from the Liberal Party's right; others thought he just said what he believed.

Ameer Ali, president of the Australian Federation of Islamic Councils, said he was concerned Australia could return to the days when immigration laws denied entry to people from non-white European backgrounds. 'Either the Government is trying to go back to the White Australia policy or to have multiculturalism minus the Muslims,' Dr Ali said.

WHAT IS HEALTHY PUBLIC POLICY?

The term *healthy public policy* was coined by Nancy Milio (1986), who reviewed the impact of particularly US government policy on human health. She found that virtually any government sector, be it economics, employment, finance, defence, agriculture, social affairs, foreign affairs, immigration, or science and technology, can positively or adversely affect health. She then contended that it is the moral, political, and economic responsibility of any government to assure the healthfulness of all its policy. A contemporary activist definition is:

> Equity, ecologically-sustainable development and peace are at the heart of our vision of a better world—a world in which a healthy life for all is a reality; a world that respects, appreciates and celebrates all life and diversity; a world that enables the flowering of people's talents and abilities to enrich each other; a world in which people's voices guide the decisions that shape our lives....

> People's Charter for Health <www.phmovement.org/en/about> accessed 6 April 2006

POLICY AS THE EXERCISE OF POWER

Harold Laswell's compelling definition from the 1930s saw politics and policy development asking the questions *who gets what, where, and how* (Lasswell 1930, 1936). These questions inescapably lead to *power*, seen by Rummel (1976) as being exerted intentionally or unintentionally. Policy research is interested in the intentional use of power, often through established institutions such as parliament, defence and police forces, and sometimes religion. These institutions have the authority to exert power, with a system of checks and balances to protect against abuse of power. However, this system is often very subtle and blends with other forms of power, such as coercion, bargaining, and manipulative actions. *Power* is the ability to impose one's will on others, even when they resist, using Dahl's (1961) list of individual and collective power resources:

- an individual's own time
- access to money, credit, and wealth
- control over information
- esteem or social standing

- the possession of charisma, popularity, legitimacy, legality
- the rights pertaining to public office
- solidarity: the capacity of a member of one segment of society to evoke support from others who identify him (or her) as like themselves because of similarities in occupation, social standing, religion, ethnic origin, or racial stock
- the right to vote
- intelligence
- education
- and perhaps even one's energy level.

As shown in Figure 14.1, Wrong (1996), asserts that the mere possession of any of these power bases does not necessarily constitute power. The potential power holder will have to be in some sort of relation to other lesser power holders and should have a sufficient interest in exerted power to consider the employment of her (or his) resources in that relation.

Figure 14.1   Forms of power

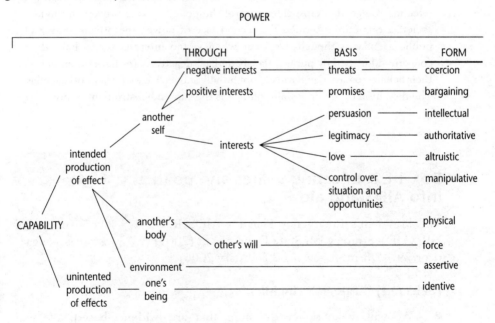

The political science literature can help health promotion by offering two related ways of exercising power in the policy debate: *agenda setting* and *network analysis*. Neither concept by itself explains power and policy, but when they are put together they help us to understand how power is exercised, and where to intervene and advocate for healthy public policy.

EXERCISING POWER THROUGH AGENDA SETTING

When the collective and ecological values behind ecological and upstream health promotion clash with the values of governments, corporations, and lobby groups that espouse individualistic and market values of economic liberalism, something has to give. Evidence is not enough to promote a policy if its value base is at odds with the values of the dominant paradigm. Yet powerful interests are unlikely to dismiss a policy proposal by citing a value clash. In the real world, the way that potential and actual policy issues are managed has been likened to the management of an agenda. Therefore, agenda setting:

> is a process in which government attempts to prevent policy issues from emerging, to influence the public perception of issues and to shape or delete issues on the current agenda of policy making (Harding 1985: 224).

Considine (1994:138) argues that although policy-makers and political scientists agree that issues do suddenly become hot, that this can be traced to the power of elites:

> Behind this notion lies another, more fundamental conviction: that through the selection of agenda items, elites control the policy making process in modern societies. Sometimes termed the second face of power, the private setting of public agendas is thought to occur when vested interests act to have their concerns addressed by public officials, and act negatively (or have others act on their behalf) to have dangerous or potentially subversive issues kept off agendas. The definition of the policy alternatives is the supreme instrument of power.

Box 14.2: Injecting values and politics into AIDS and aid

The President's Emergency Plan for AIDS Relief: US Five Year Global HIV/AIDS Strategy US State Department (2003) (<www.state.gov/s/gac/rl/or/29712.htm>, accessed 2 February 2006)

(Selected) Strategic Principles

- **We will make policy decisions that are evidence-based.** We will build on the best practices established in the fight against HIV/AIDS and bring the resources of sound science to bear in selecting and developing interventions that achieve real results.
- **We will demand accountability for results.** The President's Emergency Plan will establish measurable goals for which we will hold ourselves and our partners accountable. In the focus countries and throughout the world, effective monitoring and evaluation systems will identify

successful models for scaleup and poorly performing programs for revision or termination.

- **We will employ the prevention lessons learned from the 'ABC' model.** Uganda's success has identified the 'ABC' model (Abstinence, Be faithful, and, as appropriate, correctly and consistently use Condoms) as an effective HIV/AIDS prevention tool. We will promote the proper application of the ABC approach, through population-specific interventions that emphasize abstinence for youth, including the delay of sexual debut and abstinence until marriage; HIV/AIDS testing and fidelity in marriage and monogamous relationships; and correct and consistent use of condoms for those who practice high-risk behaviors.

- **We will encourage and strengthen faith-based and community-based nongovernmental organizations.** Faith-based and community-based organizations were among the first responders to HIV/AIDS, caring for fellow human beings in need. Their reach, authority, and legitimacy identify them as crucial partners in the fight against HIV/AIDS. We will encourage their involvement, and, in particular, we will welcome new partners with innovative ideas.

Trying to convert value based to value neutral policy

The Director of U.S. Policy and of the Health Action AIDS campaign at Physicians for Human Rights placed the President's strategy in a political context as follows:

Thanks to recent activism by conservative political and religious groups, AIDS has finally started to gain foreign policy attention commensurate with its substantive importance. Prodded by its conservative evangelical base, the Bush administration has pushed AIDS to the forefront of its international agenda, backing record increases in U.S. assistance for AIDS treatment abroad and beginning to address issues such as sex trafficking and the dangers of HIV transmission from unsafe injections and blood transfusions.

The future of U.S. global AIDS policy will be complicated, however, because the conservative groups interested in the issue have different tactical priorities than their liberal counterparts and the broader medical establishment. They have traditionally been hostile to some important AIDS-prevention strategies such as comprehensive sex education and condom distribution, and they are much more enthusiastic than others about policies such as the promotion of abstinence.

Now that the United States is finally stepping up its efforts to tackle the crisis, it would be tragic if their impact were dissipated because of ideological differences between constituencies that are vital to the struggle against AIDS. The time has come, therefore, for all interested in AIDS policy to unite behind a comprehensive strategy to combat the pandemic, one based on the most effective practices in both prevention and treatment. The tens, possibly hundreds, of millions at risk deserve no less.

The Politics of AIDS: Engaging Conservative Activists, Holly Burkhalter. *Foreign Affairs*, January/February 2004 <www.foreignaffairs.org/20040101facomment83102/ holly-burkhalter/the-politics-of-aids-engaging-conservative-activists.html> accessed 3 February 2006.

The case study of the United States's AIDS policy demonstrates how, in the policy phases of deciding to decide and deciding how to decide (Hogwood & Gunn 1984), agenda setting involves the exercise of power, influence, and advocacy by a range of people, institutions, and interests. The case shows how the President of the United States adopts the role that Milio (1988) describes a *policy keeper*: an entity that by its own initiative or by mandate holds a specific, articulated policy at any given time, and moves the policy at a pace consistent with its interests. The role of conservative religious groups in the case study shows how policy-keepers interact with organised groups whose resources, authority, status, influence, or survival is affected by a policy. Interest groups include, but are not limited to: political parties; parliamentary committees; ministerial offices and bureaucratic units; commercial enterprises; and voluntary, professional, religious, communications, or minority organisations (Milio 1988). In this case, the interest groups attempt to redefine the policy as evidence-based—one that is too important to be derailed by a discussion of values. In this way, the policy networks attempt to present a strongly value-based policy as a non-contentious strategy that should unite all interests.

Power is exercised in complex ways, as shown in Table 14.1's summary of some key techniques that these institutional policy-keepers use.

Table 14.1   The exercise of power by institutional policy-keepers using agenda management techniques

symbolism	provide symbolic rewards, reassurance, or dissuasion
tokenism	offer limited action on larger problem
new organisations	set up new organisations to deal with the problem
negativism	argue that problem is beyond governmental resolution or is insoluble
postponement	set up special committees or inquiries; demand further consultation
co-option	co-opt leaders of dissenting organisations
discredit leaders	attack leaders of dissenting organisations

discredit group	criticise dissenting organisations or affected publics
redefinition	Redefine issue in a more favourable way
displacement	shift focus of controversy to different issue or to policy response to initial issue
deny legitimacy	argue that issue is not appropriate or desirable for government action
deception	argue one thing and do another
retaliation	threaten opponents, secretly or publicly with retaliation (e.g. withdrawal of government funds or contracts) if they continue agitation
recognition	encourage groups whose policies accord with government's (e.g. place them in advisory committees)
exchange	trade concessions in less important area for cessation of group opposition in more important area
adjustment	redefine, delay, or drop collection of social indicators

Summarised from Cobb & Elder 1983; Nordlinger 1981

An important set of competencies for health promoters is to recognise ways in which policy-keepers and interest groups manage agendas while obscuring their underlying focus on values and negating either good evidence or persuasive arguments. These competencies include knowledge of theories of agenda building and an appreciation of the power that lies in networks.

Cobb and Elder proposed three models, summarised in Table 14.2, to describe agenda setting: *outside initiative, inside initiative*, and *mobilisation*.

Table 14.2 Models of agenda building

	INITIATION	SPECIFICATION	EXPANSION	ENTRANCE
Outside initiative	by outside group	general grievances to specific demands	expand issue to other groups	from public to formal agenda
Mobilisation	decision-makers put on formal agenda to get public support	few concrete details	implementation depends on public acceptance	from formal to public agenda
Inside access	decision-makers put on formal agenda avoiding expansion to the public agenda	concrete proposals	limited to decision-makers who avoid issue expansion	by power-brokers

Adapted from Cobb & Ray (1976)

OUTSIDE INITIATIVE

In this model, the central question is 'How does legitimisation of a social problem to a policy problem take place?' The basic notion is that there is a need for such a policy and, as a result of sufficient public and interest group pressure, the issue will move from the systemic or societal agenda and will find a place on the institutional agenda. This institutional agenda comprises a general set of political controversies that will be viewed at any point in time as falling within the range of legitimate concerns meriting the attention of the polity i.e. a particular institutional decision-making body (Cobb & Elder 1983: 14). Therefore, such an issue has high probability of being addressed by formal policy (although non-decisions may be policy as well). The case study below resonates with the activist, protest-movement influences on the history of health promotion.

Case Study 14.1: An outside initiative approach to policy

'Primary Health Care was and still is the correct pathway for us all. Let's listen to these communities. How many times do we allow them to be part of their development? Genuine people-centred initiatives must be strengthened to increase pressure on decision-makers, governments and the private sector to ensure that the vision of Alma-Ata becomes a reality.'

Dr Upunda, Chief Medical Officer Ministry of Health, Tanzania, April 2002, opening a People's Health Movement workshop in Tanzania; <www.phmovement.org/en/about> accessed 6 April 2006

INSIDE INITIATIVE

According to the inside initiative model, it is insiders who more or less independently place issues on the institutional agenda. These insiders are a government agency or a group that has easy access to the policy-makers and political decision-makers. To protect the interests to be served by the new policy, the insiders try not to expand range of issue conflict, but try to coalesce with groups with similar interests. In other words issue expansion is limited and controlled by homogenous interest groups. A key feature is that undesirable expansion to attentive and general publics will hinder formalisation of the issue into policy because the interests at stake are too narrow to attract a wide audience that would be required in an outside initiative model. This model therefore provides policy-makers with very concrete proposals for policy.

Box 14.3: Insiders using evidence to change policy in concrete terms (once the value and cultural changes have occurred)

Despite dramatic improvement in road safety in Australia, there are still significant problems in metropolitan Australia. Woolley (2005) reports that in 1994 initial attempts to discuss a national speed limit lower than 60 km/h were contentious and all the states could not agree to the proposal. More work was needed to convince the community and politicians. In 1996 it was decided that each state could pursue a lower limit. New South Wales trialled 50 km/h in 1997 and by 2003 all of Australia had a default 50 km/h limit, except the Northern Territory.

A number of influential studies provided the evidence base to convince the community and politicians of the scientific merits of a 50 km/h limit.

The Road Accident Research Unit at the University of Adelaide carried out groundbreaking research relating speed to the incidence of serious crashes. Results showed that on arterial roads, the proportion of vehicles that crashed doubled with each 5 km/h increment above the (then) 60 km/h limit. Woolley (2005) reports studies in New South Wales showing a 25.3 per cent reduction in crashes 21 months after the move to 50 km/h. Pedestrians and cyclists benefited most. Similar work was done in other states.

Woolley (2005: 3570) made the observation that '...an intervention aimed at the general driving population also seemed to have considerable impact on those drivers at the extreme end of the scale with very high travelling speeds'.

In this case study, research outcomes were useful in influencing politicians and the community to change policy because the evidence was persuasive and was preceded by a sustained effort to change values and cultural norms (see Marshall 2004). The case study shows how health promotion can use evidence to change policy over a relatively short time: providing that the hard work has already gone in to changing cultural and political rationalities or values. The case illustrates the value of well-designed studies, yielding local evidence, presented in ways that drive home the benefits of a relatively simple policy change. The case also demonstrates the relevance of a classic 1985 paper, 'Sick individuals and sick populations' (Rose 1985), in which Geoffrey Rose argued that universal strategies can change not only the overall average of a distribution (in this case, speed); but also the extreme values (in this case the smaller numbers of high-speed drivers). In other words, the typical approach of 'just target those at risk' is not the intervention of choice here.

MOBILISATION AND POLICY NETWORKS

The third model, mobilisation, is an extension of the inside initiative model. Here, decision-making is already finalised but policy-makers seek support from the public to realise implementation. There are also elements of the outside initiative model in that public support is needed for effective implementation of the policy. Policy is considered formal as soon as political leaders make an explicit statement on the issue. Leaders therefore seek support when the implementation of policy is dependent on voluntary adherence or change in attitude by specific groups in society. As a result, there can be expansion of the issue as it becomes known to groups previously unaware of it. The initial formal statement can thus be a starting point for public debate and discussion and pressure to induce further sharpening of the demand for concreteness, which, of course, may well be an objective of the initial decision-maker.

The mobilisation model is an appropriate tool to study development of health policies because there are many contestants in the definition of the issues and generally the government has the legitimacy to deal with health issues because the constitution makes the government responsible for protection of public health (de Leeuw 1989). Further, there are very intricate interconnections in the health system, giving rise to the influence of powerful interest groups. The nature of healthy public policy, especially the way it involves intersectoral approaches, mixes of interventions, and participation of interest groups and communities, requires negotiation rather than direction (i.e. mobilisation rather than inside initiative) and consultation rather than bottom-up pressure (i.e. mobilisation rather than outside initiative).

For health promotion to be effective, we argue that participation in making policy by all interest groups is of utmost importance for the establishment of healthy public policy and that the mobilisation model has the highest potential for adequate communication between interest groups and decision-makers.

The *agenda-setting* model presented above is a necessary, but not sufficient, condition to explain the use of power in policy-making. We generate more profound insights by adding *network theory*. Deborah Stone (1997) and John Kingdon (1995) maintain that the policy-making process is in constant flux, value-laden, and with participants drifting in and out of the policy-making realm. Their commitment to the policy-making process varies according to whether they see their interests being served by claiming or denying ownership of the policy problem and by whether they can attribute meaning within these fluctuating realms. Kingdon sees continuous streams of problems, policies, and politics. In each of these streams visible and invisible stakeholders are at work, either trying to connect streams, or endeavouring to keep them disconnected. Individuals, whom Kingdon labels *policy entrepreneurs*, try to link these stakeholders and the streams and develop new policies. Skok (1995: 326) found that other theorists have described similar roles under different names: 'social entrepreneur', 'issue initiator', 'policy-broker', 'strategist', 'fixer', 'broker', or 'caretaker'. Whatever the label, this is typically a role that health promotion or public health professionals can and should play in a move toward healthy public policy. Kingdon finds that when policy entrepreneurs communicate with stakeholders they follow a pattern of 'alternative specification' in order to 'soften up the system' so that windows of opportunity for new policies are opened.

When these policy networks are mapped, we can see why certain policy options acquire priority over others. This approach may also explain why *health* does not always gets the policy priority for which the public health and health promotion community argue. Policy network analysis is a relatively new area of research (Lewis 2005) but it holds enormous promise for more effectively guiding policy development processes towards outcomes in the spirit of the Ottawa Charter.

Recent work on health policy-making among local authorities in the Netherlands revealed that 'the' policy network does not exist (Hoeijmakers 2004). In fact, different networks operate at the same time, and changes in one type of network may have consequences in another network later in time. In Figure 14.2, the three types of networks operating simultaneously, are depicted for a hypothetical situation.

Figure 14.2 Three types of policy networks

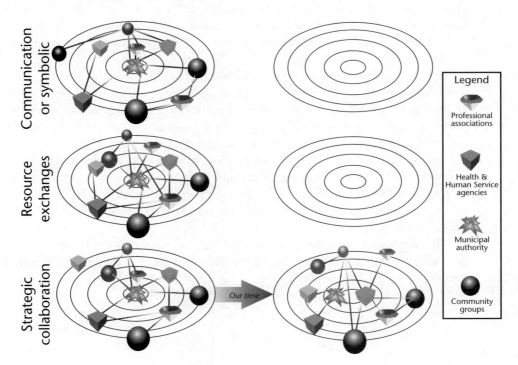

Hoeijmakers (2004) argues that participants are involved in communication or symbolic networks, but at the same time have more peripheral roles in other functions of policy development, such as strategic collaboration ('where do I want to go, and who else do I need for that?') and resource exchange ('do I share knowledge with others? Do we subsidise community groups?'). The research discovered that policy entrepreneurial action in one type of network may change network composition. In Figure 14.2 a more central role in the network for health and human service agencies arose after community groups and a health and human service agency (in this case social work) moved closer to local authority in their communication/symbolic network. As a result, responsibility for strategic collaboration to develop healthy public policy became shared between the municipality and social work. This might presumably have an impact on the capacity of the network to build healthy public policy.

SUMMARY

We make a distinction between the grand project of healthy public policy and narrower activities such as health policy and health care policy. The complexity and apparently chaotic features of healthy public policy cannot be understood as linear and technocratic approaches to solving problems. Linear, technocratic processes appeal to policy-keepers who seek to keep off the policy agenda such ideas as collective values and consideration of social determinants of health. Linear frameworks are consistent with easily measured behavioural and educational approaches to health promotion, relegating social determinants to the margins of the main agenda.

Instead, the possibilities for the intersectoral health promoter are boundless, as health promoters embark on the task of analysing complex social phenomena and act as social entrepreneurs, mapping, influencing, and creating networks for health gain. Modern theories of policy-making emphasise connectedness, cyclical, iterative, incremental changes towards windows of opportunity that inevitably involve participation in, analysis and manipulation of, and development of new networks. A crucial role for health promoters is to work with communities to help unlock their capacity so they can take part in the networks that allocate values, determine the general course of policy, and thereby change the way health promotion works.

In conclusion, we draw on Hancock (1990) to summarise the complex and demanding competencies that health promoters require if they are involved in advocating for healthy public policy.

Box 14.4: What is needed to advocate for healthy public policy

1 **Take a long-term view.** We need to learn the lessons of history so that changes of the magnitude we are discussing here do not occur swiftly.

2 **Secure political commitment.** Since public policies require political action, it is essential to secure as much political commitment as possible early on and to maintain it; where it is lost, healthy public policy will also be lost.

3 **Establish intersectoral processes and structures.** These may consist of new government structures or quasi-formal multisectoral structures involving politicians, bureaucrats, non-government organisations, community members, quasi-autonomous councils, and academic centres.

4 **Seek public support.** This requires establishing 'activist credentials' with the community, being responsive to the community, and ensuring good public relations are established and maintained.

5 **Develop a community-driven process.** People will 'speak for themselves', undertake community self-reports on health, identify community challenges to health in a variety of ways.

6 **Adopt multifaceted strategies.** There is no simple approach to healthy public policy, and public policies must address the challenges to health in variety of ways.

7 **Be credible.** Initiators and activists must be credible, have expertise in the area, and must have staff and resources to develop and implement healthy public policy initiatives.

8 **Aim for win/win solutions.** Rather than establishing confrontations that result in win/lose situations, coalitions are an important way of fashioning win/win solutions.

9 **Change organisational culture.** Healthy public policy is a dramatic departure from the old way of doing things that requires a new culture of organisational management and policy-making.

10 **Use health as a metaphor for broader human goals.** Health may be a useful metaphor for addressing issues such as social injustice and environmental deterioration.

Source: Adapted from Hancock 1999

15 HEALTH PROMOTION POLICY ANALYSIS

Helen Keleher

Key concepts

- Understanding different forms of policy is a core competency for health promotion.
- Analysis of the political foundations of health promotion and public health policies will enable practitioners to more effectively advocate to influence policy change.
- Having the skills of analysis of public policy documents from health promotion perspectives is empowering.

Key terms

- Health promotion policy
- Public policy
- Organisational policy
- Policy for advocacy

INTRODUCTION

Public policy is central to the promotion of health—after all, the building of healthy public policy has been a central tenet of public health and health promotion since the 1980s. Because policy is so critical for health advancement endeavours of governments and organisations, skills for analysing and understanding policy are, therefore, essential for health promotion and public health practitioners.

Indeed, whole courses can be taken for those who wish to study policy in some depth to develop skills for working in government and non-government sectors. Here, you will be introduced to some of the key elements of policy analysis.

In Chapter 14, you will have found discussion about the distinguishing features of policies *for* health and policies *of* health. To follow that discussion, this chapter sets out the basic concepts for the analysis of public policy for the promotion of health. The chapter is organised in two parts. The first part of the chapter is a brief overview of the main political drivers for health policy, and while you might ask why you need to know about the politics of health, my aim is to facilitate your understanding of why public health and health promotion practitioners need to have a working knowledge of the political thinking that steers funding and systems. Nonetheless, you may wish to skip over this to the sections that set out basic skills in policy analysis. Then perhaps you will see the value in returning to the first part of the chapter! The overall intention of the chapter is to assist practitioners to gain understanding of the policies that guide their work, in order to make judgments about the quality of those policies, to recognise their explicit and implicit values, their structure and design and, thus, their purpose.

TYPES OF POLICY

Public policy

Policy is a fluid term that describes actions taken by public authorities to address a given problem or an interrelated set of problems (Pal 1997: 2). A policy is a general statement of intentions, with goals, objectives, and processes that culminate in an issue or situation being defined, redefined, or changed. Public policy is made by an appropriate authority in order to tackle problems, and should be made in the interest of all people but, from an equity perspective, health impact should be analysed, particularly the impact on vulnerable groups among the general population. Policies are sometimes called Strategies (as in National Health Strategy), or Action Plans (such as the National Action Plan for Alcohol) or Frameworks. Policies address public issues identified by governments as priorities for action, and the courses for action taken to address those issues. In other words, public policy-making is a process by which governments transform political vision into programs with the intention of change, and the delivery of outcomes.

Health policy has a social purpose in that it is developed from a recognition that for people to lead healthy, productive lives, there must be appropriate structural (i.e., political and economic), environmental, and social supports in place. In Australia, we have an expectation that health policy will be guided by a values framework link that includes:

- justice and fairness
- basic living standards for all people with a decent minimum income
- redistributive taxation (i.e. Medicare) and welfare support when people need it.

Health policy is an active field of interest, and health policy is consistently on electoral agendas. However, the policies most likely to be on electoral agendas are related to the illness care system, hospitals and medical services, rather than public health and health-promoting policies that have a much lower profile in political agendas and the minds of the voting public. What does this mean for health promotion activists trying to raise awareness of issues of social determinants of health, or inequities, or prevention?

Policies are dynamic and because they are part of regular cycles of change, they develop incrementally over time and in so doing, they tell a 'policy story'. For example, researchers and activists concerned with overweight populations have been very successful in constructing a policy story about physical activity and, to a lesser extent, about nutrition, in order to persuade politicians to put these issues on their agendas. As a result, considerable funds have been committed to campaigns and programs to address physical activity, nutrition, and overweight populations. Advocates arguing for a broader approach to people's health and well-being, to link social–structural factors to issues of overweight populations, have been less successful in getting their policy story across to the media and politicians.

Policy for advocacy

Public policy should not be confused with policies for advocacy, which are developed as a lobbying tool by interest groups or non-government organisations. Yet, while public policy is usually made within government processes, it is not normally made in isolation from interest groups. There are active policy communities, usually organised around a theme, such as a disease (HIV/AIDS, hepatitis C or multiple sclerosis), or they might have a broad representative scope, such as the Australian Nursing Federation (ANF) or the Australian Medical Association (AMA), which represent nurses' and doctors' interests, or the Public Health Association of Australia (PHAA), to which members belong because they have interests in promoting and advancing public health issues.

Many of these groups are very active in the development of policy positions. For example, the PHAA has a comprehensive set of policies (available at <www.phaa.net.au>), which are essentially position statements endorsed by the members. Other non-government organisations with comprehensive policies are the Australian Council of Social Services (ACOSS), the ANF, and the AMA. Such policies are used for lobbying and advocacy but because they are developed in the non-government sector, those policies may have limited political power, although many could be said to carry a good deal of authoritative power. One of the limitations to the degree of power of any organisation is its political affiliations, so while its policies may be argued to be evidence-based and therefore authoritative they may be regarded with suspicion by governments who take into account the politics of the organisation.

The way in which interest groups and policy communities influence public policy and how they advocate for their interests was first analysed by Alford (1975) in terms of structural interests, corporate interests, repressed groups, and dominant groups. Theories to make sense of these groupings include pluralism and social structuralism.

Organisational policies

Governments and organisations develop policies, but policy should not be confused with administrative decision-making that results in protocols or guidelines for routine matters, quality assurance, or accreditation. Organisational policies are developed by organisations to govern matters such as:

- equal opportunity, staffing policies, diversity, anti-discrimination, bullying and harassment
- policies to guide practice such as health promotion or counselling services within community health services
- protocols such as those in hospitals for universal precautions or safe waste disposal.

POLITICAL IDEOLOGIES AND THEIR VALUES

Public policies are the creations of governments, and therefore they are imbued with values. Policies allocate values and are driven by the values of the political party or public authority that has designed the policy. Broadly, health policy is made by the political party in power and all political parties develop their positions in health either to guide policy (if the party in power) or influence policy development.

Values are derived from differing political beliefs (or ideologies) that steer government action (or inaction) and although some values may seem to transcend politics, such as the needs of those whose health is the worst or most vulnerable, value positions arise from political ideologies about how to address those problems. Political ideologies broadly arise from notions of the modern welfare state and capitalism and how they shape societies and government action. The links between them are critical for what approaches will be developed in health policy.

Welfarism and capitalism

The welfare state is an instrument of capitalist societies that has arisen primarily since the end of World War II, both to rebuild Western economies and national identities and as a response to social needs. In Australia, those social needs included, for example, pensions for war widows, and the aged pension. These social needs are not able to be provided by the private sector, as Teeple (2000) explains:

> (The welfare state is) a capitalist society in which the state has intervened in the form of social policies, programs, standards, and regulations in order to mitigate class conflict and to provide for, answer, or accommodate certain social needs for which the capitalist mode of production in itself has no solution or makes no provision (Teeple 2000: 15).

The aims of welfare policies are multiple, including the provision of sufficient income to enable people without employment to afford housing, food, and other basic necessities. Another intention of welfare policy is a more equitable distribution of income and wealth through progressive tax reforms. The introduction of Australia's universal health insurance (Medicare) was a progressive tax reform and a classic type of redistributive policy. The Medicare levy is collected through taxation and effectively transfers economic resources (hospital and medical care) to those who have least economic resources. In summary, welfarism describes the belief that governments have responsibility for the care and welfare of its citizens that cannot be entrusted to the private sector. Value is placed by welfarists on taxation and investment by government in structures that bring direct benefit to people.

Esping-Andersen (1990) has developed a typology of capitalist welfare states, illustrating the degree to which they support welfarism:

- Social Democratic (SD) states have high levels of government intervention— examples include the Scandinavian countries of Sweden, Norway, Finland, and Denmark. Social democratic political parties typically have greater trade union density than Liberal or Conservative Nations, greater expenditure on social security, and higher employment levels.
- Liberal Nations (LN) favour residual welfare systems—examples include the USA, UK, Canada, and Australia.
- Conservative Nations (CN) fall midway between SD and LN states— examples include France, Italy, and Germany.

Social-structuralism and neoliberalism

Within these capitalist–welfare states, there are two dominant political positions that are usually in tension:

- *Social-structuralism*—which sees that the individual does not exist in isolation of wider social influences and determinants, such as wealth distribution, education, employment opportunities, and racial conditions, and sees health status as a profound indicator of social position, especially of social disadvantage. Therefore, solutions to policy problems must be grounded in social and structural reform. Welfarists (who are akin to social structuralists) believe that governments should protect people against poverty and the extremes of market economies and economic rationalism.
- *Neoliberalism*—arises from laissez-faire or neoclassical economics and has a strong emphasis on individualism. Neoliberalists place great faith in the power of markets and see that what is in the interests of the private individual ends up being for the good of society. Neoliberalists believe that a free market is the best mechanism for efficiency and see it as providing necessary freedoms for individuals to pursue personal goals within a competitive environment.

The different kinds of states are, of course, subject to variations as their major political parties are elected to government, and then create their own social and economic policies, often under the banner of 'reform'. In doing so, governments create their own identities.

The health policies of political parties all reflect party ideologies. Each political party decides its policy focus and policy processes, and the advice it will accept or reject from consultation with communities, paid advisers, or non-government organisations. The policies of major parties demonstrate their orientation to public health and health promotion towards understanding the health of individuals and populations, as influenced by wider social forces. Remember, though, that many election campaign policies of political parties are policies for advocacy—and there is no guarantee, even if that party is elected, that the policy will be enacted.

Tensions typically arise between social-structuralists and individualism, and between those who support higher levels of government intervention and those who do not. Nevertheless, since the 1980s, Australia has experienced a rapid transformation from a welfarist to a corporatist-driven, market state.

Health policy in the market state

Traditionally, public service goals were about due process, democratic principles, equity, and service delivery. Since the late 1980s, governments have restructured the public sector and changed governance styles towards theories and models of the private sector—managerialism and corporatism. There is new emphasis on economic efficiency and performance indicators, and inputs/outputs (Considine 1997). Chapter 12 explains this history in more detail.

In today's modern market economy, strategic policy-making methods are created within the context of 'economic rationalism' and 'managerialism', both of which have an enormous effect on the direction of policy. Strategic policy-making methods include the creation of competition or competitive markets (including 'internal' markets in health), program budgeting, and a 'product' orientation. These are all concepts taken from the private or corporate sector, and adapted to the health system.

Corporatism is increasingly prominent in health policy as links are acknowledged between government, industry, private interests, and labour markets. Large and often multinational corporate businesses have become key interest groups: governments now negotiate directly with corporate health business interests including the private health insurance industry, pharmaceutical companies, and nursing home operators.

Key questions to ask include:

■   What is the government's role in policy?
■   Should a government 'steer' the policy ship or 'propel' it?
■   What is the 'public good'?

- New discourse that governments should decide and manage from a distance, rather than directly provide (referees rather than coaches).
- Focus on outcomes rather than process.
- Opening up of government 'business' to the market and, thus, to competition.

Policy and health inequalities

As discussed in Chapter 4, deepening social and health inequalities in most developed countries since the 1990s and into the twenty-first century are the result of the failure of governments to respond effectively to emerging social, health, and economic problems. The dominance of market economies has demanded greater efficiencies, accountability, and rationing of government programs. The simultaneous rise of markets with insatiable demand for increasing levels of competition is apparent in both private and public sectors. Yet deepening social and health problems suggest the need for increased access to both welfare benefits and government programs by vulnerable groups in order to tackle inequities. *Universalism* and *residualism* are both proposed as solutions to redressing inequalities.

Universalism is the provision of universal services, available to the whole population. Maternal and Child Health Services are a good example of a universal service—they are available to all new mothers, at no cost. However, universalism is often debated by residualists. A good example of the discourses about universalism is the story of Medicare (see Scotton 2000, and <www.phaa.net.au> for Medicare Fact Sheets that tell a 'policy story'). Medicare provides universal access to a decent minimum of sick care and basic hospital and medical care and the Pharmaceutical Benefits Scheme. But cost containment of hospital and medical services is sought through a range of measures, one of which is rationing.

The discourse of residualism is linked to the neoliberal critique of welfarism. Residualists believe in a contained role of the public sector (steering not rowing, purchasing not providing), and the provision of safety nets only for the very poor, indigent, and for limited periods, and often with conditions attached. What results from these reforms to welfare benefits is a residual welfare state.

However, Gardner (1997) argues that economic rationalism is not just about cost cutting, it also about effectiveness, best practice, competencies, standards, codes of conduct, benchmarking, and outcomes. Nonetheless, we should not take those goals at face value, but look more deeply at the policy's intentions and its value base because policy-making methods can be used as tools to reduce the public sector, and increase privatisation of the provision of services. This has been referred to as governments that are 'steering not rowing', whereby governments no longer see themselves as in the business of direct service delivery but have changed their modus operandi to be the outsourcer of services, with governments steering courses of action through their role of contract management.

WHO DOES WHAT ... LEVELS OF GOVERNMENT RESPONSIBILITY FOR HEALTH POLICY

In order to contribute to the shaping of health policy, it is necessary for public health and health promotion practitioners to grasp the different responsibilities of the different levels of government. These responsibilities necessarily involve the development of health policy, the development of services, and the implementation of policy through service delivery.

In Australia, there are three levels of government—Local Government Authorities (LGAs), six state and two territory governments, and the federal government—each with their own jurisdiction, or ability to make laws. All levels of government have health policy responsibilities through policy and planning units and processes. Some of those policy responsibilities are summarised in Table 15.1.

Table 15.1   Government levels of health policy responsibility in Australia

FEDERAL GOVERNMENT	LEVELS OF RESPONSIBILITY	TYPICAL HEALTH POLICIES
Main bureaucracy is Department of Health and Ageing <www.health.gov.au> Administers health responsibilities especially health insurance—Medicare (public) (administered by the Health Insurance Commission (HIC)) and private health insurance Provides advice to the Minister for Health	Policies about Medicare e.g. General Practitioner rebates, public hospital funding to states/territories Pharmaceutical Benefits Scheme ■ Approvals of drugs listed by the PBS; ■ Level of subsidy ■ Cost to consumers of prescriptions ■ Aged care Nursing homes and home nursing organisations including Home and Community Care (HACC) Subsidies for family planning and blood transfusion services (mainly through Red Cross) Food safety—e.g. GM foods, labelling of products National Health Priorities: <www.aihw.gov.au/nhpa/index.cfm>	■ National Action Plan for Promotion, Prevention and Early Intervention for Mental Health ■ National HIV/AIDS Strategy ■ National Injury Prevention Action Plan ■ National Asthma Action Plan ■ National Drug Strategic Framework ■ National Alcohol Campaign ■ Environmental Tobacco Smoke in Australia ■ Eat Well Australia: a National Framework for Action in Public Health Nutrition ■ Developing an Active Australia ■ National Environmental Health Strategy

(Continued)

Table 15.1 *(Continued)*

State/territory governments	Levels of responsibility	Some state/territory health policies
Each state/territory government has a Department that develops policy, administers funding, and provides advice to state/territory Minister for Health States/territories provide 80 per cent of costs of running hospitals and are concerned with bed numbers, staffing, capital works, quality, community-based services, workforce development, health programs, public dental health, health information systems	Disease control and health protection Epidemiological surveillance systems, identification of public health issues, intervention and monitoring of outcomes (e.g. communicable diseases such as legionella, tuberculosis, measles) Drugs and poisons Emergency responses (e.g. floods, fires, bioterrorism) Health promotion Immunisation, maternal and child health (funded by state, adminstered by LGAs) School health, dental screening	■ Active for Life Victorian Physical Activity Strategy ■ State framework for Alcohol ■ Nutrition Monitoring and Surveillance in Victoria: a Framework for Action ■ Promoting Oral Health 2000–2004 ■ Mental Health Promotion Plan
Local Government Authorities	**Levels of responsibility**	**Typical LGA health policies**
All LGAs have departments for developing local policy and by-laws, administration of programs and local development.	Legislative responsibility for administration of *Food Act 1984* (Cwlth) Administered through Environmental Health Officers—food premises, food production, food selling Environmental health, including cultural, community and recreational development Environmental hazards Provision of community services—youth, aged care (HACC—meals on wheels, home maintenance etc Land-use planning Roads, drains, footpaths	■ Food safety policy ■ Food for All policy ■ Community health and safety policy ■ Drug and alcohol policy

POLICY DESIGN

While policy design is an imprecise science, there is a series of steps and processes that contributes to a policy result that has both quality and integrity of purpose (Palmer & Short 2000). The steps include (broadly):

- problem definition
- consultation with policy actors and policy communities
- clear statements of intentions, aims, and objectives
- decisions about policy instruments
- implementation planning
- evaluation planning.

Other considerations in the policy development process include:

- the strength of the evidence
- political priorities
- community considerations
- amenability of the problem/s to intervention.

The following is a brief summary of each of the steps in policy development, but to gain a depth of understanding, you will need to read more widely—the references provided are a guide to your further reading.

Problem definition

Problem definition is about how health issues become the subject of public concern or gain the attention of policy-makers and the role of media, lobby groups, and other parties in policy processes. Problem definition gives rise to complex issues for bureaucracies and governments. The policy context of the twenty-first century is infinitely more complex than in the past. There is very little 'new' government money, so if a Department identifies a problem it must also identify a funding solution. This is similar in community-based agencies. So how priorities are set, and how problems are defined and get onto the agenda of some organisation or government Department, are of key interest to health promotion, or public health, practitioners.

Further, the media may play a dominant or negative, even an obstructive role in focusing attention on a narrow tunnel view of policy rather than a structural upstream approach. Structuralist perspectives view the state as acting in the interests of society as a collective while individually focused downstream approaches tend to see individuals as always personally responsible, if not 'blameworthy'.

Problems are not always able to be clearly defined because they can be stubborn and hard to resolve. Change can often only be incremental because of the political sensitivities of radical change; many problems are defined by prevailing norms, beliefs, and values either of government and/or community (for example, neoliberalism, socio-structuralism, welfarism, universalism etc). Because of these complexities, non-decisions may result in relation to a problem.

It can be mystifying to see a new policy idea being launched in the media or by a politician. To help understand the agenda behind a new policy problem, questions that you might ask include:

- Why has the issue arisen now?
- How did this situation arise?
- Who is affected by this issue and why?
- What are stakeholder views?
- Is there international data that suggests trends/trajectories for this issue?
- Can the problem be disaggregated?
- What programs/policies already exist in related fields? Are they working?
- If not, why not?
- Whose problem is it? And is it a problem that requires intersectoral action?
- Are the policy solutions put forward of sufficient scope to adequately address the problem?

Policy drivers can be internal, such as those arising from party political platforms or from Ministerial or governmental changes. External policy drivers (those outside government or political parties) include media attention, opinion polls, demographic shifts, and international relations.

Consultation with policy actors and policy communities

In reality, governments/local agencies have limited internal policy capacity and often just a few staff working on quite large problems. High levels of accountability and rigorous policy development are demanded by media and sometimes, but not always, by the electorate. Thus, the bringing in of expertise augments the policy capacity of internal government departments. Policy analysis is also sometimes conducted unofficially by think tanks who could be either supporters or opponents of the policy.

Consultation is linked to notions of participation because consultation facilitates forms of citizen/consumer participation in policy development.

Consultation can be characterised in various ways: it may be seen as top-down, where the information flow is one-way; there may be a use of key contacts, include meetings with interest groups and the circulation of proposals with invitation to comment and public hearings; partnership models may be developed with Advisory Committee mechanisms, inclusion of policy communities and peak bodies (which may not be so much a 'partnership' as a 'mechanism' for getting a consultation happening); or a delegation model that includes public inquiries (include Royal Commissions) and formal commission of evaluations and assessments.

Questions to ask of any consultation process include:

- Who is included in consultation processes and who is being excluded?
- Who is being represented and do they represent a wide range of views?
- Are both organised groups and unorganised 'publics' included?

- Are there attempts to 'reach' into communities?
- Are decent periods allowed for consultation and how are submissions made?

Consultation overload commonly occurs within community organisations especially if they are unfunded and rely on volunteers. So while the non-government sector may be relied upon to provide the views of various 'publics', if those NGOs do not have the capacity among their scarce resources to develop submissions, to fund their own travel to attend meetings (which are often in Canberra), then the consultation processes are weakened and those well-funded groups who receive government subsidies have greater opportunities to put their views on the table.

Why consult?

Consultation is a democratic process that provides for accountability from government. Transparency is another major reason for consultation. The electorate is often wary of secrecy in policy development, which may be regarded with suspicion by communities of interest. Any policy is likely to have enhanced legitimacy if stakeholders have a degree of ownership. Consultation also gathers in expertise and broadens the input to the processes involved, and consultation helps to gain stakeholder support for the policy.

The politics of consultation include suspicions that consultation can be used to 'structure' or control debate. This can be frustrating for the bureaucracy or stakeholders outside the bureaucracy. Policy 'control' can be delegated—including to the private sector. There is, therefore, often a need to design a consultation process that is acceptable to policy communities.

Statements of intentions, aims, and objectives

- *Policy aims* are broad qualitative statements that are general statements of intent. They narrow the process from broad global thinking to specific actions that might be listed as expressions of desired *outcomes* or *processes*. Policy aims should be distinct and generate their own objectives.
- *Policy objectives* elaborate and restate the goals *in operational terms*. They are more specific and concrete statements of the changes that are expected to occur as a result of the policy—in other words, they are statements of what the policy is meant to achieve. Objectives may be implicit rather than explicit in policies. When analysing a policy, it is useful to first look for its aims and objectives, and if they are not expressly written in this form, look for statements of intention. They will give you a sense of the scope of the policy, its understanding of the problems the policy is meant to address, and its approaches towards addressing those problems.

Policy instruments and approaches to implementation

Policy instruments are the technical means of achieving a policy goal. Policy-makers choose the most appropriate instruments to deal with the policy problem in order to achieve their goals. Instruments might include cash grants, pricing (e.g. tobacco and alcohol), price controls (e.g. petrol), tax breaks, administered contracts, and rationing (e.g. hospital waiting lists) (Bridgman & Davis). Box 15.1 below illustrates a range of policy instruments put forward in response to a debate about housing policy.

Box 15.1: Inquiry into cost of housing: policy alternatives: the solutions and their problems

■ **Remove negative gearing**: Advocated to curb property investors. Negative gearing enables the investor to rent out property at a loss and to claim the loss against other income, saving tax. When it was briefly removed in the 1980s, rents surged.

■ **Cut state stamp duty**: Supporters include the federal Treasurer, the HIA, and the Real Estate Institute. But states argue that stamp duty pays for hospitals, schools, and so on. The fear is that if stamp duty is cut, the saving will simply push property prices up, and cut government services.

■ **Raise first home owner's grant**: The Treasurer, Peter Costello says the $7000 grant has helped 482,000 people into their first homes. But the benefits were largely dissipated in higher housing prices.

■ **Boost land supply**: More land, especially for detached housing, eases demand. But Melbourne's boundary has been set.

■ **Equity finance**: It splits the cost of a property between the buyer and a financial institution. But it is hard to make this scheme work commercially.

Source: *The Age*, 2 August 2003: 2

Note that way the policy options are put briefly, with 'pros' and 'cons' to allow the reader to weigh up the alternatives.

Evaluation

Policy evaluation is managed and conducted on similar principles to program evaluation—public policy may be more about accountability for performance as well as outcomes, i.e., measurement of success and whether objectives were met, what might be done to improve impact, and so on. Policy evaluation is conducted officially by governments but they often outsource to private companies or universities.

There are different forms of evaluation such as:

- public inquiries: e.g. deaths in custody
- program reviews (ongoing, mid-term, end of program).

Evaluation reports may or may not be made publicly available, and within them there can be a blurring of policy analysis/policy evaluation. Public policy evaluation has political sensitivities as no government or its Departments want to hear bad news, while evaluation may seen as less important than designing and implementing solutions to public policies, resulting in funding not always being sufficient for decent evaluation.

Yet, there are some imperatives for policy evaluation. Accountability is increasingly demanded, with questions asked by the electorate or policy communities about what was spent—did the taxpayer get the most out of the process and resulting policy? There are also fiscal pressures with very little new money available for policy implementation. Evaluation is a component of good governance, the monitoring and assessment of outsourced (contracted) government services, and assessing of service quality levels.

Managerialism has brought increasing levels of contracting for policy evaluation, arising from an interest in better reporting of performance and measuring results. Contracts are both a tool for monitoring and compliance, which are forms of evaluation. Evaluation is still used more as a management tool than for actual health and social outcomes of government policy.

Difficulties with policy evaluation:

- isolating causal factors and effects is not easy—policy just one of many
- methodological issues for large public programs are complex
- policy can need process, impact, and outcome evaluations as well as cost-benefit
- cost-benefit analysis is not always feasible, and there is often a need to include organisational analysis as policies seek to change the way organisations think, operate, deliver, e.g. health promotion
- policy is an intervention that depends on some idea of causal connection that may not be measureable
- the evaluation may be complicated by politics!

POLICY ANALYSIS

Policy analysis is about evaluating a policy document, or a set of policy documents/proposals, which is either implemented or proposed. Policy analysis is a search for facts, logic, interpretations, political positions and values, feasibility, and process. Good policy analysis requires understanding of:

- benefits and costs of implementation
- alternatives (including the status quo) and the kind of outcomes they might yield
- paradigms: economic and political philosophies and positions

Policy critique seeks to identify the argument or the claims of the policy 'story' and the values on which it is based, the politics of this policy, and how the policy sits within the context of political and institutional systems. A policy critique needs to understand the political field(s) of interest, and then ask reflective questions such as:

(a)   What is my position? Do I share the belief system behind the policy?
(b)   Why has this policy emerged (in political terms) at this time?

When does policy analysis occur?

Policy analysis is often done concurrently with policy development. So questions being asked by those developing the policy include:

- What are our options?
- What is our position?
- What outcomes do we want to achieve?
- What are the likely outcomes of the proposed policy?
- What are the alternatives (one of which might be to maintain the status quo), and what kind of outcomes might result?
- On what criteria can policy options be compared?

Or if your analysis is retrospective, questions to ask include:

- Is this a good policy? Why? Why not?
- What was its intent and was that intent achieved?
- Can you predict an unfolding of a political dynamic? If so, what is it?
- Are you able to predict future policy developments or related scenarios?
- Does it make sense? Is it logical? Is it factual?

Does rationalism result in better decisions?

Perhaps one way to answer this question is to consider if you would use a rational model to decide a marriage partner! This illustrates that decisions actually require a balance of rationalism and reasoning but the art of policy is to assess what is the place of wisdom, experience, and intuition as well as evidence and hard-nosed political considerations. The rational model has strong concerns with efficiency (greatest results for least cost). Truly rational policy-making is exhaustive of all evidence and ALL options so it can be seen as radical but it rarely occurs in a pure form.

The incremental model assumes the rational model is unrealistic because it sees that policy is made in small steps and that change is usually the result of small regular policy adjustments. Incremental policy tends to be more amenable to politically safe, expedient, and practical policy decisions than the rational model, often using limited information, and tends to conservatism—which is common to all political parties.

Post-positivist models are critical of both rational and incremental models and their emphasis on facts and values. They emphasise the importance of conceptual frameworks, language, and the construction of reality through the policy 'story' or 'narrative'.

POLICY ANALYSIS CRITERIA

There is no definitive 'list' of criteria that an analyst might use to analyse a policy so the following summary will give you guidance in coming up with your own set of criteria. Broadly, policy analysis criteria are based on *values, interests, resources, context, institutions, and politics.* In any analysis, there will be more to say about some of these criteria than others. So you might ask of a policy: what are its value positions? Are they explicit or implicit? Is the problem narrowly defined in terms of health promotion, or does it promote a larger, more intersectoral, and multilevel vision? What are its economic implications? What processes were used to develop the policy? What was the influence of interest/pressure groups or professional bodies involved? Has the policy been evaluated and with what result?

Case Study 15.1: Proposed maternity leave policy for staff

One of the objectives of this chapter is to assist you to develop skills in policy analysis. This case study provides an opportunity for you to construct a framework of analysis, via the development of policy analysis criteria.

The following is adapted from a sample framework by Palmer & Short (2000: 25-7). Hancock (1999: 22–4) also has policy analysis criteria. There is no definitive 'list' of criteria that one might use to analyse a policy—you need to come up with your own set of criteria but the material here will give you guidance.

First, read the short document on Paid Maternity Leave in Australia: HREOC's Valuing Parenthood, by Marian Baird, University of Sydney, available at: <**www. econ.usyd.edu.au/drawingboard/digest/0206/baird.html**>. Then work through the following questions and, in the process, you will start to work out what questions you want to ask of the policy and how you might construct your own set of key criteria.

CRITERIA/QUESTIONS	YOUR RESPONSES
Identify relevant frameworks	
What different values and ideologies might guide policy development?	
What is the role of the state in providing benefits for new mothers?	

(Continued)

CRITERIA/QUESTIONS	YOUR RESPONSES
Who are the main stakeholders?	
Approaches: does the policy include a corporatist approach, where business interests are represented? Or do structuralism or welfarism dominate?	
In what ways is maternity leave policy a political issue?	
What/who might be the vested interests in maternity leave policy?	
Who and what were might be the influences on the policy development process?	
Who would be the policy-makers?	
What might be the stages and methods in the policy-making process? Who would/should be consulted? Who would not be consulted?	
What considerations about feasibility would be considered for a policy on maternity leave?	

SUMMARY

So what does all this mean for you? You need to be:

- aware of policies that influence your work (big picture)
- engaged in conversations about policy—and understand the implications of divergent and convergent views
- involved in networks
- involved in representative committees
- taking opportunities to become involved in policy development
- recognising your strengths, becoming familiar with the tools and using them
- operating with integrity.

Policy skills are not only relevant at political levels—the rules apply whether influencing policy in a school canteen, or in your own organisation. Think about an occasion when you have been close to policy or reflect on an occasion when you could have been closer. I hope you will see that policy is not dull—it has high stakes with large impacts, hence health promotion practitioners need to be in there to make a difference.

USEFUL WEBSITES

There are many policy think tank websites. Some analyse public policy, others are more focused on policy advocacy.

Australian Council of Social Services: <www.acoss.org.au>

Australian Medical Association: <www.ama.com>

Australian Nursing Federation: <www.anf.org.au>

National Aboriginal Community Controlled Organisations: <www.naccho.org.au>

Public Health Association of Australia: <www.phaa.net.au>

Royal Australasian College of Physicians: <www.racp.org.au>

16

BUILDING COMPETENCIES AND WORKFORCE CAPACITY FOR HEALTH PROMOTION

Helen Keleher & Nerida Joss

Key concepts

- Competency frameworks provide structure and uniformity to workforce capacity-building in health promotion.
- Learning about competencies and capacity-building assists practitioners to shape and determine their own career directions and to facilitate the development of colleagues within organisations.
- Reflective practitioners are able to identify the theories (knowledge) and skills that underpin effective health promotion practice.
- Reflective and effective practitioners understand what competent skills and knowledge are required to enhance health, well-being, and quality of life.
- More advanced practitioners employ strategies to build competencies and capacity with their organisations to explicitly enhance/release the capacity of staff, organisations, and communities.

Key terms

- Health promotion competencies
- Workforce capacity-building

OVERVIEW

The building of competencies for health promotion among the workforce is essential for the growth of health promotion as a discipline and for its practitioners to be increasingly effective as social change agents. Health promotion competencies are useful for staff recruitment and selection, staff development, strategic development, training courses, and quality improvement programs (Health Promotion Forum of New Zealand 2000). Throughout this book, including many of the guidebooks, there are references to skills and knowledge for health promotion but in this chapter we provide summary detail of both the Australian and New Zealand competencies. This allows you to compare and contrast different approaches to framing health promotion competencies and will help to broaden your thinking about approaches taken to framing the skills and knowledge that graduates and practitioners require. Indeed, it is useful for both students and those already employed to have an understanding of what competencies are required for successful practice and to reflect on what additional skills and knowledge you need to acquire in order to contribute to improving health, well-being, and quality of life.

WORKFORCE CAPACITY-BUILDING

In Chapter 3, capacity-building was reviewed as a key strategy for the advancement of health promotion. An important component of capacity-building frameworks is the development of sustainable skills in the workforce, which occurs through incidental learning, informal learning, and formal learning or training programs (NSW Health 2001). Fundamental to workforce capacity-building is the view that health promotion arises from a confident, skilled workforce, based on teams who work across the organisation and in partnerships with other organisations and communities.

Workforce capacity-building incorporates notions of leadership and strengthening of existing capabilities. Leadership is critical for the advancement of health promotion, at both the level of the Board and management team, as well as within staff teams, which allows for a shared understanding of the organisation's health promotion goals and strategies including the resources required.

Keleher and Marshall (2003) found that the elements of workforce capacity development could usefully be understood by the organisation in terms of best practice components that, in turn, provide outcomes for the organisation. These are summarised in Table 16.1:

Table 16.1 Workforce capacity development components and outcomes

BEST PRACTICE COMPONENTS	OUTCOMES
Capacity-building goals for workforce are included in the organisation's Strategic Plan and the HP Strategic Workplan	Recognition of value of skilled health promotion workforce
Staff audit is periodically conducted to identify particular health promotion skills and gaps	Assists workforce development plans Builds skills across organisation; promotes sustainability and quality; builds commitment to health promotion as staff confidence grows
Identify skill development opportunities such as gender and diversity training, research and evaluation, submission writing—work across regions or clusters of community health services to share resources for training in health promotion skills	Efficiency and quality in work practices
Encourage sharing of skills across multidisciplinary teams and systems of recognition at the highest level in the organisation	Efficient use of resources; sharing knowledge and skills Encourages staff to extend their practice Builds understanding at management and Board level of what integrated, multidisciplinary health promotion practice can achieve
Identify particular staff for advanced health promotion skill training Establish team leaders to take greater leadership, e.g. in identifying workforce development initiatives such as internal schemes for mentoring, information sharing, and self-directed learning	Provides leadership for complex, integrated health promotion Increases capacity of staff to influence change
Provide opportunities for staff to promote their health promotion achievements and showcase health promotion programs to Boards of Management, audits and reviews	Demonstrate that health promotion effort is recognised; provide opportunities for staff to demonstrate the effectiveness of health promotion that staff feel is undervalued and unrecognised

Source: Keleher & Marshall 2003

COMPETENCIES

Competencies define skills and knowledge that are generic to a discipline or profession. Competency frameworks bring these together to provide work-related standards to provide a benchmark of accepted skill, knowledge, and practice expected of practitioners—commonly thought of as agreed levels of performance (Health Promotion Forum of New Zealand 2000: 7). Competency frameworks also refer to outcomes: 'what people are able to do and also with the ability to do this, in a range of contexts' (NTIS 2006). They are often described as 'domains' of competence, with core competencies considered to be essential to the workforce of that discipline. Desirable competencies are often the skills and knowledge developed with experience. However, health promotion competencies are not just about the individual skills that each of us can have, but also about building competent systems and the capacity of organisations to respond to inequities, overcoming disadvantage, and so on.

Health promotion competencies

In this section, we present two sets of competencies: those from the Australian Health Promotion Association, and those of the New Zealand (NZ) Health Promotion Forum.

The Australian Health Promotion Association competencies in Table 16.2, comprise eight domains of technicality, and specific competencies under each of those domains.

Table 16.2 Australian Health Promotion Association competencies

NEEDS ASSESSMENT
(Carry out appropriate needs assessment)
**Obtain data on health needs of clients/communities/populations
**Identify behaviours that promote or compromise health of clients
**Analyse needs assessment data
*Determine priorities for health promotion
PLANNING
(Plan appropriate health promotion interventions)
**Involve clients/stakeholders in program-planning and evaluation
**Establish appropriate links and intersectoral collaboration
**Develop logical, sequenced health programs
**Formulate appropriate and measurable objectives
**Select and develop strategies
**Critically analyse literature
IMPLEMENTATION
(Implement appropriate health promotion interventions)
*Produce pamphlets, posters, and other audio-visual materials
*Carry out pre-testing procedures

(Continued)

Table 16.2 *(Continued)*

Organise sponsorships and fundraising
**Apply community development processes
Devolve programs to community
**Apply mass media strategies
**Apply group strategies
Apply individual contact strategies
Conduct health-related 'screening tests (health risk appraisals, cholesterol testing etc)
Provide health counselling to individuals
*Operate audiovisual equipment
*Produce educational packages
COMMUNICATION
(Communicate effectively with other professionals and clients)
**Write for professional audiences
*Write submissions/grants
*Write policy statements
**Write reports
Write for professional journals
**Write for lay audiences
**Write for newspapers
*Apply interviewee skills on radio
Apply interviewee skills on TV
**Communicate verbally and listen reflectively
*Apply role-play and drama to health education
*Speak to large groups
*Debate health-related issues
**Apply political advocacy skills
*Plan conferences
KNOWLEDGE
(Demonstrate appropriate knowledge necessary for conducting health promotion)
*Examine & apply knowledge of societal values in planning and implementing HP programs
**Conceptualise and operationalise components of health promotion, theories of health promotion (planning, evaluation, behaviour change, etc.), and learning theory
Apply knowledge of the structure and function of the human body to health issues and diseases
*Examine & synthesise information on different health issues/topics, diseases and prevention

KNOWLEDGE
*Apply knowledge of epidemiology to health issues
*Analyse the behavioural, political, and environmental influences on health
Examine and apply knowledge of the health care system
ORGANISATION AND MANAGEMENT
(Organise and manage health promotion interventions)
*Chair meetings
**Apply interpersonal skills (negotiation, teamwork, motivation, conflict resolution, decision-making, and problem-solving skills)
**Demonstrate leadership skills
**Demonstrate personal qualities (creativity, sensitivity, initiative, flexibility, cooperation, and professional integrity)
*Manage resources (time, funds, personnel, equipment)
Coordinate volunteers
**Liaise and collaborate with other professionals and organisations
*Organise and conduct in-service programs
*Conduct time management skills training
EVALUATION
(Evaluate health promotion)
*Select and apply assessment instruments
**Monitor programs and adjust objectives
**Interpret and report evaluation findings
*Apply and interpret statistical methods/analyses
*Choose appropriate evaluation designs
*Demonstrate use of computerised health information/resources
USE OF TECHNOLOGY
(Demonstrate the application of appropriate technology)
**Operate a PC—word processing, etc
**Create written/graphic presentation materials via PC
Manage database and spreadsheet applications
*Use computer-based statistical programs
Use computer software such as Endnote

** = Essential competency

* = Desirable competency

None = Optional competency

The NZ competency framework differs substantially from the Australian framework. The NZ framework comprises seven *knowledge-based* competency clusters and nine *skill-based* competency clusters.

For each level of the clusters, there are three levels of competence identified in this way:

■ At level 1, a health promoter will be able to:
■ At level 2, a health promoter will be able to demonstrate level 1 skills and in addition:
■ At level 3, a health promoter will be able to demonstrate level 2 skills and in addition:

We have not been able to include all the detailed competencies here for space reasons, because they are very comprehensive, but we encourage you to visit the website of the Health Promotion Forum of New Zealand to explore the detail for yourself. Health promotion practitioners will find these levels useful in understanding what might be expected of them in the workplace.

Knowledge-based clusters: The knowledge-based competencies, listed below, reflect learning from a variety of sources. They describe knowledge and theories from a range of social and behavioural sciences contributing to health promotion, while also recognising the learning accumulated by experienced health promoters in the field.

Skill clusters: Set out the skills that a health promotion worker needs to be a competent practitioner. The skills reflect ability acquired from a variety of sources. The skills might have been learnt as a result of formal training, as well as those that might have been developed on the job.

Table 16.3 Skill clusters of New Zealand health promotion competencies

1. Working with Indigenous people
Elements:
■ 1.1 Integrate the principles and provisions of Indigenous ways of knowing into health promotion practice
■ 1.2 Integrate Indigenous perceptions and realities of health into health promotion practice
■ 1.3 Consult Indigenous communities using appropriate processes
■ 1.4 Advocate by, with and for Indigenous health promotion practice
2. Program planning, implementation, and evaluation
Elements:
■ 2.1 Structure planning to achieve well-informed and sustainable programmes and services
■ 2.2 Work collaboratively when planning, implementing, and evaluating programmes
■ 2.3 Identify, use, and integrate a range of health promotion strategies
■ 2.4 Manage the expectations of a range of stakeholders

3. Contribute to the learning of others

Elements:

- 3.1 Deliver and enable learning in a range of contexts
- 3.2 Develop individual skills and knowledge
- 3.3 Develop group/community skills and knowledge
- 3.4 Train the trainers/educate the educators
- 3.5 Promote workforce development and training

4. Advocacy and political action

Elements:

- 4.1 Build intersectoral coalitions and strategic alliances
- 4.2 Inform, engage, and support community action
- 4.3 Influence local, national, and global decision-makers for healthy public policies
- 4.4 Proactively reorient health services to focus on well-being

5. Communication

Elements:

- 5.1 Communicate in written form and orally to suit a range of contexts and stakeholders
- 5.2 Develop media skills and engage the media
- 5.3 Identify and develop information and resources
- 5.4 Demonstrate an understanding of social marketing

6. Facilitation

Elements:

- 6.1 Facilitate group processes
- 6.2 Facilitate community processes
- 6.3 Acknowledge and mediate conflict

7. Research

Elements:

- 7.1 Critically analyse and disseminate relevant research and literature
- 7.2 Identify and employ a range of research approaches
- 7.3 Plan, conduct, and write up a research project

8. Professional development

Elements:

- 8.1 Critically reflect on and evaluate own work
- 8.2 Maintain professional knowledge and skills
- 8.3 Identify, develop, and maintain professional networks
- 8.4 Assist colleagues achieve professional growth

9. Health promotion management

Elements

- 9.1 Advocate for effective, healthy, and sustainable services
- 9.2 Promote and demonstrate sound health promotion principles and practice
- 9.3 Actively develop the health promotion workforce
- 9.4 Demonstrate strategic leadership

You will notice the NZ framework includes system-wide competencies including Maori health, which act as a guidance tool for workers, providing a benchmark for the level of skills, training, values, and beliefs needed in the discipline.

Table 16.4 Knowledge clusters of New Zealand health promotion competencies

KNOWLEDGE CLUSTER 1: History of Indigenous people

Elements:

- 1.1 Historical background and context
- 1.2 Content and meaning of Maori and English texts
- 1.3 Relevance and significance to both treaty partners

KNOWLEDGE CLUSTER 2: Cultural diversity

Elements:

- 2.1 Cultural awareness and responsiveness to the needs of tangata whenua
- 2.2 Cultural beliefs, norms and practices of different Pacific peoples
- 2.3 Cultural beliefs, norms and practices of Tauiwi

KNOWLEDGE CLUSTER 3: Origin and evolution of global health promotion

Elements:

- 3.1 Historical developments in health promotion philosophy and practice
- 3.2 Content, context, and significance of the Ottawa Charter
- 3.3 Current and ongoing developments and approaches
- 3.4 Relationship of health promotion to public health, health education, and disease prevention

KNOWLEDGE CLUSTER 4: Theory underpinning health promotion practice

Elements:

- 4.1 Models of health promotion practice
- 4.2 Models of empowerment and enablement
- 4.3 Diverse theories of learning
- 4.4 Group processes and dynamics

KNOWLEDGE CLUSTER 5: The health status of New Zealanders

Elements:

- 5.1 Wider determinants of health status and well-being
- 5.2 Lifestyle factors that influence health status and well-being
- 5.3 Major diseases contributing to ill health
- 5.4 Demography of health inequalities

KNOWLEDGE CLUSTER 6: Community and political awareness

Elements:

- 6.1 Community networks, agencies, and services
- 6.2 Range of information and resources available
- 6.3 Health systems and relevant structures in Aotearoa–New Zealand
- 6.4 Impact of local, national and global policies on health
- 6.5 Social movements and philosophies that influence social change

KNOWLEDGE CLUSTER 7: Research, planning, and evaluation

Elements:

- 7.1 Range of planning and evaluation approaches
- 7.2 Range of research methods
- 7.3 Ethical issues in research

SUMMARY

Competencies, capacity-building, and training are important elements in ensuring that health promotion practice is recognised for its complexity, comprehensive skill sets, and broad knowledge base. We believe that competency frameworks should be connected to an explicit value base, with a vision for ethical practice that is both generic to health promotion as well as being context-specific. For example, the framework profiled below, from the Health Promotion Forum of New Zealand (2000), combines globally accepted values for health promotion with values inherent to working in the unique context of Aotearoa–New Zealand and with Maori people. There is a real need in Australia for a similar competency framework that is specific about the competencies and values necessary for working with Aboriginal and Torres Strait Islander people.

USEFUL WEBSITES

Australian National Public Health Education Framework: <www.health.gov.au/internet/wcms/publishing.nsf/content/pherp-pdf-nphef-cnt.htm>. This site provides detailed competencies for public health practice developed by the Australian Network of Academic Public Health Institutions (ANA-PHI), 2002.

National Training Information Service: <www.ntis.gov.au>. This site provides comprehensive information about competencies for a very wide range of jobs, and levels of competence required for those jobs.

The Health Promotion Forum of New Zealand: <www.hpforum.org.nz/>. This site provides detail of the New Zealand health promotion competencies featured in this chapter.

17

REFLECTIVE PRACTICE

Anne Johnson & Colin MacDougall

Key concepts

- Upstream and intersectoral health promotion uses theory and practice that differs markedly from downstream interventions based in the health sector. These theories and practices are in early stages of development, so a reflective approach is likely to be the most effective way to approach teaching and learning.
- Learning about practice and transforming practice are key outcomes of critical reflection.
- It is essential to understand the literature on theories and processes of reflective practice.
- Reflective approaches can be part of formal studies, staff development, embedded in the culture of learning organisations, and an integral part of a practitioner's commitment to lifelong learning.

Key terms

- Reflective practice/critical reflection
- Technical reflection, practical reflection, emancipatory reflection
- Learning plans
- Mentors
- Experience + reflection = growth
- Instrumental learning, dialogic learning, self-reflective learning
- Distinguishing characteristics of critical reflection

OVERVIEW

Careers are funny things. Sometimes they are planned, most times they are serendipitous. We argue, however, that whether planned or accidental they should always be subject to reflection and critique. Otherwise, the result is not so much a 15-year career but one year fifteen times over: a career on automatic pilot flying over sectors without landing and getting to know them. We do not mean that the career should be planned with blinkers or tunnel vision, getting more and more technically focused without thinking laterally on how the world might be different. What we do argue is that modern health promotion provides a dilemma for careers and professional practice. Health promotion is frequently based within the health (or more accurately illness) sector with all the language, incentives, and disincentives that are part and parcel of those systems. The language speaks of health, illness, interventions, education, programs, early intervention, evidence, health gain etc etc. Earlier in this book we have seen ways in which there are policy, structural, and financial incentives for specialising in promoting particular lifestyle changes associated with specific diseases. There are structural and cultural disincentives for collaborating across sectors—especially with the 'determinants sectors' discussed in this book.

So it is not easy to work out what to do when we realise that we have to radically change our practices and work within and outside the health sector if we are going to make a difference to the fundamental social, economic, and cultural determinants of health and well-being. To take an example from this book, Chapter 12 by Paul Laris and Colin MacDougall critiques the role of organisations in favouring value-free and technocratic actions over deep-seated yet more messy discussions about philosophy and values. That chapter demonstrates the pitfalls faced by individuals trying to advocate for intersectoral action on the determinants of health. These dilemmas call for sustained and serious examination of our practice.

In this chapter we describe and discuss how reflective processes can be used to approach the intertwined problems of changing our practice and managing our careers, embedded as we are in organisations that so powerfully shape our destinies. We do this by exploring ways in which we can use reflective and practice-based learning to change what we do to make the reflective choice the easy choice within education and professional practice. We also address how to go about setting up and maintaining a reflective, career-long approach to practice improvement.

In the first part of the chapter we describe the rationale for, and how to engage in, reflective teaching and learning. In the second part we elaborate on theoretical and practical processes that we see as key to using critical reflection to change health promotion practice in line with upstream thinking.

PART 1: DOING REFLECTIVE TEACHING AND LEARNING

Why reflective practice?

The rationale for using reflective practice is that it provides opportunities for practitioners to demonstrate and deepen their understanding of theories and principles that underpin their practice, especially as it relates to health promotion; and re-evaluate their practice using critical reflection, appropriate theories, principles, concepts, and experience.

Paulo Freire's idea of authentic education is central, where people develop their power to perceive critically the way they exist in the world with which, and in which, they find themselves. This involves learning through doing, through problem posing, through testing solutions, and reflecting on their effectiveness. This therefore involves cycles of reflection and action. To do this, practitioners should identify the difficult areas of work practice (or intended future work practice) and develop a plan to develop skills in health promotion. Practitioners can start to formalise the process by developing a Learning Plan, where they identify an overall goal and a recommended five areas for skill development that will assist them in achieving this overall goal over a period of time.

As educators, mentors, managers, or concerned colleagues we are interested in seeing how practitioners are able to reflect on the way they work now, and how they would like to work in the future in order to be more effective.

The need for theory

Practitioners need a theoretical framework, and for some that framework against which they plan and assess their development will be primary health care principles, health promotion theory, and related theories. Therefore when goals, skill development areas, and strategies are listed, these must relate to what changes the practitioner wants to see in their practice. For example, if an analysis of their role and performance has highlighted the fact that they need to become more confident and skilled in taking a leadership role in primary health care or health promotion in their workplace, then they would identify the kinds of skills and knowledge they could further develop in this area. Mentors and colleagues assist them to identify these, and then as part of the evaluation process provide feedback on how they are progressing.

There are two important things to remember about reflective practice:

■ The journey is as important as the arrival. In other words, performance is assessed on ability to analyse issues and address them, on practitioners' willingness to be critically reflective and confront difficulties in their practice, whether or not they actually get to their final goal by the end of the available time. Therefore honesty is critical (and rewarded), especially when there are problems and they have not been able to achieve their goals.

■ Practitioners need to support their claims by reference to literature and examples. Reflective practitioners should use the literature, a reflective journal, records of meetings with mentors, feedback from colleagues and clients, and critical reflection to show where they started, how they developed, and where they have got to. These all aim to build a story of development, and a commitment to lifelong learning through critical reflection.

Box 17.1: The three stages of reflective teaching and learning

Stage 1: The development of a learning plan for reflection on health promotion practice

This involves the practitioner reflecting on their practice and career, and how they would like to further develop skills and knowledge in specific areas as follows:

- Identifying an overall goal
- Skill development areas to change practice
- How they are going to achieve this and by when
- How they are going to recognise that they have got there
- A process to identify a mentor (or mentors) and negotiate a mentoring agreement
- A framework for critical reflection
- A journal to record the critical reflection processes required to develop their learning plan.

Stage 2: Implementation of learning

This is the longest part of the process and is where the practitioner focuses on developing their skills, critically reflecting on the process, as well as incorporating other evaluation methods and reporting on progress.

Stage 3: Consolidation

In the final stage the practitioner reports on their work, using critical reflection, and feedback from mentors and colleagues as part of the evidence to support achieving their goal. They also utilise relevant theories, principles, and/or concepts to critique their findings.

Format for Developing a Reflective Learning Plan

Overall Learning Goal:

_____

_____

_____

AREAS FOR SKILL DEVELOPMENT	STRATEGIES	RESOURCES	TIMELINE	EVALUATION
(skills required to achieve overall goal)	*(things you can do to achieve the skills)*	*(people, literature etc.)*	*(plan for scheduling activities)*	*(how will you show you have achieved your areas of skill development)*

Source: Flinders University 2006

PART 2: THEORISING REFLECTIVE PRACTICE
Reflective practice

Reflective practice is about learning how to develop autonomous thinking, where practitioners learn how to make their own interpretations rather than act uncritically on the interpretations, ideas, beliefs, judgments, and feelings of others (Mezirow 1997). Developing autonomous thinking is really important for practitioners to move towards a frame of reference about practice that is more inclusive, discriminating, self-reflective, and integrative of experience (Mezirow 1997). Reflective practice is a fundamental component of adult learning and supports transformative learning, which is the process of effecting change in a practitioner's frame of reference (Mezirow 1997).

Reflection is a means of extending learning where new understandings and appreciations about practice can be acquired (Boud & Walker 1990), problems reframed (Schön 1983), and knowledge creation capacities developed (Ereut 1994). It is a way in which practitioners become aware of the much wider environment in which they operate. This includes power relationships in the organisation they work, and their networks.

Taylor (2000) states that reflection can be used for may purposes, depending on how and when it is done, by whom and why. She introduces three different categories (types) of reflection. These are technical, practical, and emancipatory reflection.

- *Technical reflection* is associated with technical rules to generate empirical knowledge.
- *Practical reflection* involves reflection on human interactions, or communicative action, which involves reciprocal expectations about behaviour that are defined and understood by the people involved.
- *Emancipatory reflection* is rooted in power and creates transformative action, which seeks to provide emancipation from forces that give people the strong impression that they are beyond their control.

Engaging in reflection on practice

Experience + reflection = growth (Posner 1989: 21). As this equation suggests, practitioners do not actually learn and grow from experience unless they reflect on that experience. Learning generally only occurs when practitioners challenge meaning and reconcile new ideas with the presuppositions of prior learning, and then use these insights to act and change (Williams 2001). Mezirow (1985) describes learning as being of three types: instrumental, dialogic, or self-reflective.

- *Instrumental learning* is about learning facts and cause–effect relationships. It is about learning 'how to', not 'why'. An example of instrumental learning would be a cooking class.
- *Dialogic learning* involves understanding meaning in the world and testing it through induction to gain greater understanding. It is about understanding the meaning of things. An example of dialogic learning would be learning about the meaning of food in different cultures.
- *Self-reflective learning* is a more personal activity of learning one's own place in the world, and understanding how prior experience influences one's ways of thinking and ability to understand and interpret the world. An example would be to learn why you associate different foods with particular emotions.

Mezirow (1985) describes learning processes as learning within meaning schemes, where more factual learning takes place; learning new meaning schemes in which these schemes are understood and applied; and meaning transformation, in which new ways of thinking about reality are understood. Learning about practice and transforming practice are key outcomes of critical reflection.

Smyth (1989) says that practitioners should introduce themselves to critical reflection, create a reflective journal, find a trusted colleague to discuss issues with, find time and space to think, and revisit journal material frequently to reflect on its meaning. He describes a four-stage process of critical reflection: describe, inform, confront, and reconstruct.

Distinguishing characteristics of critical reflection

The characteristics that distinguish critical reflection from other forms of reflection are:

- It is concerned with questioning assumptions.
- Its focus is social rather than individual.
- It pays particular attention to the analysis of power relations.
- It is concerned with emancipation (Reynolds 1998).

Critical reflection is described as bringing assumptions, premises, criteria, and schemata into consciousness and vigorously critiquing them (Mezirow 1985).

Critical reflection is an active process. It requires us to describe, question, and challenge our assumptions, beliefs, values, and theories about why things happen and explore how things may be different. It behoves us to think critically, seek feedback, and to move out of our comfort zones and individual frame of reference as we question the assumptions on which we base our practice. Posner (1989) states that critical reflection frees practitioners from mere impulsive and routine activity and enables them to act in deliberate and intentional fashion to achieve what is needed.

Schön (1987) in his now classic work on professional practice provides some challenging thoughts on what professional practice is, and why it is important to be critically reflective. Schön (1987) and Smyth (1989) both argue the importance of critical reflection in the professions as a way to guard against over-socialisation and over-ritualisation of the workforce. In health promotion practice, which is not a 'profession' as such, critical reflection can be seen to be of even greater importance in working within the principles of achieving equity, access, empowerment, community self-determinism, and intersectoral collaboration, which have strong political dimensions and goals of changing organisations and society. For those of us working within professions, and applying primary health care principles and health promotion actions to our work, this can also be a challenging task requiring critical reflection and action.

Box 17.2: Examples of moving forward using reflective practice

One way to start moving forward is to consider how to use reflective practice to deal with some of the health promotion dilemmas presented in this book.

For example, in Jennie Popay's chapter (Chapter 9) on Engaging Communities we see the problems that occur when professionals are unable to understand the need to transfer power if community engagement is to be successful. How would reflective practice help here?

Helen Keleher's Chapter 8 argues that the practice context is more important than the program in delivering outcomes. How does the reflective practitioner sort out how context affects programs, and their own role in shaping—and being shaped by—that context?

In Chapter 13, Mary Mahoney and Grace Blau aim to examine Health Impact Assessment as a policy and practice tool to address inequity and to illustrate intersectoral working. How can health promoters change their practice to incorporate these tools?

The authors of Chapter 6 describe how evidence is derived and generated from the sectors in which health promotion aims to affect change and how health promotion can contribute to the evidence base of other sectors. We argue that this is not merely technical or 'book' knowledge: new ways of working are needed to use new types of evidence. How do we change our practice to use new sources of evidence?

SUMMARY

As yet there are neither accepted, evidence-based skills or competencies for upstream, intersectoral health promotion, nor a range of skill-based teaching and learning options. In this climate, practitioners who seek to migrate from the high moral ground of didactic health education to the messy swamp of intersectoral health promotion require new theories, frameworks, and practice skills that can be developed building rigorous and critical reflection into practice.

Reflective approaches can be part of formal studies, staff development, embedded in the culture of learning organisations, and an integral part of a practitioner's commitment to lifelong learning.

Disciplines such as education and nursing have well-developed theories and models of critical reflection that have been applied to health promotion. We can draw on these theories and models to design critical reflection that both develops new skills and helps us to develop new theories to inform twenty-first century health promotion practice.

USEFUL WEBSITES

Critical reflection website links:

Critical reflection: <www.learningandteaching.info/learning/critical1.htm>

Keeping a reflective journal: <www.clt.uts.edu.au/Scholarship/Reflective.journal.htm>

Seven questions for critical reflection: <course1.winona.edu/wnelson/html/questionsforcriticalreflection.html>

A very useful article (PDF): Herrington, Jan and Ron Oliver (2002). 'Designing for Reflection in Online Courses'. HERDSA. <elrond.scam.ecu.edu.au/oliver/2002/HerringtonJ.pdf>

The Role of Critical Reflection in the Portfolio Process. <www.sitesupport.org/module1/teacherreflection.htm>

Mentoring website link

All about mentoring and coaching: <www.mentors.ca>

(All these websites were accessed 21 December 2005)

Additional reading for mentoring

Scott, K., McInerny, M. & Tye, M. (1999) *Mentoring for Women: A Guide to Finding and Using Multiple Mentors*. The Australian Federation of Business and Professional Women Inc (BPW Australia), Swan Hill, Victoria.

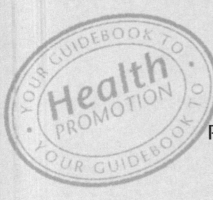

GUIDEBOOK 5:
HEALTH PROMOTION
PROGRAM PLANNING AND
EVALUATION RESOURCES

Nerida Joss

NAME	ORGANISATION	WHAT DOES THIS RESOURCE OFFER?	WHERE TO FIND IT
Evaluation in Health Promotion— Principles and Perspectives	World Health Organisation	This online book reports on evaluation as a tool to achieving program goals, provides a wealth of guidance on how to undertake them, and calls for greater investment in the evaluation of health promotion.	\<www.who.dk/ eprise/main/WHO/ InformationSources/ Publications/ Catalogue/20010911_ 43\>
Program Management Guidelines for Health Promotion	Central Sydney Area Health Service (CSAHS)	A user-friendly guide to program planning and evaluation. The guidelines are divided into discrete sections including checklists and case studies to make sure that you have considered all aspects of each process.	\<www.health.nsw.gov. au/pubs/p/ pdf/pmg_hp.pdf\>
The Project Planning and Evaluation Wizard	South Australian Community Research Unit (SACHRU)	A colourful online 'map' to easily navigate yourself through planning and evaluation steps. Designed for project officers working in primary health care and health promotion, this tool is ideal for community health workers.	\<www.sachru.sa.gov. au/pew/index.htm\>
The Bush Book	Department of Health and Community Services (Territory Health Services)	Written for practitioners working with Aboriginal communities in the Northern Territory. The book contains straightforward information to assist planning and evaluating health promotion programs.	\<www.nt.gov.au/ health/healthdev/ health_promotion/ bushbook/bushbook_ toc.shtml\>
Evaluating Health Promotion Programs	The Health Communication Unit (THCU)	A workbook based on a simple nine-step process for health promotion evaluation. The resource includes worksheets so that you can monitor your progress through the stages and make sure that your evaluation is rigorous.	\<www.thcu.ca/\>

(Continued)

(Continued)

NAME	ORGANISATION	WHAT DOES THIS RESOURCE OFFER?	WHERE TO FIND IT
An Evaluation Guide for Community Arts Practitioners	VicHealth	Evaluation guide for practitioners working in the area of community arts with an express guide for the time-savvy worker.	<www.vichealth.vic.gov.au/Content.aspx?topicID=239>
Framework for Program Evaluation in Public Health	Centre for Disease Control	A six-step framework for conducting an evaluation of a public health program. The framework has been designed through the collaboration of ninety public health representatives to ensure effective evaluation processes.	<www.cdc.gov/mmwr/preview/mmwrhtml/rr4811a1.htm>

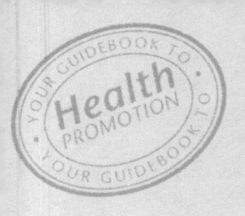

GUIDEBOOK 6: RESOURCES ON HEALTH EQUITY

Nerida Joss

NAME	ORGANISATION	WHAT DOES THIS RESOURCE OFFER?	WHERE TO FIND IT
Four steps to equity: a tool for health promotion practice	NSW Health Promotion Directors Network	This tool is written specifically for health promotion practitioners and other relevant workers to consider and integrate health equity into their work rather than including it as an 'add-on'. It consists of a four-step process using principles, questions, a planning cycle, and website support based on research findings.	\<www.health.nsw.gov.au/pubs/f/pdf/4-steps-towards-equity.pdf >
Health equity audit: a self-assessment tool	Department of Health (UK)	Through the use of visual models this tool aims to help services narrow the gap in health inequalities. It allows you to rate the current management of health equity and assist in assessing the readiness to use HEA.	\<www.dh.gov.uk/assetRoot/04/07/55/39/04075539.rtf>
A health equity assessment tool (equity lens) for tackling health inequalities in health	New Zealand Ministry of Health	A straightforward set of questions that has been developed to assist you in considering how particular inequalities in health have come about, and where the effective intervention points are to tackle them.	\<www.moh.govt.nz/moh.nsf/0/ 24474c74 64606a5acc25700b0 009d6f8? OpenDocument>
The concepts and principles of health and equity	World Health Organisation	A brief discussion paper that outlines the importance of equity in health and the key concepts and principles that underlie it. The paper looks at the links between health status, socio-economic factors, and social justice to give you the basic understandings of this complex issue.	\<ftp.who.dk/Document/PAE/conceptsrpd414.pdf>

(Continued)

(Continued)

NAME	ORGANISATION	WHAT DOES THIS RESOURCE OFFER?	WHERE TO FIND IT
The Centre for Health Equity Research and Promotion	The Centre for Health Equity Research and Promotion	This website offers myriad information and links that are current and continually updated.	<www.cherp.research.med.va.gov/index.php>
The Gender and Health Equity Network	The Gender and Health Equity Network	The Gender and Health Equity Network is a partnership of national and international institutions concerned with developing and implementing policies to improve gender and health equity, particularly in resource-constrained environments. On this site you can see who the partners are, read summaries of the country case studies, and find out more about resources on gender and health equity.	<www.ids.ac.uk/ghen>

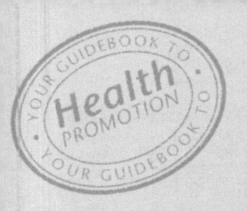

Nerida Joss & Helen Keleher

NAME	ORGANISATION	WHAT DOES THIS SITE OFFER?	WEBSITE ADDRESS
Capacity building	NSW Health	The comprehensive webpage presents capacity-building in a simple manner by providing a definition and links to key documents produced by NSW health including a user-friendly framework and indicators that are beneficial for practitioners at all levels. The site also links you to case studies and FAQs. This site should be a first stop to learn about capacity-building.	\<www.health.nsw.gov.au/public-health/health-promotion/capacity building/index.html\>
Health Promotion Interventions and Capacity Building Strategies	DHS Victoria	This site gives an overview of integrated health promotion (IHP), the health promotion framework and capacity-building, which clearly illustrates their connections. It also links you to the Integrated Health Promotion Resource, which is a complete guide to health interventions and capacity-building.	\<www.health.vic.gov.au/healthpromotion/hp_practice/interventions.htm\>
Community Capacity Building Tool	Public Health Agency of Canada	A planning tool that will help you to build community capacity in health promotion programs. It covers nine important components for capacity-building and will enable you to see where you are and where you can go to build your capacity further. It is clearly presented and easy to complete providing useful results.	\<www.phac-aspc.gc.ca/canada/regions/ab-nwt/download.html\>
HealthLink Newsletter	Health Promotion Journal of the ACT	This is an online newsletter that has been dedicated solely to capacity-building. Comprehensive yet uncomplicated, it includes theory-based articles written to enhance your understanding but also complemented with community examples.	\<www.healthpromotion.act.gov.au/research/journals/files/healthlink_winter_2002.pdf\>

(Continued)

(Continued)

NAME	ORGANISATION	WHAT DOES THIS SITE OFFER?	WEBSITE ADDRESS
Community Builder	NSW Government	The site is an interactive clearing house for everyone involved in community-level social, economic, and environmental renewal. Community building contains practice resources (guides, toolkits, hand-books, and articles); case studies, a discussion forum, events calendar, and featured organisations as well as the opportunity to join an email list called Newswire.	<www.community-builders.nsw.gov.au>

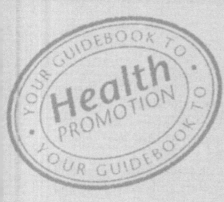

GUIDEBOOK 8:
PREPARING FOR A MEDIA
INTERVIEW—TEN-POINT
CHECKLIST

Berni Murphy

The following 10-point checklist is designed to help novices prepare for a media interview.

1   Call the interviewer by name and look him/her in the eye. This will help you stay focused and will reduce the risk of developing 'bunny in headlight syndrome', characterised by darting eyes and a panicky demeanor.

2   Annunciate clearly and calmly. Use plain language—absolutely no jargon. For instance, terms such as *infrastructure*, *stakeholders*, and *intersectoral collaborations* are commonly understood within the health sector, but are likely to disengage you from the general public.

3   Dress to look and feel professional yet comfortable. Avoid wearing anything that is likely to flare on television, including predominantly white clothing, loud prints, or shiny jewellery. Sunglasses or spectacles with lenses that darken outdoors do not work well on television either.

4   Avoid sounding long-winded—instead prepare short punchy statements. (If being interviewed by news reporters be aware that most news sound bites on television or radio last 5–10 seconds at most. Don't talk faster, just be concise. Sentence stems are acceptable. If the interview is live to air then make your responses more conversational. Before going to air, ask the interviewer what the first question will be so you can mentally prepare a response and hopefully get off to a good start.)

5   Don't *ever* raise your voice or get hostile even if baited by the interviewer. Remain in control of your emotions. Remember your primary task is to *use the medium to get your message across*, not to get sidetracked into a heated debate with the interviewer.

6   If you cannot answer a question, say that you don't have that precise information on hand and offer to follow up and provide it as soon as possible. Make sure you honour this promise.

7   Have two or three key points that you want to get across prepared in advance. If you are not happy with a particular question, respond with '*I think the real issue here, James, is …*' and then include one or more of your key points. (This diversionary tactic is commonly used by politicians when being interviewed by reporters. Learn from the good media performers on television and radio.)

8 Rehearse being interviewed in both standing and seated positions in front of a mirror and then settle on what feels and looks comfortable for you.

9 Finish the interview with a prepared take-home message such as: *'It's time we gave this issue the attention it deserves. This initiative will help these children have a much better quality of life.'*

10 Review your performance after the interview. Ask yourself what went well and what you would do differently next time? Rate each experience and learn from it. Don't be too hard on yourself!

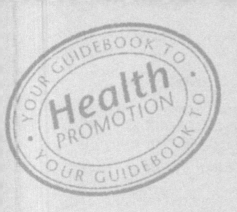

GUIDEBOOK 9: DEVELOPING TRAINING, FACILITATING, AND PRESENTING SKILLS

Berni Murphy

This checklist will help you recognise the attributes of highly skilled trainers, facilitators, and presenters. Professionals typically focus on four main aspects, namely the environment, content, relevance to the audience, and method/s of delivery. Use this checklist to help you identify three to five potential aspects for development. Write an action plan for building these skills (e.g. attend a course; find a mentor).

FOCUS	A HIGHLY SKILLED PROFESSIONAL TRAINER/FACILITATOR/PRESENTER:	SKILLS TO DEVELOP ☑
Credibility, engagement, and adaptability ... creating the right learning environment	■ establishes credibility and rapport from the outset through competence, confidence, credentials, and an engaging training style ■ is articulate, enthusiastic, and exhibits highly developed interpersonal communication skills ■ is participant-focused, flexible, and able to be spontaneous ■ is organised and able to present information in ways that make sense to participants ■ is passionate, empathetic, and sensitive to participant reactions ■ is curious about participants' opinions and experiences ■ self-perception is that of a facilitator of learning rather than an authority figure and controller of content/knowledge ■ can respond appropriately to unexpected events ■ is able to create a safe yet challenging atmosphere in which participants feel motivated to engage and willing to take risks ■ is able to pace, lead, and build (i.e. can work the space/time/resources/group/activities) through appropriate pacing of the delivery; by leading debate and encouraging participant contributions; and by building knowledge, skills, and confidence ■ is skilled in managing the dynamics of the group and is able to handle difficult interactions with integrity ■ recognises and responds positively to uncertainty or confusion	

(Continued)

(Continued)

FOCUS	A HIGHLY SKILLED PROFESSIONAL TRAINER/FACILITATOR/PRESENTER:	SKILLS TO DEVELOP ☑
	■ is aware of the importance of the training space or environment in facilitating the learning process ■ is responsive to participant needs with respect to breaks, room climate, furniture setup, lighting, access to audio-visual aids, refreshments, etc.	
Attention to content	■ is sufficiently familiar with the content to achieve the learning objectives ■ is well prepared and has thoroughly researched the content prior to delivery ■ is able to incorporate case studies and exemplars relevant to the group ■ is able to diverge from the script in order to better meet the groups' needs ■ recognises that administration and process issues are as important as content in optimising outcomes	
Ensuring relevance	■ constructs meaning for the participants by contexualising, illustrating, demonstrating, including ■ recognises that learning occurs when participants identify relevance to their own contexts ■ seeks opportunities to draw on the experiences of participants ■ does not feel threatened by the knowledge, skills, and experiences of participants	
Training methods	■ can employ and adapt a range of methods (e.g. group processes; case studies; audio-visual demonstrations; problem-solving; brainstorming; nominal group technique; role play; modelling; scenarios; didactic presentations; participant reflections; interactive challenges; other) ■ identifies which methods best suit the content, the group, the training space, the time available, and the learning objectives ■ is not unduly reliant on formulaic training techniques (e.g. ice breakers, gimmicks for gaining attention, or dividing participants into groups)	

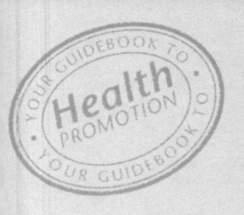

GUIDEBOOK 10: PREPARING A PRESS RELEASE—TEN-POINT CHECKLIST

Berni Murphy

The following ten-point checklist is designed to help novices prepare a press release. A press release is a brief article covering information that might have some news value to the media, whether locally or nationally. It is usually issued by an organisation.

ESTABLISH THE PURPOSE

1   Be clear about **what you want to say** and **why you want to say it**. Are you certain you have the approval of your organisation before you proceed?

2   **Who is your intended audience** for this story? What **impact** are you trying to create with your audience by releasing the story? For instance, are you trying to raise awareness, influence public opinion, or influence decision-makers? Is your story really newsworthy?

WRITING THE STORY

3   **What angle(s) will you take**? Most news stories are constructed around one or more of the following angles:

(i)   Is this story **current** news or about a current event?

(ii) Does this story have far-reaching **consequences**? How many people will be affected?

(iii) Is this story **close** to home? Occurring in the local area?

(iv) Does this story have **novelty** appeal? Does it involve a bizarre or extraordinary person or event?

(v)   Does it involve **prominent** organisations, persons, or celebrities?

(vi) Is there a **human interest** aspect to the story?

(vii) Is there an element of **conflict** or **controversy** evident in this story? (adapted from Lupton 1994).

4   Your story needs to include the five Ws: what, why, who, where, and when.
     (i)   What happened or is about to happen?
     (ii) Why? Convey the perspective of your organisation here.
     (iii) Who is/was involved and how are they involved/affected?
     (iv) Where?
     (v)   When?
5   Your press release must be concise, well written, *absolutely accurate*, professional in appearance, and formatting. Sentences should be punchy. Have you included a quote from a credible person?
6   It should be accompanied by a **FACT SHEET**, a 1–2 page document providing *absolutely accurate* background facts, statistics, and other details that are referenced where appropriate.
7   Have you included an eye-catching **title**? While this title might not make it to print, it can nevertheless be useful in grabbing the attention of the journalist and therefore increasing the chance of your story being published.
8   Have you considered suitable **photo opportunities**? Who will this involve? Where? When? Will you be available to speak to the journalist about your story? Have you provided your contact details on the press release including your after hours phone number?

WHO TO CONTACT

9   Find out about the newspaper you are targeting:
     (i)   Who is the most appropriate journalist for your story? Is there a dedicated health reporter?
     (ii) What is this paper's production schedule? Deadlines? Good days/ bad days to contact them?
     (iii) Contact can initially be made by phone to introduce yourself and your story. Rehearse what you intent to say and be very brief as the journalist will be working to deadlines. The personal approach is preferable to faxing or emailing, as some journalists are likely to view hundreds of press releases a day.
     (iv) Once you have established a relationship with the journalist, become a reliable source. Follow up with further information as requested and on time.

EVALUATION: MEASURING YOUR SUCCESS

10 Keep a record of all press clippings and any media spin-offs (e.g. radio broadcasts of the story). Keep a record of the contact details of the journalist for future reference. Assess the following:

(i) Where was the story positioned? (i.e. front page or as a page 27 filler?)

(ii) Was the coverage favourable?

(iii) Was the story accurate?

(iv) What reaction did the story generate? (e.g. spin off stories in this paper or other media channels, letters to the editor, talkback radio, an editorial response in the next edition.)

(v) Any opportunities to follow up this story with further stories? If the answer is yes, return to point 1 of this checklist and commence the checklist process all over again. (Adapted from Deakin University Health Communication course materials 2005)

GUIDEBOOK

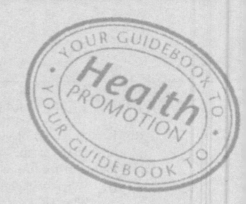

GUIDEBOOK 11:
CROSS-CULTURAL
COMMUNICATION

Berni Murphy

This guidebook emphasises the importance of cultural sensitivity when seeking to promote a health agenda with groups in the community. The word *culture* in this context is typically used to refer to ways of thinking and acting. It encompasses history and a world view, values, beliefs, and religion. Implicit here are notions of socialisation, education, enculturation, language, and non-verbal communication (Mohan et al. 2004). This guidebook provides a useful comparison of Australian communication styles and behaviours with that of other cultures.

A comparison of cross-cultural communication styles and behaviours

BEHAVIOUR AND COMMUNICATION STYLE	AUSTRALIAN CULTURE	IN OTHER CULTURES
Written communication	Using a standard written document is often seen as an integral part of engagement. Reports, memoranda, and letters have a standard recognisable format. Emails on the other hand are often more conversational and informal.	Written communication is not universally seen as the medium of interaction or business. The content or writing style of Western documents may be viewed as too direct or bold and therefore offensive to some cultures.
Communication subtleties: non-verbal	Australians tend to exhibit confidence in stance, body language, and gestures.	Stance, body language and gestures can be interpreted very differently in other cultures, e.g. pointing a finger may be perceived as being very rude, while in Australia it might simply be used to emphasise a line of reasoning.

BEHAVIOUR AND COMMUNICATION STYLE	AUSTRALIAN CULTURE	IN OTHER CULTURES
Communication subtleties: verbal	Australians are sometimes unaware of linguistic subtleties such as tone, inflection, and word selection evident in other languages such as Vietnamese.	Amateurish attempts to communicate in a different language can be welcomed as an endearing willingness to engage in some cultures. In other cultures such attempts can be more problematic; particularly with languages that have subtle inflections and tone variations.
Formality	While ostensibly conformist with respect to dress in a business context and formal social occasions, Australia is regarded as one of the least formal cultures in the world.	Other cultures may have strict rules governing dress, language usage, and behaviour.
Appearance	Rules and expectations about appearance and dress can vary dramatically depending on the circumstances in Australia.	Dress and other appearance expectations may not be the same in other cultures.
Humour	Australians often use humour to break the ice when meeting people. Humour is also commonly used to relieve pressure in tense situations, and is becoming more popular in online interactions.	Other cultures may view the Australian version of humour as being disrespectful or inappropriate.
Social customs	Australians tend to be forgiving of violations of their own social customs by foreigners.	Other cultures may be less forgiving than Australians (e.g. a gift may be interpreted as a bribe in some cultures; informal attire may be viewed as disrespectful).
Use of space	Australians generally prefer lots of personal space.	Other cultures may not require the same amount of personal space.
Use of time	Australians generally prefer to be on time and quickly get down to business in a meeting.	Other cultures may view time more flexibly. They may start meetings slowly with social discourse.

(Continued)

(Continued)

BEHAVIOUR AND COMMUNICATION STYLE	AUSTRALIAN CULTURE	IN OTHER CULTURES
Friendships	Australians often try to make friends quickly and regard business acquaintances as possible friends.	Other cultures may view all business acquaintances with a degree of social distance and regard some social interactions by Australians as being too familiar and therefore inappropriate.
Class systems and social hierarchy	Class is not a predominant issue in Australia and social hierarchies are not necessarily evident.	Other cultures may have a strict social hierarchy that cannot be violated.
Religion	Many Australians are not deeply religious and lack knowledge of other religious or spiritual beliefs.	Other cultures are likely to be more religious or spiritual than their Australian counterparts.
Equal opportunity	Australians have a long way to go but are closer to equal opportunity than many other cultures.	Many other cultures openly practise discrimination based on gender, religion, ethnicity, and age.
Legal contracts	Most contracts are viewed in Australia as legally binding.	Contracts may not always be regarded highly, and may not be enforceable.
Communication competence	Communication competence is valued in Australian society, particularly in verbal and written forms relevant to our specific work contexts.	Communication competence may not be valued as highly as tradition, kinship, honour and respect.

(Adapted from Sprinks & Wells 1997)

While Chapter 11, Strategic Communication, clearly positions strategic communication as a tool for promoting and enhancing health, it is nevertheless important to recognise that communication competence in written and verbal forms is very much a Western concept. In reality, more damage can be done by cultural insensitivity than can be gained through Western notions of cultural competence. In this context, strategic communication is more about sensitivity and respectful engagement than about functional written and verbal communication skills.

CULTURAL AWARENESS WHEN WORKING WITH INDIGENOUS COMMUNITIES

The need for cultural awareness and sensitivity is sometimes overlooked when working with Indigenous communities. Non-Indigenous health professionals might set out with the noble intention of working collaboratively with an Indigenous community to build capacity to address the factors that improve or compromise the health of that community. However, failure to recognise and pay due respect to the community's cultural values and beliefs can quickly become an insurmountable barrier to achieving such an objective. Curran (2006) contends that notions of 'wellness and illness in aboriginal communities are based on cultural beliefs and values. Such beliefs and values create obligations, responsibilities, and establish an order that binds individuals, families and communities together. As a result the culture of the community is integrated into the daily lives of individuals and groups' (p. 17). Tilmouth (2006) cautions health promoters against only 'seeing health through white man's eyes' when seeking to build knowledge and capacity within Indigenous communities. Curran joins other commentators in encouraging health professionals to become more culturally aware in such situations. This often involves being prepared to set aside one's professional role as a health promoter with theoretical knowledge and skills, and instead let the community become one's teacher. Box G11.1 provides insights into working with Aboriginal communities from the perspectives of four very experienced and respected Aboriginal health workers from the Northern Territory in Australia.

Box G11.1: Cultural awareness when working with Aboriginal communities

(As shared with Berni Murphy in Alice Springs 2006 by Aunty Gwen Walley, Team Leader, Alcohol and Other Drugs Service, Alice Springs; Jennifer Kitching, Aboriginal Health Promotion Officer, Maternal, Youth and Child Health Team, Tennant Creek; Lynette Windsor, Senior Health Promotion Officer, Alice Springs; and Marlene Liddle, Coordinator 'Strong Women, Strong Babies, Strong Culture' Program, Darwin)

Respect

- Respect is everything.
- This means respect for the land ... respect for the elders ... respect for our traditions and our culture.
- Recognising, acknowledging, and valuing differences also matter to us.
- Don't be judgmental and don't impose your values on us.
- The Aboriginal people will be your best teacher—go with an open mind.
- Always tell the truth. This is very important.

Protocols for visiting communities

- Make sure you understand the protocols about *when* and *how* to visit communities. You will require permission and a permit to visit some communities. Factor in plenty of time for this to be arranged.

- Check travel arrangements the day prior to visiting a community to make sure the visit is still appropriate. Plans might change unexpectedly within communities so it's wise to check before setting out.
- Find out who the most appropriate person is to speak to in the community. This will depend to some extent on what it is you want to talk about. Is it women's business, men's business, family, or community business?
- It is very important to acknowledge the traditional owners of the land. Pay your respects and thank them for inviting you to their beautiful land.
- If planning to talk to Aboriginal students at a school about sensitive issues such as reproductive health, seek permission first from parents or grandparents with an endorsed consent form.
- Any form of community consultation is likely to require any or all of the following to attend: community elders, Aboriginal health worker, traditional owner (TO), Aboriginal teacher's aid, CDEP workers and as many community people as possible.
- Avoid getting involved in the local politics of the community. Always remain neutral.

Building knowledge about community

- Develop knowledge of black history. Good sources are the Institute of Aboriginal Development, the Menzies School of Health Development, and the Bush Book available online through the Northern Territory website <http://www.nt.gov.au>.
- Do your homework on the community you are intending to visit *before* you get there. Find out about the community's profile, the location, language groups, and issues of interest to this community. This information is usually readily available in the public domain through the local government, health department website, libraries, and other sources such as the Department of Planning and Infrastructure. Other sources include the Central Land Council and NPY Women's Council.
- There are reportedly over 500 languages and dialects. You should be aware of what the main language is for the community you are visiting, but also realise that many other languages might be represented in that community due to intermarrying.
- Be aware that *Grandmother's Law* is strong in some parts of the top end of Australia, particularly in Darwin and Alice Springs. If visiting these areas, take the time to learn about Grandmother's Law and avoid inadvertent or subtle disrespect of cultures and traditions.

Building relationships

- Don't expect to fly in and fly out. Spend time and build a relationship.
- Ask politely how to address someone. For instance, if others present are calling someone 'aunty', politely introduce yourself by name and ask if you may use that term as well.
- Adopt a two-way approach to learning … don't present yourself as the expert. Instead, take your lead from the community. Let people know that your cultural knowledge is limited and look to them for guidance.

Presentation and greetings

- Wearing casual clothes is acceptable but nothing too cheeky. No makeup. No bare shoulders, bare midriffs, or short skirts. Wear long pants or skirts. Hats are acceptable. Wear enclosed footwear.
- Hand contact such as a handshake is acceptable if offered. Take your lead from the community rather than being too forward in this regard.
- Read the body language and follow the lead of community members. In some communities eye contact is not particularly welcome. In these instances look over the shoulder of the person you are talking to. Alternatively, look down or focus your eyes on a map, resource materials, or other items pertinent to the conversation as a way of avoiding eye to eye.

Protocols for engaging with communities

- If unsure of how to behave or act, ask 'Is this OK?'
- Don't take photos without permission.
- Don't approach children, touch, or pick up babies without permission.
- Don't point or wave your finger. This is considered very rude.
- Females should not approach males unless invited to do so.
- Females should expect to talk to other females in the community about 'women's business' and should always be accompanied by an Aboriginal health worker or someone identified by the community.
- When invited to join a group, sit quietly, observe, and wait to be invited to participate in discussions. Don't be too pushy or eager. Instead, take your lead from the community members. Don't make assumptions and clarify that you have understood information correctly.
- Realise that the camp dogs are considered part of the family. Don't disrespect them by shooing them away or kicking them even though they might appear sick or snarly. Instead calmly walk around them.

GUIDEBOOK

- Seek community approval to document any information you are given.
- Never make a promise you can't keep.
- Involve the people in all stages of your work and value each person's contribution. Set realistic directions and monitor progress in conjunction with identified community people.

Participating in community activities

- Don't go wandering around—stay within the confines of the community unless invited to join community members on a walk or expedition. Failure to do so might cause offence, particularly if you wander into sacred sites.
- Be prepared for the unexpected. For instance you might be invited to sit on the ground with community members in a riverbed. Accept the invitation and follow the lead of the community. Listen and learn.
- Take every opportunity if invited to join in activities such as hunting or searching for bush tucker. Saying no to such invitations might cause offence. Consider this a valuable learning experience. Don't be too forward. Be patient, listen, observe, and learn. Ask questions quietly if invited to do so.
- Be flexible as situations can change overnight. A death in the community may result in you being asked to leave earlier or stay longer but keep a low profile.
  And finally, Aunty Gwen Walley's words of wisdom:

'You were born with two ears for listening, two eyes for observing, but only one mouth. Use them in that order and in that proportion!'

Berni Murphy offers her sincere thanks to these wise and generous women for sharing their insights.

PART 3
MULTISECTORAL ACTIONS

Part 3 includes seven chapters written from the perspectives of various sectors that have central importance to both health promotion and the social determinants of health. Of course, this is a selection of the possible chapters that could have been written to illustrate the ways in which the promotion of health is the business of a wide range of sectors.

One of our concerns, introduced in Part 1, is that the language of health promotion is not necessarily the language used by sectors other than health, even though those sectors are engaged in active and purposeful actions to promote health. Thus, there are many 'languages' used to explain what is core business for each sector. The sectors represented in Part 3 include environments, healthy cities, community arts, geography, physical activity, and sport. We invite you to consider the language, theories, and practice skills presented in the book and incorporate multisectoral (or intersectoral) skills into your practice. We also invite you to reflect on the knowledge, beliefs, and actions that determine your practice, and to ask whether they are conducive to respectful partnerships, multidisciplinary work, and multisectoral action.

ENVIRONMENT AND SUSTAINABILITY APPROACHES TO HEALTH PROMOTION

18

Ian Lowe

Key concepts

- Just as a healthy body is needed to support a healthy mind, healthy individuals need healthy communities, which in turn require healthy ecological systems.
- Unsustainable futures pose a range of direct and indirect threats to human health.
- The present development path is clearly not sustainable, so a sustainable future will involve fundamental changes in technology and social institutions.
- Principles of a sustainable future can be clearly defined and elaborated into practical guidelines.
- The next step in the evolution of health promotion is the development of these guidelines for healthy future communities.

Key terms

- Sustainability
- Ecological health
- Environment
- Resources
- Equity
- Alternative futures

OVERVIEW

Healthy individuals and healthy communities require healthy ecological systems to provide clean air, potable water, nutritious food, cultural identity, and spiritual sustenance. Since the current lifestyle in the industrialised nations is clearly unsustainable, some fundamental changes need to be made if we are to achieve that goal. The HEALTHIER society of the future will be Humane in the sense of providing equitable access to its material benefits, take an Ecocentric Approach, use a Long Time Horizon for planning purposes, be Informed about the consequences for natural systems of our choices, be Efficient in its use of natural resources, and be Resourced by having made the transition from fossil fuels that are either limited (oil) or unacceptably polluting (coal) to the abundant flows of renewable energy. Some steps toward this sustainable and healthy future society are described.

WHAT DOES SUSTAINABILITY MEAN?

There is now a widespread view that we should be aiming to achieve sustainability or sustainable development, but equally widespread confusion about the process for achieving such a goal. In discussions of the issue at conferences, meetings, and informal gatherings since the 1980s, I have been struck by two things: the enormous support for the principle of sustainability and the uncertainty about the steps towards it. If we accept as a minimalist position the Brundtland view (WCED 1987), that sustainability involves meeting our needs in ways that do not reduce the capacity of future generations to meet their needs, there are clearly at least three dimensions to sustainability: resources, environment, and social stability. We should not be eroding the resource base, since that reduces the resources available to future generations. We should not be damaging the natural environment in ways that affect the capacity of future generations to meet their needs for potable water, breathable air, food that is adequate in quantity and quality, the spiritual sustenance we obtain from the natural world, and our cultural identity. In those terms, changing the global climate in substantial ways is clearly problematic. Finally, we should bear in mind that sustainability requires a stable social system. So we need to ensure more equitable access to the material benefits of modern society, since real or imagined injustice is always a source of tension and social instability.

The 1996 report on the state of the environment (State of the Environment Advisory Council 1996) concluded that progress toward sustainable development requires integrating ecological thinking into all social and economic planning. Traditional thinking is still based on the pig-headed model, which sees the economy as the main game, with social and environmental issues peripheral (Kelly 2001; Lowe 1994, pers.com.). A more appropriate way to see the world is the concentric rings model. This recognises that the economy is an important part of society, but only a part; we all expect from society important things that are not part of the economy, such as our cultural identity, security, companionship, love, and a sense of place. Similarly, our society is totally enclosed within natural ecosystems, on which we depend for essential support services of breathable air, drinkable water, and food, as well as less tangible benefits. So economic planning should be seen as a part of social planning, meaning that such social goals as reducing poverty cannot simply be assumed to follow inevitably from economic growth, and our social planning must be contained within a context of the sustainability of the natural systems of our region. That is the basis of sustainable development. Australian studies (ABS 2002; Krockenberger et al. 2000; Yecken & Wilkinson 2000) show that the present approach is not sustainable. Global analyses (NRC 1999; UNEP 1999) conclude that a transition to sustainability will involve significant changes.

THE RESOURCE BASE

We are clearly eroding the resource base of future generations. As one extreme example, our transport system is almost totally dependent on a non-renewable resource that is now expected to decline in availability from about 2010 (Fleay 1997). There is room to be sceptical about our ability to model something as complex as the amount of oil we will eventually extract, as it is affected by technology and the price people are prepared to pay, but there is no realistic prospect of ever again finding oil deposits like the massive fields in the Middle East, which have fuelled our transport this century. We should be planning now for the transition out of the age of cheap and abundant oil, as is recognised by some oil majors and leading motor vehicle companies. This will be both a physical and a mental transition. Remarkably, we had such little concern for this at the time of writing that there was active competition between major political parties to guarantee lower prices for petroleum fuels, at a time when those prices are already lower than anywhere in the OECD except North America. In fact, Australians pay less per litre for petroleum fuels than they pay for beer, or cask wine, or orange juice, or milk—all of which can be produced sustainably at present levels. There is no absolute shortage of energy resources. The solar energy hitting Australia in one summer day is of the same order of magnitude as the total world energy use for a year (Lowe 1993). There is, however, a limited stock of the energy resource that has unique properties as a transport fuel because of its very high energy density. Our profligate use of oil is quite irresponsible and is certainly closing some options for future generations.

Australia is the driest inhabited continent, so we should be concerned about water resources. The current level of approved extraction from the Murray–Darling system is over 80 per cent of the average annual flow to the sea (State of the Environment Advisory Council 1996). Because Australia also has the most irregular rainfall of any inhabited continent, we have an unusually low level of run-off. The Murray–Darling Basin is roughly the same area as the Mississippi and Amazon basins, which have respectively about ten times and about one hundred times the flow of the local river system. A large fraction of Australia is dependent on groundwater, but the peak of extraction from the Great Artesian Basin was reached more than 80 years ago, and we now only extract about one-third of that peak level (State of the Environment Advisory Council 1996). So many of our inland communities do not have sustainable water resources.

There are other significant resource issues. While Australia is currently a large exporter of food and fibre, the production process is not sustainable. We live in an old and heavily weathered continent with very low rates of soil formation, but past practices of using the land have caused high rates of erosion. With about 5 per cent of the world's land area, we account for about 20 per cent of the world's soil loss (Ibid). To express the same problem another way, we are losing soil at about one million times the rate of soil formation. As well as losing soil, we have also degraded a significant fraction of our rangelands by over-grazing and the introduction of exotic species (Ibid). In that sense, we are not using our productive land sustainably.

BROAD ENVIRONMENTAL ISSUES

Australia has some very serious environmental problems that require urgent attention (State of the Environment Advisory Council 1996). Probably the most fundamental is the loss of biological diversity, mainly caused by the destruction of habitat. We have a very bad record of mammal extinctions and significant fractions of other kinds of native plants and animals are endangered. This is not just a local problem but also a global issue. An unusually high proportion of our native species are not found anywhere else on the planet, so the local loss of biodiversity is also a global loss. The health and resilience of local ecological systems is now seriously threatened, as is especially clear in the case of our inland rivers (Ibid).

Our serious environmental problems do not have simple causes. They are the combined effect of the growth and distribution of the human population, our lifestyle choices, the technologies we use, and the demands they make on natural systems (State of the Environment Advisory Council 1996). That conclusion could be paraphrased by saying that our communities are not interacting in a sustainable way with the natural systems of this country. The problem is getting worse because we are not just expanding the size of our population but also increasing the resource demands and environmental costs per person, causing a compounding cascade of impacts on natural systems. For example, water use per person is much greater now than it was 30 years ago, as is the level of waste produced per person (State of the Environment Advisory Council 1996). So we are putting inexorably increasing pressure on natural systems that are already clearly under stress.

SOCIAL ISSUES

Many of our communities do not appear to be socially sustainable. A sustainable community would be secure, healthy, and equitable, with a clear sense of place. Our human settlements are often inequitable, insecure, and unhealthy, with no sense of place. These are very serious problems.

One hundred years ago, Australia was one of the world's most equitable societies. A recent inequity index ranked Australia as the fourth worst in the developed world. The change has been achieved by the steady but systematic erosion of public education, health care, and other services. The old system was not equitable, because the standards of such services as education and health care varied from place to place, so that Jones (1982) was able to observe that the best indicator of an Australian child's life chances was the postcode of its parents. But the erosion of public provisions in favour of a private-purchaser model has systematically increased inequity.

Insecurity is manifest in higher levels of crime, calls for greater levels of public spending on police services, and higher levels of defensive expenditure on alarm systems, guard dogs, and private security officers. The extreme evidence of insecurity was the growing level of ownership of guns, eventually leading to political pressure to curb the worst excesses of the move to an armed society. The extraordinary move to gated communities is one of the most bizarre demonstrations of the growing insecurity, leading people to voluntarily impose on themselves the sort of sanctions that are normally only imposed on convicted criminals.

Globalisation has directly caused the withdrawal of many services once routinely provided in local communities, such as banking and postal services, reinforcing a spiral of decline. It has indirectly eroded the sense of Australian identity as media outlets dispense a crass Californian materialism, the effects of which are evident in the dress, speech, and values of young people. The decline of traditional religions has left a moral and spiritual vacuum, which can hardly be a secure foundation for sustainable communities. A new moral and spiritual base may be developing around our growing respect for nature (Lovelock 1988), but that certainly does not yet have a secure place in our society. Cleveland and Luyckx (1998) argue that the world is in transition to a 'trans-modern' way of thinking that combines intuition and spirituality with rational analysis. This suggests that the crucial conflicts of this century will not be between cultures but within them, between the pre-modern, modern, and trans-modern views.

Finally, a sustainable community needs economic security. Some areas of economic activity have disappeared (whaling), declined (forestry), or are in decline (some types of agricultural production) because they used natural resources unsustainably. Other activities are in decline because of changes in world demand (wool) or ideological choices by governments (textiles, clothing and footwear, electricity supply, provision of telecommunications). Technological change has dramatically reduced the labour demands of some types of economic activity, obviously including farming. All these changes have reduced the economic security of many rural communities.

THE ECONOMIC BASE

As discussed above, the economic base of many rural communities has been eroded by a combination of technological change, unsustainable resource use, and ideology.

As a fundamental point, a secure economic foundation will only be possible if it is based on sustainable use of natural systems. While that is a necessary condition, it is not sufficient to ensure a solid economic base. A community that used few natural resources and produced nothing of economic value could be living within the limits of its natural systems, but would not have a secure economic future. The most important economic resource for any community today is the education and skills level of its workforce.

I therefore believe that the best investment any community can make in its economic future is to educate its young people to the full extent of their abilities. This is a principle we abandoned some time ago in Australia. A related requirement for economic security is innovation, a product of a solid research and development base, and a culture of innovation. We are not seriously committed to either (Jones 1996). Recent calls for a new approach (Batterham 2000) have fallen on deaf ears.

Australia's enduring economic problem is the trading pattern of a Third World country, exporting raw materials and importing value-added goods and services. The inevitable direction of technological change is that steadily smaller and smaller quantities of raw materials are transformed by increasing amounts of ingenuity and inventiveness into more and more expensive products. Those firms and countries that sell raw materials and buy the products are swimming against the economic tide of history. If we were serious about our economic future we would be trying to become what a former Prime Minister called 'the clever country' by investing in education and innovation, as well as providing incentives for the sorts of economic activities that might be sustainable. Instead we are steadily running down our universities and research organisations, while continuing to provide large public subsidies for activities that are not sustainable. It is hard to see how that could form the basis for a sustainable community.

COMMUNITY HEALTH AND THE IMPACTS OF ENVIRONMENT

We have systematically improved community health by eliminating the infectious diseases that were the major cause of death 100 years ago, and dietary changes in the last 30 years have significantly reduced the problem of coronary heart disease among middle-aged men (Hetzel & McMichael 1985). But a new range of health problems has arisen—accidents and suicide are killing large numbers of young people, while cancers are now a serious problem among older people (Baum 1998). It has been recently suggested that as many as 70 per cent of deaths under the age of 75 are preventable, being due to lifestyle choices such as aggressive driving, drink-driving, smoking, poor diet, and lack of exercise (McElduff & Dobson 2000; Tobias & Jackson 2001). Mass media actively promote the lifestyle choices that impose these needless health risks.

Attention to our environment has produced dramatic improvements in health and well-being. Cleaning up water and air led directly to the increasing life expectancy of the last century. A hundred years ago, about 30 per cent of all Australian deaths were due to infectious diseases, many caused by the state of drinking water (Hetzel & McMichael, 1985). Fifty years ago, many parts of Australia and New Zealand still used primitive methods of handling human waste. More recently, ocean outfalls still allowed excrement to pollute some of the most celebrated surfing beaches until the public outcry forced authorities to invest in better waste treatment. In recent years, regulators have turned their attention to aspects of air pollution that had serious health impacts: hazardous industrial emissions such as asbestos, lead retarding the intellectual development of children, depletion of the ozone layer leading to increased levels of ultra-violet light, as well as various pollutants that affect respiratory function; particulate matter, oxides of nitrogen and sulphur, and the precursors of low-level ozone production. Phasing out lead as a petrol additive directly eliminated one environmental health problem. It also enabled use of catalytic converters to clean up the exhaust gases of motor vehicles, reducing the emissions of carbon monoxide and other pollutants. Concerted action to stop the release into the atmosphere of chlorofluorocarbons has halted the thinning of the ozone layer; the consensus of scientific opinion is that the layer will recover over the next 50 years. In the intervening period, ultra-violet levels will remain above those that had already established Australia as the skin cancer capital of the world.

While catalytic converters have reduced the pollution per vehicle per kilometre travelled, the number of vehicles is increasing and the average distances travelled are also growing, so the total pollution released into urban air is still increasing. Particulates are especially problematic because recent research shows a clear link between particulate levels and respiratory distress. One reason for concern is that diesel engines release much greater quantities of particulates than petrol-driven vehicles. Government policies that provide financial incentives to use diesel rather than petrol are increasing particulate emissions. While some transport authorities, such as Brisbane City Council, decided some years ago to replace diesel buses with vehicles powered by compressed natural gas, in other cities increasing numbers of diesel-powered vehicles are releasing increasing amounts of particulates. We should be very concerned about the health impacts of urban air quality. Projections show a worsening of particulate levels and consequent respiratory distress in the next decade.

Life expectancy among Australian Indigenous communities is appalling, more like that in the poorest Third World countries than the figures for Indigenous people in New Zealand or Canada. Environment plays a major part, with many remote Indigenous communities not having clean drinking water or adequate sanitation. The situation remains a national disgrace in Australia, demanding a concerted response.

Indoor air quality is an emerging environmental health issue. The EnHealth Council (2004) released *Healthy Homes*, a guide to indoor air quality. Some of the problems the report identifies have been around for decades. For example, a study funded by the National Energy Research, Development and Demonstration

Council and published more than 15 years ago showed that unflued gas heaters can produce dangerous levels of nitrogen dioxide in poorly ventilated homes. That led to tighter controls on emissions from newer models of gas heaters. The problem has not been solved, however. Some of the older models are still in use, producing higher levels of pollution. More seriously, Australian Commonwealth Scientific and Research Organization (CSIRO) tests show some new appliances do meet the Australian standard, but still emit as much as three times the limit suggested by the World Health Organisation. Nitrogen dioxide can cause breathing difficulties, especially for people who already have respiratory problems.

Unflued gas heaters also emit carbon monoxide, which reduces the capacity of the blood to hold oxygen. It is effectively poisonous and can kill—carbon monoxide from gas heaters has killed several people in recent years. It has been estimated that about 600,000 Australian homes use unflued gas heaters in winter. As use is concentrated in lower income groups, this is also an equity issue. As is often the case, poorer people are exposed to greater environmental health risks. Health authorities are now warning people who use gas heaters to ensure the room is well ventilated, but the cold nights that bring the heaters into use inevitably increase the probability that windows will be closed to keep the cold air out (EnHealth Council 2005).

There are other pollution sources in the home. Such materials as plywood and particle board often release formaldehyde. High concentrations have been found in caravans and other mobile homes, as they have many of these products. A wide range of volatile organic compounds (VOCs) can also be found in the air inside houses, or new cars in the first six months after manufacture, according to CSIRO tests. Such compounds as benzene, ethyl benzene, and toluene are found in several products used in the home such as solvents, paints, floor adhesives, and cleaning products. A study recently published in *Thorax*, a UK-based journal of respiratory medicine, found that levels of VOCs in the homes of asthmatic children were significantly higher than in a control group of dwellings where unaffected children lived. There was a clear link between the levels of exposure and the risk of asthma. Children exposed to total VOC levels of 60 micrograms per cubic metre or more were four times more likely to have asthma than a control group. These levels are lower than the current recommended thresholds for intervention (EnHealth Council 2004).

The research seems to support the theory that exposure to indoor pollutants early in life might have an important influence on the subsequent development of asthma. That conclusion was strengthened by another study reported in the same issue of *Thorax*. A Sydney group found that children exposed to the fumes from unflued heaters during their first year of life were nearly 50 per cent more likely than a control group to have wheezing or narrowing of their airways. Though these two new studies involved relatively small groups, the statistics are persuasive. They confirm the need to tighten the standards relating to indoor air quality.

There are other issues arising from indoor air. Outbreaks of Legionnaires' Disease have drawn attention to the health risks of inadequately maintained cooling systems. Dust mites, biological allergens from pets, and mould spores are also found inside many homes. There remains the problem of cigarette smoke, such a serious health hazard that it is now banned in most public buildings, but still released into the indoor air of many homes. All these add up to the conclusion that indoor air is often worse than the standard we allow for outdoor air, even in quite dirty city areas.

The report of the Australian Climate Group (2004), *Climate Change— Solutions for Australia*, warned of the potentially serious health impacts of climate change on the scale now being projected. Intensified summer heatwaves will have the direct effect of increasing mortality; it has been estimated that about 14,000 people died in Paris alone as a result of the August 2003 heatwave. Increasing temperatures will also have indirect health effects. For example, as the ACG says, 'rates of food poisoning and diarrhoeal disease will increase in hotter conditions, especially in poorer, rural and remote communities' (Ibid). Vector-borne diseases such as Ross River Virus and Dengue Fever are expected to spread across a wider area, as the changing climate allows the wider spread of the carrier mosquitoes. Urban air pollution is expected to worsen as higher temperatures increase the rate of formation of ozone. Extreme weather conditions will increase the health risks from bushfires, floods, and severe storms. Finally, as a result of the impacts of climate change it can be expected that 'morale and mental health will be adversely affected in ... many rural communities' (Australian Climate Group 2004).

That observation raises the most general consequence of environmental deterioration: its effect on mental health and general well-being. We do not just depend on the natural systems of the planet for breathable air, potable water, and nutritious food. Our natural and built environment also provides our cultural identity, a sense of place and spiritual sustenance. Just as there are 'sick buildings', there are also seedy suburbs, toxic towns, and sick cities: places in which the deterioration of the natural or the built environment reduces well-being, increases stress, and swells the levels of mental illness. Although much of this decline in mental health is neither diagnosed nor treated, it nevertheless represents a real and serious environmental health impact. Some forward-looking urban design now considers such aspects of the physical environment as sunlight, shading or water flows, as well as such features of the biological environment as native vegetation and habitat corridors. We still don't design *social* environments to produce healthy communities.

PLANNING A SUSTAINABLE FUTURE

If we want to have sustainable communities, we need to take conscious steps to achieve that goal, rather than hoping it will be produced by the magic of market forces. The notion of planning has fallen into disfavour as a result of a particularly blinkered view of economics, essentially a naïve infatuation with market forces. The allocation of limited resources by a market leads to *economically* efficient outcomes. However, there are serious limitations to this approach. Markets take no account of ability to pay, so they take no account of equity; indeed, the allocation of any scarce resource by a market is almost certain to increase inequity. Markets take no account of the social impacts of the distribution of resources, unless the social impacts are severe enough to influence consumer behaviour. Market economics systematically discounts the future, for the economically rational reason that a dollar today is more valuable than a dollar in five years time. The problem that results is that costs and benefits 10, 20, or 30 years down the track are systematically discounted, leading to resource allocations that are not optimal. As an extreme example, it has been seriously argued that it made economic sense to hunt whales to extinction rather than killing them (or 'harvesting' them) at a sustainable rate because the net present value was greater! Even if this anthropocentric argument were morally acceptable and we saw whales solely as an economic resource to be 'harvested', it is a ludicrously short-sighted conclusion.

The same logic makes it appear sensible to impose huge financial costs on future generations, for example by producing nuclear waste that will have to be stored for hundreds of thousands of years, by discounting those costs to negligible present values. This discussion illustrates the fundamental flaw of the market approach to natural resource decisions. There are two groups crucially affected by our choices that cannot even in principle express their preferences in today's market: *all other species* and *all future generations*. Leaving the use of natural resources to the market implicitly presumes that the wishes of this generation are more important than the needs of all future generations and all other species. That is a morally untenable position—and clearly in conflict with even the Brundtland definition of sustainability. If we go further and define sustainability either in fundamental terms, as the ability to be sustained, or in such operational terms as meeting the needs of the human population while maintaining the life support systems of the planet (NRC 1999), the market approach is ludicrous.

REFINING THE KNOWLEDGE BASE

As many of the present problems we face are the direct consequence of applying what had previously been expert knowledge, it is clear that the transition to sustainability will require improved understanding of the interactions between natural and social systems. The need has led to the emergence of the new field of sustainability science.

> A growing body of evidence and experience suggests that the needed understanding must encompass the interaction of global processes with the ecological and social characteristics of particular places and sectors. The regional character of much of what sustainability science is trying to explain means that relevant research will have to learn how to integrate the effects of key processes across the full range of scales from local to global. It will also require fundamental advances in our ability to address such issues as the behaviour

of complex self-organising systems, the responses, some irreversible, of the nature-society system to multiple and interacting stresses, and the options for combining different ways of knowing and learning so that social actors with different agenda can act in concert under conditions of uncertainty and limited information. (Kates et al. 2001).

The move toward sustainability science calls for new approaches to scientific inquiry, such as inverse approaches that start from outcomes that should be avoided and work backwards to identify relatively safe corridors of action, or semi-qualitative representation of entire classes of dynamical behaviour. The crucial point is that our present knowledge base does not enable us to identify with any confidence courses of action that are certain to be sustainable, so the goal of sustainability will require a significant investment in improving our understanding of the complex interactions between social and natural systems.

SUMMARY

If you were booked on the *Titanic* and knew what was going to happen, you would have had two rational choices. One option would be to live well, eat expensive food, and drink the best vintage champagne on credit, secure in the knowledge that your cheque would never reach the bank. A more ethical choice would be to try to persuade the captain to change course, enlisting the support of other passengers if the captain resisted your argument. In ecological terms, we are booked on the *Titanic* and heading for the iceberg. Some people who understand this are simply enjoying the good life while they can, while others are effectively urging the engine room to move us faster forward. If we accept that we have a responsibility to future generations to try to achieve sustainability, we need to change course. We need to take account of resource demands of our choices, to be aware of the impacts on natural systems, and to take the hard decisions in our personal and professional lives that will produce communities that are sustainable in social terms. A healthy future community will have to be based on healthy ecological systems, as well as a secure resource base and social systems that are sufficiently equitable to be stable.

I have argued that we should be aiming for a HEALTHIER future society. This acronym stands for:

■ Humane
■ Ecocentric Approach
■ Long Time Horizon
■ Informed
■ Efficient
■ Resourced

It will be Humane in the sense of providing equitable access to its material benefits, so it would develop technologies and approaches that can, at least in principle, be applied to all humans, rather than a privileged small minority in a minority of countries. As discussed above, it would take an Ecocentric Approach, seeing as the primary goal maintenance of the health of the natural systems that support us and all other species. It would use a Long Time Horizon for planning purposes, recognising that the decisions we take about urban structure, transport systems, economic emphasis, and energy supply will structure our choices for many decades into the future. It will be Informed about the consequences for natural systems of our choices, as a result of serious investment in sustainability science. It will be Efficient in its use of natural resources, having dramatically improved on today's primitive and wasteful technology; a realistic goal, suggested by the Wuppertal Institute and since adopted by some European countries, is to use one-tenth of the materials and one-quarter of the energy we now use. Finally, it will be Resourced, by having made the transition from fossil fuels, which are either limited (oil) or unacceptably polluting (coal) to the abundant flows of renewable energy. That should be both our vision and our goal as responsible global citizens; in terms of the notion advanced by Finnish futurist Pentti Malaska and developed for use in higher education by Patricia Kelly (2004), we should become *Globo sapiens*, wise members of the global community, aware of our responsibility to the entire human family, to all other species and to all future generations.

HEALTHY CITIES AND COMMUNITIES

19

Iain Butterworth & Len Duhl

Key concepts

- Intersectoral collaboration is a natural and necessary way to build health into communities, as exemplified by the Healthy Cities approach.
- Intersectoral collaboration is necessary to build health into communities.
- To drive intersectoral collaboration, healthy public policy across all sectors and government portfolios must be identified as a key goal.
- High-level political endorsement is crucial to ensuring a viable and sustainable intersectoral approach.
- Practitioners need skills as social entrepreneurs, to communicate across sectors and bring different people, perspectives, and organisations together into a coordinated approach.
- Intersectoral collaboration is part of a broader community capacity-building effort, and can be evaluated using a social ecology framework.

Key terms

- Healthy cities and communities
- Intersectoral collaboration
- Municipal public health planning
- Ecological public health
- Social entrepreneurship
- Catalytic leadership

OVERVIEW

Healthy Cities is an approach that seeks to place health on the agenda of cities around the world, and build a local constituency of support for public health (Tsouros 1995). Projects are characterised by a broad-based, intersectoral political commitment to health and well-being in its broadest ecological sense, a commitment to innovation and democratic community participation, and healthy public policy. However, intersectoral collaboration may require the overturning of entrenched, fragmented ways of seeing and working among stakeholders and sectors. In order to promote intersectoral collaboration, Healthy Cities projects found that they needed champions, skilled in acting as catalytic leaders and social entrepreneurs, to elevate health to become everyone's core business, find creative ways to bring people together from different sectors, help them learn to understand issues from other people's perspectives, and seize opportunities to broker more effective political relations. This chapter will outline the history, philosophy, and principles of Healthy Cities, explaining core concepts and using two case studies to illustrate their application.

HISTORY

Promoted since 1986 by the World Health Organisation, Healthy Cities projects are characterised by a broad-based, intersectoral political commitment to health and well-being in its broadest ecological sense, a commitment to innovation, and an embrace of democratic community participation, with a focus on creating healthy public policy (WHO 1995). The roots for this new ecological, intersectoral approach were actually sown some decades earlier. Duhl (1963) offered an early systems perspective on the links between urban design, politics and policy, health, education, and personal security. In recognition that multiple perspectives help to provide a glimpse of the complexity of urban systems, this work was innovative in arguing for holistic solutions involving all the community; to move from illness to wellness; to orient towards social action and policy development; and participatory, democratic, and integrated planning. Duhl's recommendations for systemic, intersectoral collaboration on urban mental health provided the foundations for the international Healthy Cities program, developed some twenty years later.

The Healthy Cities concept was born at the 1984 Toronto 'Beyond Healthcare' conference and then championed by WHO Europe in 1986. Since then, the movement has spawned over 7000 projects worldwide. The concept is evolving to encompass healthy villages and municipalities, and has a close relationship to municipal public health planning (National Civic League 1998).

A healthy city has been defined as 'one that is constantly creating and improving those physical and social environments and expanding those community resources which enable people to mutually support each other in performing all the functions of life and in developing their maximum potential' (Hancock & Duhl 1988, p. 24). The Healthy Cities movement is based on the recognition that city and urban environments affect citizens' health, and that healthy municipal public policy is needed to effect change (Ashton 1992). Health and well-being must be planned and built 'into' cities; this process is presented as everyone's business. Political endorsement is seen as crucial to ensuring intersectoral collaboration. Systems for participatory decision-making must be developed to ensure that all voices are heard, especially those of marginalised people (Baum et al. 1993). In many ways, Healthy Cities has provided a practical guide for implementing the Ottawa Charter, and has developed a framework for intersectoral collaboration by which programs can be evaluated (Dooris 1999).

KEY PARAMETERS FOR HEALTHY CITIES AND COMMUNITIES

Hancock and Duhl (1988) proposed eleven elements as key parameters for healthy cities, communities, and towns, listed in the box below. The parameters are as relevant today as they were then:

Box 19.1: Key parameters for healthy cities, communities, and towns

1   A clean, safe, high-quality environment (including housing).
2   An ecosystem that is stable now and sustainable in the long term.
3   A strong, mutually supportive and non-exploitative community.
4   A high degree of public participation in and control over the decisions affecting life, health, and well-being.
5   The meeting of basic needs (food, water, shelter, income, safety, work) for all people.
6   Access to a wide variety of experiences and resources, with the possibility of multiple contacts, interaction, and communication.
7   A diverse, vital, and innovative economy.
8   Encouragement of connections with the past, with the varied cultural and biological heritage, and with other groups and individuals.
9   A city form (design) that is compatible with and enhances the preceding parameters and forms of behaviour.
10 An optimum level of appropriate public health and sick care services accessible to all.
11 High health status (both high positive health status and low disease status).

(Hancock & Duhl 1988)

These parameters show how health and well-being have many determinants that are influenced by policy and activity in many different sectors and institutions, including infrastructure planning, urban design, architecture, the business sector, developers, environment, art, and culture. A robust engagement with the higher education system is also crucial, to establish research partnerships and foster an informed civic democracy (Ashton 1992; Freire 1970; Mouffe 1992). This endorsement of the parameters by WHO (1995) has been useful in persuading government officials both inside and outside the public health arena of the importance of integrated planning approaches that consider the overall well-being of the whole person and the whole community (Department of Human Services 2001; Hay, Frew & Butterworth 2001).

WHO (1995) offers a systematic strategy for progressing through three phases of development of a Healthy Cities project in their document, *Twenty Steps for Developing a Healthy Cities Project*. As depicted in Figure 19.1 below, the three main phases are: start-up, project organisation, and areas for action and strategic work.

Figure 19.1 Three phases of development of a Healthy Cities project (WHO 1995)

| Phase 1 Getting started is the informal phase of project development. It comprises seven steps:
Steps:

1 Build support group
2 Understand ideas
3 Know the city
4 Find finances
5 Decide organisation
6 Prepare proposal
7 Get approval | Phase 2 Getting organised begins after city council approves a project proposal and continues until the project has the capacity to be an effective public health advocate:

8 Appoint committee
9 Analyse environment
10 Define project work
11 Set-up office
12 Plan strategy
13 Build capacity
14 Establish accountability | Phase 3 Taking action begins when the project has sufficient leadership and organisational capacity to be an effective public health advocate and continues as long as the project lasts:

15 Increase health awareness
16 Advocate strategic planning
17 Mobilise intersectoral action
18 Encourage community participation
19 Promote innovation
20 Secure healthy public policy |

Phase 1, step 3, 'Know the city' (WHO 1995: 22–23), contains a series of ten questions that should be answered as the project team builds up its initial momentum, because they show the value of locally valid knowledge that intersectoral perspectives can bring to data collection. These can only be answered in any depth through the combined intelligence of multiple sources from multiple perspectives. These include:

(i)   questions about the major health issues facing a city and their causes
(ii)   the impact of social and economic conditions

(iii)   the kinds and sources of support that would be needed for the Healthy Cities project to succeed

(iv)   a detailed analysis of how city politics works

(v)   how the city administration functions

(vi)   the concerns of the health care system

(vii)   the role that citizens' groups play in city life

(viii)   where information for project development can be found

(ix)   how national or regional programs might affect the project

(x)   how business, industry, and labour might support the project.

Intersectoral action can be achieved through a range of approaches. By establishing steering committees with diverse membership, discussion plays an essential role in achieving shared understanding of differing perspectives and encourages building alliances. Intersectoral action provides opportunities for senior executives and professionals to compare their experiences and develop an action learning approach to testing new policies. Health impact assessments (see Chapter 13) also provide an opportunity for senior executives outside the health sector to consider the impact of their decisions on health, and for all parties to consider the health, social, and economic impacts of proposed initiatives.

Strategic planning is a core function of intersectoral planning (WHO 1995: 48). Financial incentives for policy change are a core means to promote intersectoral action. For example, a budget allocation can be made to fund changes in policy and programs that will to strengthening their contribution to health. Community participation strategies are also seen to assist intersectoral action, by providing citizen perspectives on changes that are needed and strategies for enhancing intersectoral action. Accountability mechanisms, in which reports on the state of play are made public, create strong political and managerial impetus for intersectoral action.

APPROACHES TO DEVELOPMENT OF HEALTHY CITIES

Of course, different approaches are needed in different countries, which take account of political, cultural, and administrative systems. The European Healthy Cities approach involves the establishment of a peak intersectoral working group comprising senior personnel from key organisations. A project team assists the working group by: conducting community diagnosis; developing strong links with education bodies at all levels, for educative purposes as well as to collect data; assisting participating agencies to examine ways of engaging in health promotion; helping to generate public debate, with a view towards fostering city-level health advocacy; developing and evaluating targeted health promotion interventions. The project team works across sectors to break down the barriers between them and develop better linkages (Ashton 1992; WHO 1997).

The approach developed in the United States, by contrast, has been driven more at a grassroots level, reflecting the realties of an individualistic cultural tradition of 'life, liberty and the pursuit of happiness' and small government (National Civic League, 1998: 287), from which the collective notions of the Ottawa Charter may be viewed by some with suspicion (Baum et al. 1993). Furthermore, with a somewhat chaotic private health care system, much government attention in the US is focused on ensuring access to basic health care, rather than the upstream prevention advocated in Healthy Cities. Intersectoral collaboration has frequently been harder to achieve in the US than in countries such as Australia or Canada, in which government is expected to provide some sort of leadership (Twiss & Duma 2003; Wolff 2003).

Another approach from Australia is outlined in Case Study 19.1. This illustrates that institutional change towards intersectoral collaboration requires top-down and bottom-up support for more integrated practices. Decision-makers need to be provided with clear evidence supporting a paradigm shift in thinking and practice, although champions for change can still meet with inertia, passive resistance, and sometimes hostility (Innes & Booher 1999; Kuhn 1970). In order to achieve progress across often disparate organisational and jurisdictional boundaries, social entrepreneurs are needed to 'analyse, to envision, to communicate, to empathise, to enthuse, to advocate, to mediate, to enable, and to empower' (Catford 1997: 3). They need to help translate the social paradigm of health into concepts and approaches that can be embraced by stakeholders from various backgrounds and disciplines.

LEADERSHIP FOR INTERSECTORAL ACTION

Despite the crucial role that strategic leadership plays in intersectoral health promotion, little public health research has been published about what makes a good leader, and how to strengthen leadership in this sector (Catford 1997). Nevertheless, discourse on social entrepreneurship and catalytic leadership is filling this gap. As leaders, social entrepreneurs need to have the ability to see things holistically, to be proactive, to be reflective, and be able to seize opportunities to broker more effective political relations that might help foster enhanced decision-making that results in policy improvements. They must be able to act as boundary-spanners—navigating the strong and weak connections in the network of information and influence, making use of the ambiguities and windows of opportunity that exist within and between organisations (Duhl 2000). They have to be able to connect the streams of policy problem-solving, politics, and inherent policy flux (de Leeuw 1999; de Leeuw, Abbema & Commers 1998). De Leeuw (1999) pointed out that the most successful Healthy Cities programs had institutionalised the role of social entrepreneur. As a result, cities that had connected the urban planning and social change paradigms to a broad understanding of health were able to initiate and maintain intensive community-based health promotion programs.

In many ways, social entrepreneurs are acting as agents of social change within the health promotion paradigm by attempting to address sociopolitical issues of power, social structure, and social processes (Bunton 1992; Freire 1970; Huygens 1988). Baum (2002) argued that Healthy Cities advocates need 'to combine the skills of sophisticated bureaucratic negotiation and radical community activism' (p. 38). Otherwise, the perception will take root that Healthy Cities programs are constrained by the bureaucracies that frequently fund them. Baum argued that Healthy Cities programs need to be independent of those organisations whose very approach might need to be changed. The task facing any social entrepreneur, therefore, is to form an independent, broad-based coalition of support that works to convince key stakeholders of the benefits of intersectoral collaboration and become its champions.

At their most effective, social entrepreneurs are providing a form of 'catalytic leadership' (Duhl & Sanchez 1999), which can help build up a critical mass of support for integrated planning through a series of strategic actions targeting systems change among and between sectors. These are outlined in the box below.

Box 19.2: Components of catalytic leadership

- Focusing attention on the social determinants of health by elevating the issue to the public and policy agendas.
- Engaging people in the effort to address the social determinants of health by convening the diverse set of individuals, agencies, and interests needed to address the issue.
- Providing enabling mechanisms for health promotion to be developed and evaluated through healthy public policy and increased public accountability.
- Breaking down vertical structures and barriers and obtaining better horizontal integration for working together.
- Stimulating multiple strategies and options for action.
- Enhancing relevant innovative knowledge development and research.
- Improving data collection.
- Sustaining action and maintaining momentum by ensuring that communication is effective and feedback rapid.

(Duhl & Sanchez 1999)

When working with communities, its obvious and hidden assets need to be understood for the ways they can be put to use in solving problems. For example, worldwide, leadership is often in the hands of women. Women are thought to hold a complex interrelated worldview throughout their life, whereas in many cultures, men often are uni-directional in their thinking and, thus, their approaches. Women are often found to have an innate understanding of intersectoral collaboration, without having to learn it (Duhl 2000).

Case Study 19.1: Encouraging local governments to make health and well-being a whole-of-council concern

Promoting intersectoral collaboration is a key objective of the Local Government Partnerships Team in the Victorian Department of Human Services, Australia. Beginning in 2000, the Local Government Partnerships Team developed and then disseminated the municipal public health planning policy framework, 'Environments for Health' (Hay, Frew & Butterworth 2001). Drawing on the social model of health, this Framework provides an ecological approach to local government planning that considers the overall impact on health and well-being of factors originating across any or all of the built, social, economic, and natural environments. The Framework clearly demonstrates the link between urban planning and health, and the need to integrate these planning approaches.

The Policy framework was developed through an exhaustive, iterative, and open process of systematic research and development through questionnaire, feedback, and stakeholder consultation on draft content. Several hundred people participated in the development of the Framework, and, since then, its implementation. A range of approaches was undertaken to encourage enhanced integrated planning outcomes among health planners and urban planners, and developing links between state policy-makers in the areas of public health and urban planning. A culture of participatory enquiry has been developed among representatives from the sectors involved.

Forming an intersectoral reference committee early in the development of the Framework was integral to the success of the project. This committee, comprising representatives from across local government, health policy, and health promotion, ensured a strong external and internal coalition of support and theoretical and practical relevance. Several other factors enhanced the success of *Environments for Health:*

- The Minister for Health at the time was also the Minister for Planning. This provided symbolic and political support for a policy framework that integrated these portfolios.
- The Director of Public Health within DHS was a key champion of the Framework.
- Key to the success of the process was the three Local Government Partnerships Team members' concerted efforts to employ the catalytic leadership and social entrepreneurship discussed in this chapter.

The Framework was showcased at the 2002 World Summit on Sustainable Development in Johannesburg. This example shows that intersectoral collaboration can be made to work, even from within the confines of a large bureaucracy.

DOCUMENTING INTERSECTORAL COLLABORATION

The Ottawa Charter (WHO 1986) and Healthy Cities initiatives call for nothing less than systems change across multiple levels of analysis and between multiple sectors. As a community empowerment strategy, fostering intersectoral collaboration is a long-term, labour-intensive, and transforming process achieved through many actions and 'small wins' (Kieffer 1984; Perkins & Zimmerman 1995; Weick 1984). One way to gain support for intersectoral collaboration is to document evidence on how it can benefit communities. To have ecological validity, our monitoring and evaluation strategies need to attempt to reflect the complex reality of the social system by tracking the multiplicity of actions taken to enhance intersectoral collaboration, and the related ripple effect of change across and between levels of the social system (Rappaport 1987; Reppucci 1990). Case Study 19.2 describes the powerful social ecology framework that Kegler, Norton, and Aronson (2003) employed to monitor and evaluate efforts to promote community capacity. This analysis included changes to inter-organisational—and thus intersectoral—networks.

Case Study 19.2: Collecting evidence of intersectoral collaboration

In a detailed evaluation of twenty projects funded through the Californian Healthy Cities and Communities program, Kegler et al. (2003) examined the process of community development undertaken by the projects, and the changes resulting from these initiatives. Community capacity was defined as the 'characteristics of a community that enable it to mobilize, identify and solve community problems' (Goodman et al., cited in Kegler et al.: 3). Drawing on the work of Norton, Kegler et al. identified several components of community capacity, which included: (i) civic participation; (ii) mechanisms for community input; (iii) mechanisms for the distribution of community power; (iv) skills and access to resources; (v) sense of community and social capital/trust; (vi) social and inter-organisational networks; (vii) community values and history; (viii) capacity for reflection and learning.

The authors used a detailed social ecology framework to assess changes in community capacity across five social levels:

- changes in individuals
- changes in civic participation
- organisational development
- inter-organisational activity
- community-level changes.

Empowerment research shows how community capacity 'radiates' between levels (Butterworth & Fisher 2001; Rappaport 1987). While intersectoral collaboration could be most easily documented through inter-organisational activity, all the different components of community capacity are considered to complement it—and be enhanced by it. Kegler et al.'s (2003) social ecology framework shows how intersectoral collaboration influences, and is influenced by, a range of changes, from the individual to the community level.

Through analysis of program documentation, participant surveys, and in-depth interviews, Kegler et al. (2003) showed that various organisational representatives on Healthy Cities and Communities projects formed a range of new partnerships in which they: exchanged information with many partners; co-sponsored events; coordinated services; undertook joint initiatives or programs; and shared resources. Coordinators from across the twenty projects reported at least one, and up to seven, new or expanded partnerships. In decreasing order of frequency, new partnerships were formed mainly: (i) to operate programs; (ii) for limited or specific purposes; and (iii) to promote information exchange. A minority of partnerships were formed to: (iv) form a coalition broadly to improve community health; (v) give and receive technical assistance; and (vi) engage in advocacy. Governance team members across the twenty projects represented a range of community sectors, including: education; interested resident; community-based organisation; social/human services; health care; business; faith; political/elected officials in public health; recreation; criminal justice/safety; neighbourhood/civic group; housing; and media. Partnerships with agencies external to the community sector resulted in strengthened relationships and enhanced funding and other resources, proving the worth of the Healthy Cities and Communities investment of time and effort in intersectoral collaboration.

SUMMARY

Through working with the Healthy Cities and Healthy Communities model, people are learning to usher in a new paradigm: from an epoch of growth, individuality, lack of interest in conserving resources, and greed, to one of collaboration, cooperation, and the awareness of resource use. As part of this new paradigm, we deal with issues in a multisectoral way, with active community participation, and the need for equity and social justice. However, Healthy Cities is a community and individual learning program. People progressively learn how to promote health and community capacity in a new way. We say 'progressive', because once people learn on simple matters, they can deal with the more complex. This in effect is social learning and the building of social capital.

But, Healthy Cities is truly not a program. It is a process. More than that it is a template, or what we might call *open software*, which can be used differently, and modified by each community. Like Linux it is both open and revisable, as long as changes are fed back to the system. Meetings that are constantly taking place all over the world are places to share experience and educate each other from across the sectorial divide. We have learnt that cities have helped cities, that the original consultants are not needed to get the process going. It is in some ways a pseudo anarchic non-controlled organisation, despite the fact that WHO was the first facilitator and initiator of a program whose ideas were developed over many years. Social entrepreneurs have driven this intersectoral collaboration, both from inside and outside the health and community sectors. As a result of this effort:

■ Healthy public policy across all sectors and government portfolios becomes identified as a key goal.
■ High-level political endorsement ensures a viable and sustainable intersectoral approach.
■ Intersectoral collaboration becomes part of a broader community capacity-building approach.

The paradigm has shifted and Healthy Cities has played a role in this. We do not claim that Healthy Cities is unique. Indeed, throughout several decades many people have thought in this manner but now the time is right. One can use the story of the Exodus from Egypt as a way of explaining the need for time. The 40 years on the desert were required for the old to die with their ideas, the new generation to experiment with alternative views of the world, and then finally to cross over to the Promised Land. Indeed, as Duhl's (1963) text attests, the idea of Healthy Cities has taken that long to germinate.

USEFUL WEBSITES

International Healthy Cities Foundation: <www.healthycities.org>. 'The International Healthy Cities Foundation was created to assist people and groups from many different sectors. The mission of the IHCF is to facilitate linkages among people, issues and resources in order to support the development of Healthy Cities initiatives. The IHCF will both link people, organizations, and networks currently working to advance Healthy Cities goals and provide linkages with others dealing with significant and related areas of work. All aspects of health planning, promotion and prevention activities are needed for a balanced health system and will be included. All issues of community organization and governance will be involved. And finally, special interests, often regarded as separate areas of concern will be integrated into the ongoing work and goals of the IHCF.' Managed by Prof. Len Duhl, the site contains material in English, Spanish, and Portuguese.

Healthy Cities and Urban Governance: <www.who.dk/healthy-cities>. This site, maintained by WHO Regional Office for Europe, contains an extensive range of documentation covering the entire process of Healthy Cities initiatives in Europe since their inception. This site also lists a wide range of urban health-related topics, and their related links to relevant WHO programs and associated organisations and resources.

Local Government Planning for Health and Wellbeing: <www.health.vic.gov. au/localgov>. This site, maintained by the state government of Victoria, Australia, provides the latest online version of Environments for Health municipal public health planning policy framework and supporting documentation. A great deal of information is contained about local government efforts to implement this framework, and the Local Government Partnership Team's efforts to document progress and highlight issues.

The Center for Civic Partnerships, California: <www.civicpartnerships.org>. 'The Center for Civic Partnerships is a support organization that strengthens individuals, organizations, and communities by facilitating learning, leadership development, and networking. The Center provides technical support, educational programs, products and services which emphasize participatory governance and a systems approach to healthier communities. Center projects include conducting California Healthy Cities and Communities ...' This site contains a wealth of useful information, not least the profiles of all Californian Healthy Cities and Communities initiatives—the longest running in the USA. A detailed evaluation report by Kegler, Ronson and Aronson (2003) is also available, which employs a capacity-building framework to document change among initiatives.

FURTHER READING

Ashton, J. (ed.) (1992). *Healthy Cities*. Open University Press, Milton Keynes, UK.

de Leeuw, E. (1999). 'Healthy Cities: Urban social entrepreneurship for health.' *Health Promotion International*, 14, 261–9.

Duhl, L.J. (ed.) (1963). *The Urban Condition: People and Policy in the Metropolis*. Basic Books, New York.

Duhl, L.J. (2000). *The Social Entrepreneurship of Change* (2nd edn). Cogent Publishers, Putnam Valley, NY.

Hay, A., Frew, R. & Butterworth, I. (2001). 'Environments for Health: Municipal Public Health Planning.' *Environmental Health*, 1 (3), 85–9.

Kegler, M. C., Norton, B. L. & Aronson, A. E. (2003). 'Evaluation of the five-year expansion program of Californian Healthy Cities and Communities (1998–2003): Final report.' Sacramento CA: Centre for Civic Partnerships. Available online: <www.civicpartnerships.org/files/TCEFinalReport9-2003.pdf>. Accessed 13 March 2005.

ART AND COMMUNITY-BASED HEALTH PROMOTION: LESSONS FROM THE FIELD

Christine Putland

Key concepts

- The past few decades have seen a proliferation of initiatives linking art and cultural activities to the promotion of mental and physical health and well-being for individuals and communities in many parts of the world. The term 'Arts and Health' is used here (as opposed to Art in/for Health) to refer to this broad and varied field of practice.
- Community-based Arts and Health activities commonly involve practitioners from health and human services fields working together with arts and cultural development workers. In this sense it is a definitively intersectoral field, with initiatives designed and delivered by people and agencies with differing backgrounds, assumptions, skills, and expectations.
- Examining practice offers particular insights about the field of Arts and Health as well as generic lessons for intersectoral health promotion. It underscores the need for articulating a theory of practice reflecting the relationship between art and health, and explicates a new and challenging role for health practitioners based on an understanding of social determinants.
- The diversity of the Arts and Health field means that no single example can be taken as representative—there are as many different approaches as there are practitioners. The case studies included below are drawn from Australia and the United Kingdom to illustrate particular points in the discussion.

> ### Key terms
>
> - Community-based health promotion
> - Community arts/community cultural development
> - Transformational versus instrumental views of art
> - Rationale or theory of practice
> - Intersectoral action

OVERVIEW

'Arts and Health' is emerging as a broad and diverse field of practice, commonly involving collaboration among workers from health and human services as well as the arts. There is a growing body of literature documenting the many different approaches to Arts and Health work and presenting the case for incorporating community art into health promotion practice (McQueen-Thompson & Ziguras 2002). Rather than revisit well-trodden ground, this chapter presents community-based Arts and Health practice as a revealing case study of intersectoral action for health promotion. The discussion is framed around two central questions: 'Why Arts and Health?' and 'What lessons can be learned for intersectoral practice?' The first question draws our attention to the need for a theory of practice articulating the underlying rationales for arts-based practice in advancing health. The second focuses on the practitioners and sectors that comprise the workforce in this field and the nature of the relationships involved. Each question is addressed by reflections on theory and practice, in particular seeking out lessons to be learned from the field.

PART 1: WHY ARTS AND HEALTH?

Box 20.1: Personal reflection: scoping the field

In 2002, while designing a course in 'Art, Well-being and Public Health' at Flinders University, South Australia, I undertook a study tour in the UK, examining approaches to community-based Arts and Health projects. On hearing of my plans, several colleagues offered encouraging comments along the lines of: 'I was visiting a friend in hospital the other day and I noticed the new art works on the walls in the corridor—is that what you mean by Arts and Health?' The tone of the enquiry suggested: 'is that *all* you mean, and if so, what's to study?' Having worked in public health for some time I was accustomed to the ways our understanding of 'health' has been dominated by treating illness, but this kind of reaction also reminded me that as a society we promulgate a very narrow, individualised interpretation of what constitutes art. Meanwhile we take for granted the fact that 'art' is a 'good thing', though its precise value is hard to articulate. I determined that my investigation should therefore illuminate the myriad ways in which practitioners understand both art and health, and the links between them, while attempting to develop an orderly and accessible typology.

This idea provided my first salutary lesson. How to develop a typology when faced not by 'typical' examples, but by seemingly infinite variety? Even confining my focus to community-based activities concerned with health promotion, and thereby sidelining areas like 'medical humanities' and 'art therapy' as peripheral to my study (though in practice often overlapping), the field appeared vast. Apart from sharing basic elements of involving art in some form and either implicitly or explicitly addressing some aspect of health and/or well-being, diversity was the defining characteristic—diversity in terms of:

- art media—whether the medium was photography, rap dancing, or interactive theatre
- health issue or social determinant that was being addressed—whether concerned with social isolation and poverty in an urban regeneration project, or the mental health of people who experience long-term unemployment
- organisational or sectoral drivers—whether projects have been initiated by the arts or health or other sectors such as local government, housing, and urban development, or justice
- setting—whether hospitals, community centres, remote communities, housing estates, or prisons, for instance.

This list was a useful starting point for differentiating initiatives from each another. What was missing, however, was the one thing that practitioners continually wanted to talk about: *why* they were doing it. The question of 'Why *art?*' began to dominate conversations; and more specifically, 'Why art *in relation to* health?' What is it about making/experiencing/sharing art that they were convinced had a profound impact on people's health and sense of well-being? What changes could they see occurring in people's views of the world, attitudes, relationships, and decisions as a result? Unsurprisingly, there were as many answers to these questions as there were places, people, art forms, and 'health' issues to be addressed.

Common sense tells us that art and cultural practices are not only part of what makes us human, but also important ingredients in a healthy, fully functioning society. Just as most people accept that being physically active is 'good' for us, so too participating in art and cultural experiences is often assumed to have positive effects on our mental, physical, and spiritual well-being. But for a health promotion practitioner interested in fostering these effects it is necessary to go beyond mere acceptance. Designing, implementing, and evaluating initiatives involves developing an understanding of what we mean by health and art in a given context and the relationship between them. This may seem obvious; however, a number of commentators have observed that despite the rapidly expanding field and increased government investment in arts-based initiatives, practice is frequently built on tacit, rather than articulated assumptions about these essential elements (Angus 2001; Jermyn 2001). There remains a lack of rigorous evaluation and robust evidence for practice (Hamilton et al. 2003).

There are many reasons for this trend. On the practical side is the issue of short-term funding for arts-based projects and the inadequate resources for undertaking comprehensive evaluation. At a more profound level, however, is the difficulty of moving beyond the wealth of anecdotal data documenting outcomes for individuals and communities to providing convincing 'scientific' evidence of health effects (McQueen-Thompson & Ziguras 2002). It is not within the scope of this chapter to address the subject of evidence in detail since it opens up complex debates that go beyond Arts and Health and relate to competing views about community-based health promotion more generally (Gibson 1994). Notwithstanding these debates, the question of evidence does not excuse a lack of clarity about goals and purposes: the kinds of health effects that are expected to result, and the anticipated contribution of art.

The role of art in relation to health cannot be simple given that art, like health, is a contested concept. We are familiar with the fact that 'health' carries its particular social, cultural, and professional baggage, with multiple and conflicting meanings (Baum 2002: 4). Problems, after all, do not arrive on our health promotion doorstep 'pre-packaged'. We bring to bear our knowledge of the determinants of health in defining issues in health terms, as the result of social structures or inequitable living conditions for instance. Similarly, art does not carry the same meanings across time and place, but must be understood within its social and cultural context. Ideas about what to include and exclude from the category 'art' have been changing rapidly throughout the last century (Zolberg 1990). The idea of 'the arts' as a specialised domain, meaningful to only a few, is a comparatively recent (post-industrialisation) development (Horne 1988), and one that may be at odds with a more democratic view of art as an expression of human experience. The following case study illustrates the different ways in which understanding about determinants of health are translated into arts-based health promotion, reflecting different theoretical assumptions about the role of art.

Case Study 20.1: Comparative case study

Trongate Studios

In 1994 the Trongate Studios opened, using the visual arts as a catalyst, to combat the demoralising effects of mental ill health for people who are returning to the community after a period of hospitalisation. The philosophy behind Trongate Studios is that through positive encouragement and support, members will develop a sense of self-esteem and confidence, assisting their reintegration into society. People who are interested in joining the Studios are referred by a contact in health care or social work. Individuals are seen as artists and members of the Trongate Studios rather than clients within the mental health system. Studio space and materials are provided free of charge and there is a regular program of workshops run by the studio's coordinator and visiting artists who receive in-house training related to mental health. Media include drawing, painting, ceramics, photography, printmaking, textiles, video, and digital art. The Trongate Studios has an active exhibition program and is constantly seeking commissions and other opportunities for its members to engage in. It is firmly established within the social care, health care, and cultural community of Glasgow and has growing links throughout Europe.

The Studios encourages the development of individual artistic abilities in a creative environment. By actively participating and engaging in dialogue with professional artists, members may experience a range of benefits that will positively affect their mental health:

'For me the studios is (sic) a little piece of sanity in a world gone mad' (Studio member).

Source: Trongate Studios Art Worker, 2002.
<www.project-ability.co.uk>

South Tyneside Arts Studio

South Tyneside Arts Studio (STAS) aims to provide the environment and resources that enable people from South Tyneside, both with and without established mental health needs, to participate in creative and artistic activities where 'mutual creativity can foster personal growth'. STAS is open to the whole community: it is an arts project with a priority free service to people living with established mental health needs, as opposed to a mental health project using art as a therapeutic vehicle. STAS works closely with carers and other voluntary organisations. Studio facilities are available for members to use on a drop-in basis and people come and go as they please. Workshops are run daily within the studio and accredited courses in art are also available. STAS is managed by practising artists and sessional artists are self-employed and subcontracted. Members follow their own ideas and artistic journeys, while professional artists are on duty to work with and support members in whatever they choose to do. Media include painting, drawing, printmaking, sculpture, photography, digital media, and crafts such as silk painting, etc. Exhibitions are held each year for Studio members, featuring both groups and individuals, and members' work is also shown outside the Studio.

'The community as a whole has benefited from the Studio's presence through provision of affordable and accessible facilities and increased understanding of mental health issues. As a direct result of attending the studio, people are finding their way back into education at all levels.'

'Indirectly, and harder to quantify, are effects such as lower admissions to hospital for people using mental health services, less need for crisis intervention ... and fewer people living in isolation.'

Source: STAS Arts Worker, 2002.
<www.southtynesideartsstudio.co.uk>

The two examples comprising the comparative case study (Case Study 20.1) are similar in many respects. Both address mental health issues by providing studio-based visual arts facilities staffed by professional artists in a community-based setting. Starting from the specific needs of individuals with experience of mental health issues to move from a state of ill-health to a state of wellness—TS in particular is concerned with the return pathway from living in an institution to living in the wider community—they also represent an awareness of the wider social determinants of health including social networks, social and economic participation, and community attitudes, norms, and sanctions. The role of art in relation to these determinants is multiple: as a catalyst and motivation for participation, a productive and creative individual activity in itself, a pathway to economic independence and, in the case of STAS, as a conduit to wider democratic processes. Notably, in both instances participants are regarded as practising artists rather than clients of the health system.

Broadly, the initiatives reflect the argument that people suffering mental health issues are likely to have experienced 'damaged or precarious' self-image and community perception; arts involvement is argued to mean that they are 'often for the first time, appreciated for their talents rather than deficits' (VicHealth 2003a). Whereas TS defines itself as part of the 'social care, health care, and cultural community' of Glasgow, stressing the development of individual professional practice in a supportive environment, STAS has aligned itself more explicitly with non-health sectors including voluntary agencies and education. Reflecting its focus on improving community awareness, STAS has opened the studio to carers and the wider community and in this sense represents a broad understanding of social determinants and responsibility for promoting health (Keleher & Murphy 2004). This taps into one of the unique characteristics of working through the arts, according to Matarasso (1997): 'What matters so much about participation in the arts is not just that it gives people the personal and practical skills to help themselves and become involved in society—though it does—but that it opens routes into the wider democratic process and encourages people to want to take part'.

Figure 20.1   Health and arts discourses

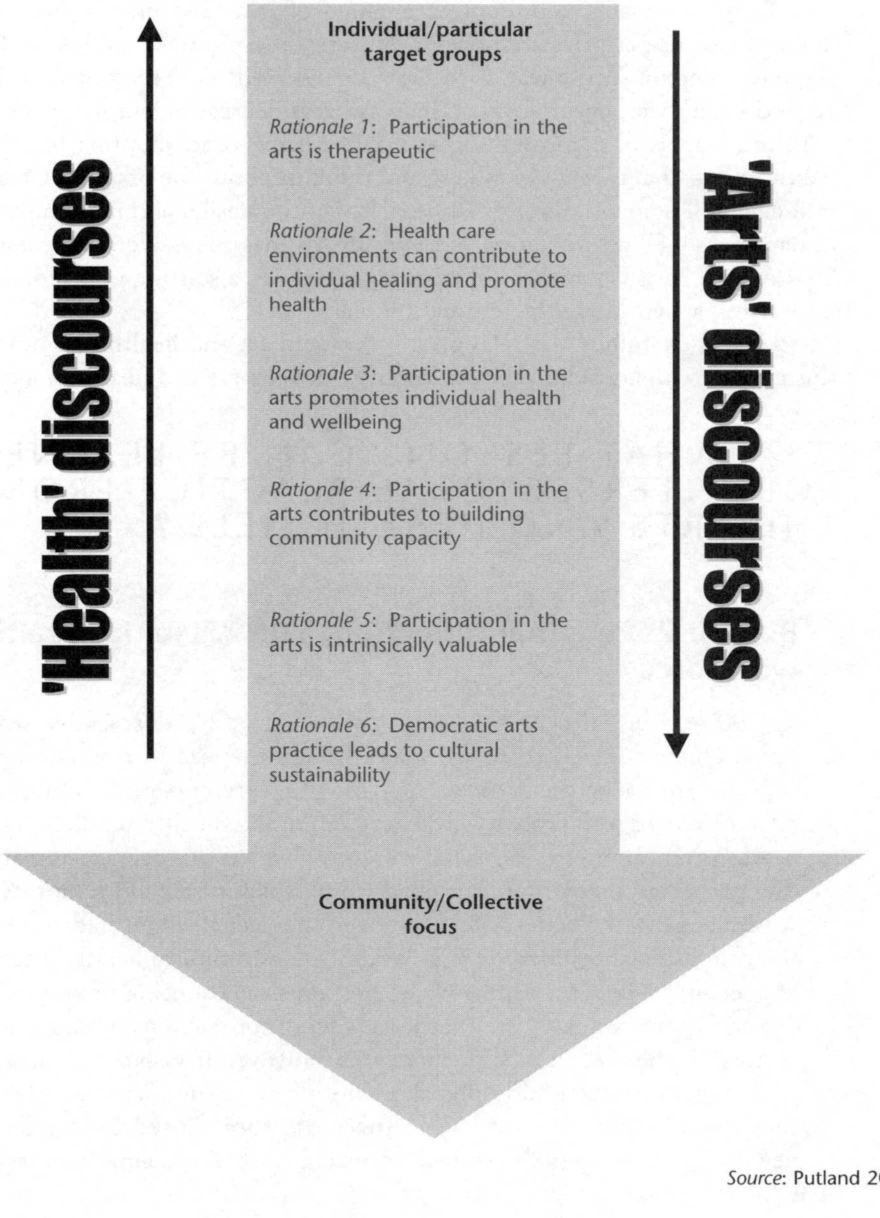

Individual/particular target groups

Rationale 1: Participation in the arts is therapeutic

Rationale 2: Health care environments can contribute to individual healing and promote health

Rationale 3: Participation in the arts promotes individual health and wellbeing

Rationale 4: Participation in the arts contributes to building community capacity

Rationale 5: Participation in the arts is intrinsically valuable

Rationale 6: Democratic arts practice leads to cultural sustainability

Community/Collective focus

'Health' discourses

'Arts' discourses

Source: Putland 2003

The question 'why arts and health?' is shorthand for thinking about transparency of purpose and developing a theory of practice that identifies the determinants of health relevant to a given initiative together with the proposed role of art in relation to these determinants. As part of daily practice Arts and Health practitioners reflect on their work, review decisions, and analyse effects. A theory of practice simply calls for explicit attention to this process. A useful starting point is to consider the broad rationales that are evident in the field, as identified in Figure 20.1.

These rationales, representing a range of intended effects, are neither a definitive or prescriptive framework, nor are they mutually exclusive. They are presented here in such a way as to show the very different relationships between art and health that ensue from an increasing or decreasing emphasis on working with individuals or communities, and at the same time adopting health or arts 'discourses'—that is, ways of talking and thinking about the practice. Clearly each rationale will demand different approaches to the design and implementation of initiatives as well as evaluation of their effectiveness. The overall framework can be used as a basis for analysis of existing initiatives, a starting point for designing initiatives, or hypotheses for evaluation planning.

Having examined the relationship between art and health, the next part of this chapter will consider the relationship between art and health practitioners.

PART 2: WHAT LESSONS CAN BE LEARNED FOR INTERSECTORAL PRACTICE FROM THE ARTS AND HEALTH FIELD?

Box 20.2: Personal reflection: The Arts and Health workforce

In 2002–03 a series of workshops was held at Flinders University for practitioners committed to working through the arts to promote health. The diverse backgrounds of participants was striking: artists, community arts/cultural development workers, community health workers, nurses, health promotion officers, social workers, hospital managers, occupational therapists, and many more travelled from urban, rural, and remote South Australia as well as interstate. Moreover, the agencies that had supported them to attend included local government, community health, arts, drug and alcohol services, youth services, hospitals, and housing projects.

All participants were keen to learn more about working across sectors. In the course of the workshops, however, it became evident that their practical and philosophical points of departure were as varied as their backgrounds. The key differences are summarised here (albeit in necessarily over-simplified form) according to the principal sectors with which they identified:

SUBJECT	HEALTH (AND RELATED SECTORS) PARTICIPANTS	ARTS-ORIENTED PARTICIPANTS
Views about health and health promotion (in context of Arts and Health)	Awareness of different models of health and health promotion Familiarity with and commitment to social determinants model Health sector has a central role	Commitment to broad understanding of well-being that includes health 'Health' language regarded as too restrictive and limited to medical model Health-sector role depends on context
Views about the role of art and art workers in initiatives	Instrumental—one tool among many for promotion of health Art workers contribute art skills	An end in itself—intrinsically valuable Art workers also play community development role
Characteristics of the 'system' they are part of	Inflexible administrative processes and accountability requirements Workforce in medium–long-term contract positions	Short-term funded projects Workers on fee-based contracts with no fixed hours; casualised and freelance labour force
Evaluation measures they identified as indicators of success	Changes in health status and/or wider social determinants Extent to which the social issues have been addressed Participation levels Participants report improved health and well-being	Evidence of quality of art work and creative process; Participation levels Participants report improved well-being

As an indication of the Arts and Health workforce, these workshop participants (Box 20.2) depict a broad field of interest rather than a cohesive sector, and one that is definitively intersectoral in nature. The particular characteristics of the sectors involved in this relationship and the understanding they bring are worthy of examination for the insights they offer about intersectoral health promotion more generally. The first thing to note is that Arts and Health practice represents the coming together of sectors that are intrinsically complex and multidisciplinary.

As we know, the workforce engaged in public health increasingly encompasses broader aspects of human services concerned with housing, local government, education, transport, and urban planning (Keleher 2004). Many health promotion workers may be well-schooled in the social and economic determinants of health and strive to work collaboratively with other sectors in response. Nevertheless, government priorities and the powerful professions that make up the health sector conspire to ensure that the influential view of 'health' in the wider community is one dominated by a focus on disease and individual behavioural change, and informed by the rationalist sciences and medical and technical expertise (see Chapter 1). In contrast, art is concerned with symbolism, metaphor, and the creation of value from precisely non-rational qualities: 'the strength of art-making is its capacity to communicate in multisensual or emotional domains' (Stafford 1998 cited in Thiele & Marsden 2003). From the perspective of many arts workers, therefore, the 'transformational' qualities of art (Mills 2003) can be seen to be at odds with an idea of art as merely instrumental (for example as a 'tool', 'aid', 'means') to health-defined goals.

In Case Study 20.2, for example, art represents many different things: a 'medium' (recycled instruments creating music), 'approach' (creative workshops), 'outcome' (youth leaders and lobbyists), 'product' (musical performance), 'catalyst' (continuing involvement of young people in music and musicians in community), and an 'indicator' of successful health promotion practice (all of the above). Rather than a utilitarian relationship with health, art is valued on its own terms.

Case Study 20.2: Music Recycles

This was a project involving young people from the western suburbs of Adelaide and the Adelaide Symphony Orchestra (ASO), making music with percussion instruments made from recycled metal scrap.

A community consultation process undertaken in conjunction with the development of a community cultural plan by the City of Port Adelaide Enfield identified the need for greater opportunities for young people living in the industrial suburb of Kilburn to participate in arts and cultural activities. Through the Adelaide Symphony Orchestra's Community Partnerships Program, a percussionist was engaged to provide workshops for young people from a range of cultural backgrounds. A local company, Metalcorp Recyclers, supported the proposal by opening its yards to the young people, providing them with hard hats and the chance to rummage for suitable scrap metal to use as percussion instruments. This collaboration between local government, the private sector, an incorporated arts industry body and young community members was aimed at addressing social exclusion. It featured:

- a community performance where the young people proudly showed off their creative skills to families and friends
- some young people emerging as leaders and lobbying successfully for facilities such as a youth centre in their community
- other young people continuing to work with the percussionist on developing music theory and technique
- more ASO musicians becoming involved in the next phase of the project and developing a sense of engagement with the wider South Australian community
- community members developing a sense of local identity beyond the heavy industries and rail yards for which their neighbourhood was known.

As a professional artist, working in the community requires new approaches:

'You have to communicate, you can't pre-empt how participants will respond and in
that sense it is not like playing in an orchestra program. You can't be stuck in your ways.
You have to listen and allow them to express themselves ...'

(ASO musician)

Meanwhile the Community Cultural Development Officer described how she
had to learn to act as 'interpreter' to explain the purpose of the project to her local
government colleagues:

'I would be asked "when is the orchestra coming to play?" It is so hard to explain, you
almost have to see it to understand what it means.'

Source: ASO Musician in conversation with Community Cultural Development Officer, 2003.
(Video: Flinders University Art and Health 2004)

It is apparent from the case study that artists and arts workers are a
heterogeneous group bringing a wide variety of skills and training, and reflecting
different views and ways of practising 'art'. In other words, just as not all health
practitioners appreciate the social determinants of health, not all artists are
experienced in community arts and community cultural development. Hence
not only is it unsurprising to discover variations in understanding, experiences,
and expectations in the Arts and Health workforce, but very often these may be
based on overly narrow interpretations or stereotypes of 'health' and 'art'. In such
a field, negotiated partnerships and collaborative action appear to be inherent
rather than discretionary features of practice; however, the relationships involved
are characteristically complex and unpredictable:

> Very few organisations have expertise in the combined fields [of Arts and
> Health] or combine these areas in their organisation ... The arts and health
> intersection promotes partnerships across sectors that do not have a history of
> working together (VicHealth 2003a).

The implications of this for practitioners include a requirement to relax
their customary professional boundaries and to confront the need for new skills
and new kinds of relationships.

Intersectoral action offers the promise that through collaboration
practitioners can expect to achieve outcomes that surpass their individual
capacities (Gray 1985, cited in Delaney 1994). For this promise to become a
reality, however, requires of practitioners the development of considerable skills

over and above those inherited from their immediate sector. 'Music Recycles', for example, clearly presented challenges to all of the practitioners, involving the adaptation of practice to meet different expectations and ways of working. For the health sector, moreover, it raises another set of questions. Nutbeam and Harris (2004: 53) note that the World Health Organisation (WHO) defines intersectoral action as 'a recognised partnership between part or parts of the health sector with part or parts of other sectors which has been formed to take action on an issue to achieve a health outcome'. 'Music Recycles' reminds us that insofar as Arts and Health initiatives may be instigated by 'non-health' sector partnerships, they unsettle a notion of the health sector as necessarily the driver in action to promote health. Thus social inclusion, an acknowledged determinant of health and well-being, is addressed directly as opposed to being mediated by health-oriented discourses. There is no 'health sector' partner in the collaboration, and rather than a specified 'health' problem, the starting point is a belief in the intrinsic value of art and young people's rights of access to art-based activities.

Just as we asked in Part 1 of this chapter 'what is the role of art?' this observation begs the question of 'what is the role of the health sector in arts-based health promotion founded on an understanding of social determinants?' Once we have understood and accepted the idea that responsibility for the key determinants of health lies outside the formal health sector (see Chapter 1), effectively a relinquishing of control, we must also consider the implications of this for its leadership role. The case study of 'Music Recycles' highlights one of the possible ways forward.

The theory of effective partnerships tells us that a 'healthy alliance' must be based on equality, which means respecting the contributions of all partners and learning from different ways of working (Gibson 1994). A barrier to achieving this has been 'the way that people from different knowledge systems tend to position themselves at the centre of the universe' (Mills 2003). From their respective viewpoints, both the musician and the local government worker in 'Music Recycles' acknowledge the need to shift their practice in order to communicate across professional and sectoral boundaries. For the professional musician this takes the form of a new kind of relationship between practitioner and participants, based on 'listening'. In the case of the local government officer, it is the necessity to act as 'interpreter', to find ways to explain this different conception of art to colleagues. This alerts us to one of the most challenging implications of intersectoral practice: the need to develop a shared vocabulary, one that is meaningful to and respectful of all of the partners involved, and which will enable dialogue across sectors. This challenge is being recognised by both health and arts practitioners:

> '...[Health promotion needs to] become more creative in making the connections between health and the language and agendas of other sectors' ...
> in order to 'create more permeable boundaries' (Sindall 1997).

Artist practitioners working alongside other non-arts professionals in fields such as criminal justice, health or welfare need to be able to explain the effectiveness of their practice to those other professionals. Furthermore they need to be able to do this without compromising or overly simplifying what is effectively a highly structured and complex practice (Thiele & Marsden 2003).

Insofar as such a vocabulary relates to the ways in which issues are framed as well as the ways in which the value of Arts and Health initiatives is expressed, it has the potential to contribute greatly to evaluation approaches in terms that are convincing and meaningful. Consider, on the one hand, the call from the public health sector for more scientific approaches to evaluation, prioritising evidence-based practice that goes beyond 'anecdote and opinion' (Hamilton et al. 2003). On the other hand, we have an arts sector that is justifiably fearful of the reductive nature of health methods, and evaluation in particular, and wary of being tied to prescribed social outcomes (Thiele & Marsden 2003). What would have to change for the elements of 'artistic function and outcome' to be respected and represented alongside the principle of 'evidence-based practice'? What would it mean for intersectoral relationships if such elements were integrated into a new, democratic way of expressing the value of the work in this field? If this sounds unrealistic, consider Matarasso's (1997) observation that 'if social and aesthetic value systems can be opposed, they do not have to be ... It is perfectly possible to combine high aesthetic standards with lasting social value'.

The notion of a peculiarly intersectoral language suggests a different role for the health sector that takes it beyond the dilemmas identified in Chapters 2 and 3. No longer having to choose between being the driver of health promotion or merely one of the passengers on the train, health practitioners can play a critical 'inaugurating' role in starting conversations of this nature. Perhaps this chapter has played its part by crafting some of the opening lines.

SUMMARY

- There is a range of approaches to Arts and Health, assuming different understandings about the role of art in health promotion; consideration of 'why Arts and Health?' or articulating a theory of practice is an important component of effective practice. A useful starting point is to identify the underlying rationales for particular initiatives.

- The contemporary field of Arts and Health comprises activities that are initiated and delivered by people and agencies with differing backgrounds, assumptions, and skills. This implies that the field is inherently multidisciplinary and unavoidably intersectoral. Therefore the ability to collaborate effectively across sectors is clearly an additional layer of skills demanded by this relationship.

- Partnership theory tells us that a 'healthy alliance' must be based on equality, which means respecting the contributions of all partners and learning from different ways of working. In Arts and Health this means valuing the transformational role of art and not just its instrumental use for health-defined goals. One of the difficulties currently inhibiting the realisation of such a relationship is the lack of a common language on which intersectoral action can be based.

■ Despite appearances, there is much common ground between community-based health promotion and community arts or cultural development approaches, which augurs well for the development of a healthy alliance that respects the different contributions.

■ Art represents to health a challenge to do things differently. In exchange health is well-placed to play a critical role in starting conversations about a genuinely intersectoral relationship based on social determinants.

USEFUL WEBSITES

The following websites are a source of information about 'Community Cultural Development' (ccd) approaches and examples of practice in Australia.

Community Cultural Development in Australia: <www.ccd.net>

Community Cultural Develoment New South Wales: <www.ccdnsw.org>

Community Arts Network Western Australia: <www.canwa.com.au>

In the United Kingdom the National Network for the Arts in Health gives a good overview of the wide range of activities that can be found under its umbrella: <www.nnah.nhs.uk>

The Australian Network for Arts and Health is also a useful starting point for learning about the field: <www.anah.org.au>

VicHealth, the Victorian Health Promotion foundation based in Melbourne, Australia, is a strong supporter of community arts programs. There are a number of publications that describe the links between community arts and health and well-being as well as many examples of initiatives to be found on the website: <www.vichealth.vic.gov.au>

FURTHER READING

Health Development Agency (2000). 'Art for health: a review of good practice in community-based arts projects and initiatives which impact on health and wellbeing.' HDA, London: <www.hda-online.org.au>

Mills, D. & Brown, P. (2004). *Art and Wellbeing*, Australia Council for the Arts, Sydney.

Williams, D. (1995). *Creating Social Capital: a study of the long-term benefits from community based arts funding*. Community Arts Network of South Australia, Adelaide.

SPACE AND PLACE: GEOGRAPHY IN HEALTH PROMOTION

21

Lisel O'Dwyer

Key concepts

- Health promotion efforts have a spatial context and a spatial impact—everything happens somewhere.
- Geography provides a framework and tools to understand how space and place influence health and how health promotion can account for that.
- There's more to interpreting maps than looking at the picture.
- 'Location' is more than a place on a map—it includes distance, area, adjacency, accessibility, environment, travel, density, and scale.
- We need to choose the right scale and the right place for a health promotion effort, or tailor health promotion to the necessary place and scale.
- 'Place' is not just where something or someone happens to be; it has emotional/cultural/personal significance.
- We can take advantage of the benefits of place for health promotion using concepts such as therapeutic landscapes.

Key terms

- Location
- Scale
- Place
- Accessibility
- GIS
- Boundaries
- Human geography

OVERVIEW

Why should health promotion consider and account for space and place? Space and place in part determine life chances, including health. Health promotion and human geography are both concerned with populations and groups. Geography pays explicit attention to physical location and what this means for health outcomes, health interventions, and policy-making. Location is a major determinant of many factors related to health, such as type and quality of housing, access to employment, access to services such as schools, shopping, and hospitals, and the quality of social and physical environments. Geography is also concerned with the patterns and distributions of social processes and demographics over physical space—geographers ask 'What is where and why is it there?' A spatial perspective of health promotion provides a context that can improve understanding of the incentives and barriers to the health of individuals and communities. Because social (and political) processes operate at various spatial scales, health promotion policy-makers and practitioners need to understand how scale can inform understanding of a phenomenon and influence the impact and success of an intervention.

INTRODUCTION

Health geography? What's that?

What's geography got to do with health?

Geography is a misunderstood discipline with an image problem. The popular perception of 'geography' is that of knowing the capital cities of various countries, what soil type is found in the south-western tablelands of NSW, or the main imports and exports of Slovenia. This perception is common even within the social sciences. Most health scientists and practitioners don't think about geography at all, let alone incorporate or use any geographical concepts or methods in their research or practice. This is unfortunate, because human geography, and its subfield of health geography, offers many useful ideas and methods to health promotion. This chapter aims to open new doors for health promotion by showing the ways in which geographical concepts can be harnessed and exploited.

Assuming that you, the reader, are unfamiliar with the joys of geography, we will begin with a brief description of both human geography and health geography.

WHAT IS GEOGRAPHY?

The discipline of geography can be seen as two connected parts—physical and human. Physical geography is concerned with the distribution of elements in the natural environment and encompasses such subfields as geomorphology and environmental management. Human geography, on the other hand, is concerned with the distribution of elements in the social and built environment. It includes such fields as urban and housing studies, population and demography, economic and regional development, political geography and, of course, health geography (sometimes also referred to as 'medical geography' or the 'geography of health'). Human geographers work within the broad theoretical paradigms common to most of the social sciences.

Geography investigates everything in its context. Context encompasses the social and the physical, but it generally involves more precise considerations such as the operation of housing and labour markets, the role of demographic factors (e.g. education level, ethnicity, family types, age, and so on), local environments, pertinent public policies, and public and private attitudes and perceptions, and group and individual behaviours. Understanding how these processes operate is an important part of enabling action in the five priority areas identified for health promotion in the Ottawa Charter for Health Promotion (WHO 1986), particularly those of building healthy public policy and creating supportive environments for health.

Within health geography there have been two main focuses: disease ecology (the study of the distribution of diseases and their correlates), and accessibility to health care and services. The boundaries between them have become permeable, especially with the increasing use of Geographical Information Systems (GIS) as a research tool able to integrate many different sets of data. Health geographers also study how people experience different states of health and illness in different places and how the place where they live or work influences their health.

There is also a role for physical geography in being prepared for and managing natural disasters such as bushfires or earthquakes, and understanding how physical processes involved in land degradation are ultimately related to human health. Such processes include desertification, rising water tables, salinisation, deforestation, wind and water erosion of soil, and the role of climate and terrain in providing a habitat for disease vectors.

All subfields of geography are concerned with location and spatial distribution—not just identifying and describing a distribution but explaining why it is the way it is, why something is in a particular place or location, and what this means for equity, quality of life, social and public policy, and in this case, health and health promotion.

Geography is a very practical field of study. Like health promotion it is oriented towards making a difference in the human condition, not only by providing evidence for public policy-making by describing and analysing, but by helping to decide where things should happen (i.e. targeting) and understanding why some things happen where they do. It offers new ways of viewing old problems. We all know that sometimes a different perspective makes all the difference.

It is not so much 'what' is studied that is of interest here—it is 'how' and 'why', and sometimes also 'when'. This chapter aims first to show health promotion practitioners what geographical concepts they need to be aware of and consider, and then gives some tips on how to put these ideas into practice.

COMMON THEMES IN GEOGRAPHY AND HEALTH PROMOTION

By now the reader might see that there are many common themes between human geography and health promotion, such that the twain can meet quite easily.

Geography and health promotion both deal with:

- populations, subgroups, and collective outcomes
- lifestyle, behaviour, and environment
- change over time
- human experience and interaction with wider social structures, processes, and institutions (economic, social, political, cultural)
- human experience and interaction with the natural environment
- diversity, difference, and differentials: inequality juxtaposed with ideals of inclusion and social justice
- access (and unequal access) to resources
- quantitative and qualitative research methods
- diffusion of social processes and policies over time and place
- understanding the role of wider context—neither can be understood as either solely physical processes, or solely social processes.

Geography and health promotion both link with or draw on other disciplines. Indeed, most of the social determinants of health as identified by the WHO (Wilkinson & Marmot 2003) are themselves the focus of some subfield of geography. For example, social and population geography examines the distribution of income, education, occupation (also known as class gradient or socio-economic status), family structure, and access to transport over space and time. Environmental management focuses on issues such as sanitation, natural hazards, and sustainable development and exploitation of natural resources. Environmental perception and cognitive geography draws on behavioural psychology to understand both individual and group behaviours and actions in different environments.

BASIC GEOGRAPHICAL CONCEPTS RELEVANT TO HEALTH PROMOTION

Particularly when dealing with large groups of people, as happens in health promotion, a project might require the input of various bodies of knowledge and expertise not residing in any one discipline. Multidisciplinary collaboration does not require extensive training in the 'other' fields, but it is important nevertheless to have at least some grasp of the other field's (or fields') basic concepts for many reasons:

- so that you know them when you see them
- so that you do not overlook or underestimate their relevance to the problem at hand

■ so as not to inadvertently misuse (or abuse) them
■ so that you know how much more there is about the field that you don't know.

Using the techniques or theories of other fields without fully appreciating them is risky. The main risks are that

■ outcomes do not reach their potential
■ future multidisciplinary collaboration is less likely
■ the user's opinion of the unfamiliar discipline's value in future work is unfairly tainted.

Two common misuses of geographical methods by other disciplines are, first, producing and using maps despite having little knowledge of cartography, and second the inappropriate use of GIS. The first usually results in misleading or even meaningless patterns, while the second is reduced to producing pretty maps without utilising the powerful analytical tools.

The following section introduces the basic concepts of location, scale, and place in the hope of promoting good geographic practice for non-geographers and for the benefit of geographical approaches for research, analysis, and planning in health promotion.

Location

Location may seem a straightforward concept but in fact there are two types of location. These are known as 'areas' and 'points'. Both are forms of spatial data.

Areas

Areas can be real but can also be abstract and have a two-dimensional concept. In all cases, they consist of space enclosed by boundaries and they have the dimensions of size and shape. In both real life and geographical investigation, we use areas as a way of simplifying and organising reality.

In the social sciences, areas are almost always abstract because they are defined for administrative purposes and do not physically exist in the real world. We cannot actually see the line denoting where Queensland ends and New South Wales starts unless we look at a map. Physical boundaries defining an area—like a fence around a house or the coastline of a country—obviously exist but most of the areas we work with in health geography and health promotion exist on paper only. This is because we need to use a variety of different-sized areas to summarise information, depending on the information and our purpose (discussed below in the section on scale).

One area represents one value. For example, in Adelaide, South Australia, 2.7 per cent of persons in the labour force in the Local Government Area (LGA) of Burnside are unemployed, while 7.4 per cent of the Playford LGA labour force is unemployed. Each LGA in the metropolitan area, state, or Australia will have a value indicating the percentage of its labour force that is unemployed.

Areas are also a mental concept used by people to move within or between in their everyday life and to describe particular places, such as their residential neighbourhood. In this instance areas as conceptualised in people's minds may have fuzzy or undefined boundaries that may vary greatly in size and shape between individuals.

Case Study 21.1: Conceptions of neighbourhood

A study of the relationships between health and place in South Australia asked a wide range of people to draw how they see their neighbourhood on a map that showed their home in the centre of the map. Some people drew very small boxes enclosing the house on either side of their homes. Some people drew large, rough circles denoting neighbourhoods spanning several kilometres or more. Still others drew a series of discrete, geographically unconnected points indicating specific places they considered to be significant in their daily lives. There was great variation in the shape, size, and geographical orientation of neighbourhoods, and also in the attention given to defining boundaries (O'Dwyer et al. 2004).

The way people conceptualise their neighbourhoods may offer useful insights for health promotion given that many health promotions, particularly those relating to exercise and social networks, operate at the neighbourhood level.

Attributes

Areas and points also have 'attributes', the term for the information (data) relating to each individual area or point. Attributes for an area might include information on its size in square kilometres or metres, the number of people living in the area, rate of overweight, percentage of persons aged 15–24, whether it is urban or rural. Points will always have a geographic reference expressed as a 'coordinate', which is the latitude and longitude. The degree of the coordinate's accuracy (whether it is accurate to within a kilometre, metres, or centimetres of the entity's real location) depends on how many decimal places the coordinate has. Other attributes of a point could be a code for the type of house it represents (e.g. 1= townhouse, 2 = detached house), the age of the entity (whether person or building), the date an event occurred, or the number of people using a service in a specified time period.

Sometimes we may only have data for an area when we need to know what the value is for a specific point in that area. Assuming that all points in an area will have the area's value, which has been averaged or aggregated from the values of the individual points, is unrealistic (and an example of what is known as the 'ecological fallacy';) but sometimes can't be avoided in area-based analyses. Nor can we assume that an area will have the same value as some individual points within it—this would be the 'atomistic fallacy' (Tunstall et al. 2004).

Box 21.1: Significance of spatial relationships for health promotion

Areas and points can both be characterised, described, or referenced by specific locational features such as 'adjacency', 'containment', 'proximity' (distance from something), 'overlap', and 'intersection'. In other words they have inherent spatial relationships with other areas or points. These relationships can be highly significant for health promotion because:

- they influence how quickly new ideas can penetrate or diffuse through a community
- they show the optimum place for a new service with a view to reaching as many people as possible
- environmental or structural factors might determine behaviour in certain areas.

Note that some things, like parks, can be expressed with maps as either areas or points, depending on the scale or detail you need (resolution) and whether it is relevant or necessary to do so. For example, if we want to find out how far it would be for people to walk to their nearest bus stop from their homes, we do not need to know the shape or size of their house. We only need to know its point location. If we wanted to find how much green space there is in within a larger area such as a suburb or neighbourhood, we would need to know the area of a park. But if we wanted to know how far that park is from a school, we would need point level data. We could use the centroid of the park's area as the point from which to base the distance measurement, or a point on its closest edge.

Scale

What is geographic scale?

Scale is a way of conceptualising location, size, and distance. Like time, height, weight, or age, geographic scale is a continuous variable, ranging from the precise point where you are sitting reading this book, which can be identified and labelled with coordinates, accurate to the nearest millimetre (or even less, if you really need it) to the global.

How is scale relevant to health promotion?

The scale at which data are collected or a health promotion program is implemented has major implications for the quality and success of your efforts. You need to target health promotion efforts at the appropriate geographic scale to maximise efficiency and effectiveness. Geographic scale also affects individual stakeholders' perceptions and their ways of knowing. For small-scale areas, stakeholders' ways of learning and knowing tend to be subjective, relying on diverse personal experiences and specific place features. For large-scale areas, stakeholders rely more on scientific analyses and symbolic abstractions.

Geographic scale combines with factors such as expert–versus–layperson tensions and organisational identity to affect working relationships in a collaborative stakeholder participation process (Cheng & Daniels 2005). Such relationships are a key part of health promotion. Yet a recent systematic review of area-based interventions into health inequalities found no discussion or acknowledgment of the relationship in the public health literature either between geographic scale and stakeholder views, or between the scale of interventions and their outcomes (O'Dwyer et al. under review).

Spatial units

For ease of analysis and utility, scale is divided into hierarchical structures, each with a range of different classes or levels, known as spatial units. Spatial units are to scale what physical measurements like metres or miles are to length. There are many ways of dividing scale into spatial units, like the way length can be measured using various systems such as the imperial or metric systems.

Most spatial units have idiosyncrasies the user needs to be aware of. For example, the Australian Bureau of Statistics has postcodes comprising Census Collector Districts agglomerated to match the postcode boundaries designated by Australia Post as closely as possible. Unfortunately, they are not always a good match. Suburbs can be a useful scale at which to collect data and to operationalise a pilot program, as they are not too big (like local government areas) or too small (like Collector Districts) but they only exist in metropolitan areas, and so do not cover the whole country seamlessly. Like postcodes, they consist of the best fitting Collector Districts rather than locally known boundaries. The boundaries of Local Government Areas and electorates in particular are subject to frequent change, which can make time series comparisons difficult.

Choosing the right scale

The trick is knowing which size spatial unit, or scale, to use for your purpose. Sometimes you might need to use several scales at once. To select the right scale, you need to consider the geographic size, extent, or bounds of the issue you are addressing.

We need to give more attention to conceptual underpinnings about the scales at which social and policy processes work. Some issues are better addressed at the local level, others at larger levels. Some are influenced by processes operating at two or more different scales. Housing status is a good example of an important influence on health which is affected by local, state and national forces.

Community stakeholders' knowledge and participation in decision-making also tends to be enhanced at smaller geographic scales (Cheng & Daniels 2005; Fleming & Henkel 2001; Harker & Natter 1995). Conversely, some issues most visible at local geographic levels are caused by factors operating at much larger

Case Study 21.2: Using the right geographic scale

An example of a successful neighbourhood-level project is the Moving to Opportunity program in the US (Fauth, Leventhal & Brooks-Gunn 2004). This program hinges on the presence and role of social capital—a neighbourhood or small area phenomenon (Kawachi & Berkman 2003). Randomly selected households in deprived areas were moved to more advantaged areas, where they were able to develop social networks with their new neighbours, gain access to local resources such as safe playgrounds, and adopt local social norms. Households who moved to better neighbourhoods had improved health relative to the households who stayed behind. Such results would not occur if the hsouseholds had moved to locations chosen at the level of the city, state, or country—they are too large for the operation of localised social processes like building social capital.

scales. For example, unemployed persons and part-time and casual workers with low incomes tend to locate in specific suburbs and parts of cities—but their shaky position in the labour force is really related to national or global industrial restructuring. Their residential location in turn is related to the spatial allocation processes inherent in housing markets, which can operate at the local, metropolitan, state, and even the national scale. Action to improve both the economic and housing positions of low income people and thereby their health, is therefore best addressed at the national or state scale. This falls outside the scope of most health promotion efforts unless there is multidisciplinary collaboration between government departments and between tiers of government.

Smaller scales can sometimes be used to test new approaches. However, 'scaling up' from local place-based interventions to larger regional scales can be difficult, because geographic scale affects the delegation of responsibility. Another potential problem when the scale is too small is dependency on program funding. Local organisations and communities are key stakeholders in small areas but if funding for local programs dries up, such groups can be left without alternative means of support. That can undermine any positive outcomes that may have been achieved.

On the other hand, scaling down a successful regional level intervention is possible in some circumstances, if a good example has been set to the local stakeholders. By initially focusing on regional or national scales, interest groups can mobilise broad public support for policies that may otherwise fail when considered at smaller scales (Taylor 1984: 4, in Cheng & Daniels 2003).

Place

The concept of place has long been a key focus for geographers and we are pleased that its importance is now being recognised in other areas, especially health promotion. Place is more than just a physical location—it refers to emotional or ontological attachment to and feelings towards a specific location or area. Place is somewhere that has a meaning to individuals or populations, perhaps because of events that have happened there in the past, physical beauty, culture, religion and tradition, or significant personal experience. Place can be just a single house, or even a room in a house—or it can be a beach, a town, a neighbourhood, a mountain range, a forest, a building, an expanse of land. Places can be hidden, private, public, shared, or sacred. As Tunstall et al. (2004: 6) put it, 'Place is to space as history is to time and home is to house'.

Case Study 21.3: Places of stigma

Every town or city has its places where no one really wants to live. These places have a popular image of disadvantage, hopelessness, barren environments, and poor access to resources and facilities. They are often located far from the city centre—out of sight. People who live there can't afford to live anywhere else, and their poverty engenders a whole range of other social and even physical ills. The media and popular culture reinforce negative perceptions of these places in many subtle and not so subtle ways, but sometimes these images lend their residents a unique strength of character and sense of community (Peel 1995).

The idea that areas or neighbourhoods affect health is not really new to health promotion. However, the concepts of 'community' and 'place' are often blurred, as are 'community', 'neighbourhood', and 'area'. In geography, these terms are all (albeit arguably) conceptually distinct and it may be useful for health promotion to recognise the distinctions. 'Neighbourhood' has a spatial dimension and refers to the area surrounding a residence—it may or may not have any special meaning to the resident, whereas 'community' consists of people who interact with each other on some basis (which is usually, but not always, the area they live in). The (understandable) confusion arises from the fact that communities and neighbourhoods are physically located somewhere and tend to be described using their location. 'Place' can also be described using a physical location, but it refers to the relationship between a person or group and the location, not the relationship between persons or groups in the same community. It has been used, however, in recent public health research to mean the contextual environment for health outcomes, without necessarily considering emotional attachment or individual meaning.

Place is not just the domain of geography. Depending on the type or scale of place, disciplines such as architecture, psychology, and philosophy have different approaches and insights to how people live and perceive place. Both health geographers and now public health researchers, practitioners, and policy-makers, however, see it as an essential element in the development of identity, health, and overall well-being. This is the logic underlying the health benefits of local programs and policies such as urban regeneration and tenure mix (avoiding the creation of public housing estates geographically concentrating disadvantaged households). There are also larger scale official efforts to define, create, change, or identify places by giving them descriptive labels. Thus we have the Festival State, the Garden State, the Sunshine State, and so on.

Maps and GIS

A map is a graphical display of spatial data that describes the distribution and location of objects or phenomena over space. Just as charts can distort information depending on the scale of the axes and categories used, maps can present the same data differently depending on the spatial scale and classification system used. It can be very easy to impress and mislead unsuspecting non-geographers with maps. Similarly, with the variety of software packages now available it is very easy for people not trained in cartography to produce maps that inadvertently give the wrong impression. However, when done properly, maps are a very useful tool for communication—data are more readily understood when mapped and significant patterns or outcomes are more visible.

A GIS is a computer system for storing, manipulating, analysing, and displaying spatial data. It is the manipulation and analysis capacities that separate it from mere mapping software. GIS can be used to query spatial data. For example, you may wish to find a site for a new health centre that meets a set of requirements, such as being within five kilometres of a major hospital, in a low socio-economic status area, with a minimum land area of 500 m². All sites meeting these criteria can then be listed or displayed on a map, and investigated further. GIS can be used to find the distance or travel time along roads between two or more points, or the shortest routes between them. Many 'layers' of data can be overlaid or combined to reveal new insights. GISs are becoming increasingly sophisticated in their analytical capacities, and fortunately are now more user-friendly than in the past. There are often training courses available tailored specifically for the health field. While there may be a steep learning curve, health professionals can gain enormous benefits from using GIS in their work. The benefits of understanding what GIS can do is worth it.

Case Study 21.4: Confusing mapping and GIS

A health geographer working in a public health department with colleagues from different disciplinary backgrounds occasionally uses illustrative (descriptive) maps in research, team conference presentations, and reports where appropriate. In conversations about current work with outside personnel such as visiting researchers and government bureaucrats, reference is made by other team members as to how 'GIS' was used, because of: the increasing profile of the term 'GIS' in public health; the connotations of GIS as cutting edge and 'hi-tech', and the misconception that mapping and GIS are the same thing.

SUMMARY

- Geography covers a wide range of subject matter, even within the subfield of health geography.
- Geography is concerned with explaining location and distribution and the implications of these for health.
- Health geography shares some ground with health promotion.
- Spatial relationships between factors in the physical and social environment can determine people's health outcomes and the way health can best be promoted.
- Geography has a range of tools and frameworks that can further the aims of health promotion, particularly in terms of planning and evaluation.
- It is important to understand how to use another discipline's specialist concepts and techniques properly.
- Location can be described as an area or point.
- We need to remember that boundaries of areas are artificial when interpreting patterns in maps showing different values for areas over space, and also that we need to consider the reliability of the data they are based on.
- The Australian Bureau of Statistics is the best place to find demographic and other social data for large areas; the census has demographic data for smaller areas.
- All area data is aggregated and therefore less precise than point level data—but point data is usually difficult to obtain.
- We need to match health promotion efforts for specific issues to the right scale.
- The concept of place may be a useful avenue for health promotion.
- Maps can be a useful way of summarising and describing information with a spatial dimension.
- GIS is more than just mapping.

USEFUL WEBSITES

Using Geographic Information Systems Mapping across the Disciplines: <www.geog.buffalo.edu/ncgia/pdf/Housel_Miller.pdf>. This paper is an easy to understand explanation of what GIS is and how it can be used in a range of disciplines outside geography.

Centre for Spatially Integrated Social Science: <www.csiss.org/>. This is an excellent resource for downloadable literature about the relevance of space to the social sciences. It also provides information about spatial analysis software, including links to downloadable free software.

Centre for research into sustainable urban and regional futures (cr-surf): <www.uq.edu.au/cr-surf/>. This website documents the beginning of the Australian equivalent of CSISS (above), the ARC Research Network for

Spatially Integrated Social Science. It lists the members of the network, what they are working on and the activities of the network in promoting spatial awareness and methods for social research and policy making.

Research on Place and Space: <pegasus.cc.ucf.edu/~janzb/place/>. This site lists the key names and publications on the subject of place and is oriented towards people unfamiliar with the concept who want a good introduction or overview.

FURTHER READING

Andrews, G. J. & Moon, G. (2005) 'Space, place and the evidence base', *World Views on Evidence-Based Nursing* Second Quarter, pp. 55–62.

Cromley, E. & McLafferty, S. (2002) *GIS and Public Health*. Guilford, New York.

Curtis, S. E. (2004) *Health and Inequality: Geographical Perspectives*. Sage Publications Ltd.

deBlij, H. J. & Murphy, A. B. (2003) *Human Geography: Culture, Society and Space* (7th edn). John Wiley, New York.

Gatrell, A. C. (2002) *Geographies of Health: An Introduction*. Blackwell, Oxford.

Milligan, C., Gatrell, T. & Bingley, A. (2004) '"Cultivating health": therapeutic landscapes and older people in Northern England.' *Social Science and Medicine*, 58, pp. 1781–93.

Williams, A. (ed.), (1999) *Therapeutic Landscapes: The Dynamic Between Place and Wellness*, University Press of America.

22

REFRAMING PHYSICAL ACTIVITY

Colin MacDougall

Key concepts

- In the 1950s, evidence emerged showing exercise helped in the treatment of heart attack.
- Between the 1970s and 1990s, lifestyle approaches and counselling theories combined to shape the research and interventions aiming to promote physical activity.
- Lifestyle approaches, by themselves, are unable to make population-level increases in physical activity.
- New frameworks and research designs are needed to promote physical activity using intersectoral strategies.
- The socio-environmental approach to physical activity promotion aims to improve participation in physical activity by enhancing our understanding of its social, cultural, and environmental determinants.
- Reframing physical activity to acknowledge social determinants requires a combination of social epidemiology, qualitative research, community participation, and intersectoral collaboration.

Key terms

- Physical activity and inactivity
- Medical, lifestyle, and socio-environmental approaches to health promotion
- Research design
- Community participation and ordinary theory
- Collaboration
- Local government agenda

OVERVIEW

We know that in developed countries, governments are expressing increasing concern that physical inactivity is increasing steadily, in both children and adults. The health sector has taken a strong lead on this issue, leading to such newspaper headlines as:

Walk away your Cancer Fears (*The Australian*, 24 June 2002)

30 mins A Day Keeps the Doctor Away (*Australian Financial Review*, 6 May 2004)

Go for Your Life—Make healthy living the norm (*The Age*, 11 November 2004)

Clearly these headlines frame physical activity as a health issue, and locate the responsibility for getting active and avoiding illness with the individual. Over the years millions of dollars have been spent on campaigns to change lifestyles. Yet why is physical activity decreasing despite community-wide, targeted, and other health promotion interventions designed to improve health by increasing physical activity? Are we using the best interventions? To help think through such questions this chapter examines why promoting physical activity was first framed within the medical model, and how it then developed into a behavioural or lifestyle approach. Then, the chapter shows what it takes to reframe the debate to acknowledge the power of the social determinants of health and well-being— including physical activity.

MEDICAL MODELS OF PHYSICAL ACTIVITY IN THE 'GOLDEN AGE' OF CARDIOLOGY

A 1947 British textbook of medicine had this to say about the treatment of heart attack:

After he has been confined to bed for two months, an extra pillow may be allowed; a week or so later the bed may be gradually more raised and during the last two weeks passive graduated exercise of the body and limbs and breathing exercises may be employed. After the period in bed the patient should be moved to a couch to which he should be confined for at least two weeks (Reader 1996: 158).

The text goes on to say that patients should be told to live within the limits of their diminished cardiac reserve for the rest of their lives. The prevailing view was that:

There was very little that the individual in the community could do to avoid the perils of heart disease and little basis for a community education program (Reader 1996: 5).

All this was happening just at the time when Heart Foundations were established in developing countries, including the National Heart Foundation of Australia. The Heart Foundation's initial task was to advocate for the rehabilitation of heart attack patients, aiming to assist early return to work and a normal lifestyle. The case study below is an example of the way the National Heart Foundation established rehabilitation centres that were successful in getting people back to work.

Case Study 22.1: Changing a life through exercise

A 46-year-old married man who attended the rehabilitation unit in Hobart had spent the last seven years since the heart attack at home and was receiving a pension. He was anxious and depressed. Tests showed evidence of the heart attack but no residual physical impairment. A normal result in a vigorous exercise tolerance test surprised and delighted him. He began working by doing light gardening work and went on to find a permanent job. This was typical of the experience of many patients who were able to return to work, continue working and to resume a more normal lifestyle (Reader 1996).

It was this period of medicine that Reader (1996) describes as the 'golden age' of cardiology, and one of its key components was supervised physical exercises after heart attack, which revolutionised medical interventions and health promotion following heart attack. This is an exemplar of a *medical approach* to health promotion (Baum 2002), whereby a professional prescribes a procedure, in this case supervised exercise, to a patient with an existing cardiovascular disease. At the time it was revolutionary because it changed many lives of sick people, led to new research on the pathways and possibilities of physical activity and health, and opened the scientific and general communities' eyes to new understanding of a disease that was viewed with fatalism, dread, or stoicism. This is a great example too of the argument in Geoffrey Rose's classic paper 'Sick individuals, sick populations' that interventions making large changes in individuals do not change population health (Rose 1985). In this case the reason is clear: it is health promotion that occurs after the onset of a disease that has developed over many years.

THE DISCOVERY OF LIFESTYLE MODELS OF PHYSICAL ACTIVITY PROMOTION

Running alongside the research linking exercise to the treatment of heart disease was the landmark Framingham study in the United States. This longitudinal study, starting in 1948, aimed to identify men and women between the ages of 30 and 39 years who showed no evidence of coronary heart disease and to report all details of their health and lifestyle and to re-examine them every two years for occurrence of heart disease. The study revealed hitherto unknown lifestyle factors that were associated with risk of coronary heart disease, including increased blood pressure, elevated blood cholesterol, cigarette smoking, being overweight, and sedentary living. These results were confirmed by continuing data from the Framingham study and from other studies in America, England, and Europe. By the mid 1960s it was accepted worldwide that coronary risk factors could predict the probability of developing coronary heart disease; in other words it was not simply a matter of ageing (Yeatman 1990).

These changes were important for health promotion. The National Heart Foundation, at its inception, had no real message to offer about prevention and very little about treatment of coronary heart disease. Now, it could promote both modifications in lifestyle and advances in treatment (Reader 1996).

The link between exercise and cardiology was typical of many ways in which the impact of lifestyle on health was 'discovered' internationally in the 1970s as personal behaviours and responsibility for health were placed alongside medicine, health services, biology, and environment as influences on health and illness (Baum 2002). This led to the influence of psychological theory, particularly behavioural psychology, on community programs and campaigns designed to change risk factors that were associated with illness by epidemiological studies. These discoveries led the state to invest not only in funding for medical procedures carried out by experts, but also for self-help procedures that were the responsibility of individuals under the guidance of experts (Baum 2002).

Experts in physical activity adopted lifestyle interventions enthusiastically and mixed behaviour therapy and social learning theory with counselling strategies. What is now known in physical activity circles as the stages of change model has its roots in a warning of a crisis in psychotherapy as a result of the unprecedented pace at which new therapies were being created. There were fears that diverse models would give an impression to the community of fragmentation, confusion, and chaos and as a result there would be a retreat from the talking therapies to chemotherapy (Prochaska & DiClemente 1982). One movement towards a comprehensive theory of change, transtheoretical therapy, emerged from a comparative analysis of eighteen therapy systems and identified critical processes of change during therapy.

They rejected a linear model in favour of a revolving door schema presented as a circle whereby people started at different stages, stalled at different stages, and re-entered the model at different places and times. The stages of change model has been applied in a range of health education programs, and strongly to physical activity (Sallis & Owen 1999).

This mix of psychology, epidemiology, and social marketing campaigns exemplifies the behavioural approach's (Baum 2002) attempts to change the lifestyles of high-risk target groups by encouraging greater participation in leisure or organised physical activity in order to reduce the risks associated with particular diseases.

Case Study 22.2: The rise of the lifestyle professional

In the 1970s and 1980s many people with experience in psychology and epidemiology moved into the health promotion workforce and applied their skills to health issues— including physical activity. Bringing their experience in areas such as behaviour therapy and counselling, they developed education-focused approaches with individuals or groups, self-help books, and telephone advice lines.

One example is Professor Neville Owen, who is currently Director of the Cancer Prevention Research Centre at University of Queensland. While in South Australia, his interest in physical activity started in the early 1980s when he applied his background in learning theory and clinical psychology to physical activity and community-based health promotion. At a meeting with Tony Sedgwick from the Institute for Fitness, Research and Training (IFRT) they discussed the high drop-out rate from organised exercise programs and the disappointingly low proportion of people who maintained their new exercise regime after the classes finished. Owen resolved to apply techniques from the psychological literature to improve the generalisation and maintenance of change in behaviour following an intervention program. He concluded that his theoretical perspective on behavioural persistence could provide insights into the high rate of drop-out from fitness classes and the poor maintenance of exercise habits following exercise interventions. Owen's association with IFRT was an opportunity to examine how altering fitness program structures and teaching self-regulatory skills to participants might improve program adherence and maintenance.

In his early work, Owen used social learning theory from his training and experience as a behavioural psychologist as a framework to understand how environmental settings, social influences, and people's actions influence behavioural change and persistence. He began to view exercise as a primary prevention strategy and, with IFRT, studied participants in community fitness courses to see the effects of changing program structures and teaching self-regulatory skills on program adherence and maintenance. At that time, Owen was influenced by systematic approaches to exercise he saw while on study leave in 1982 at Stanford University in California. His later work involved the translation of the stages of change model to the problem of initiating and maintaining behaviour change in physical activity, smoking, and diet. With the National Heart Foundation he collected epidemiological and exercise data from population samples before and after the 1990 and 1991 Heart Week exercise campaigns and played a major role in designing a population survey on behaviour, knowledge, and attitudes related to cardiovascular disease and its prevention.

Source: MacDougall 1995

SEARCHING FOR SOCIAL DETERMINANTS

We have seen that the medical approach to promoting physical activity works well for individuals with an existing disease, and therefore cannot be expected to improve health at the population level. We have also covered the rationale for the lifestyle approach. The critiques of the lifestyle approach (Blaxter 1990; Wass 1994; White 1996) argue that it downplays social factors, overemphasises the power of providing information, lacks persuasive evidence of success and adopts an ideology of individualism that cannot adequately underpin explanations of patterns of health and illness. This is also a critique offered by those who use a lifestyle approach and who document poor results from mass reach campaigns (Sallis & Owen 1999), and who note that in developed countries physical inactivity and associated health problems are increasing (Bauman et al. 2002). Authors who have contributed to the adoption of the behavioural approach are arguing for ecological approaches (Sallis & Owen 1999) and for the appreciation of socio-environmental approaches (Bauman et al. 2002). There was little success even in the Multiple Risk Factor Intervention Trial in the United States, where men in the top 10% risk for coronary heart disease (who would seem to have the most motivation for change) were persuaded to make only minimal changes in eating and smoking despite six years of intensive programs (Syme 1996). Even if lifestyle programs do meet with some success with high-risk people there will be others who adopt risk behaviours because '… we have done nothing to influence those forces in society that caused the problem in the first place' (Syme 1996: 22).

However, a perusal of conference abstracts and articles about physical activity still show a high proportion of lifestyle interventions—albeit with some attempt to broaden the scope to include environmental and settings factors.

Box 22.1: Sample abstracts from the 2005 National Physical Activity Conference (Australia)

SESSION: Exercise and Ageing Free Papers

The relationship between oxygen consumption and muscle oxygenation during a ramp test to exhaustion in well-trained young and masters cyclists.

Physiological and biochemical variables affect 30-minute time trial performance in well-trained young and masters cyclists.

Muscle soreness after downhill running: a preliminary study into the influence of age on perceived soreness.

The UPLIFT study: Using progressive resistance training to promote the mental health of older people in the primary care setting.

A comparison between the effects of respiratory muscle training and exercise training in older females.

Circuit training to improve daily function in the elderly.

SESSION: Physical Activity Free Papers: Innovative Interventions with Adults; Predictors of increased physical activity levels following participation in a general practice-based intervention

Have a try! A community-based progressive resistance training program designed for older Australians.

The dissemination of a community-based physical activity intervention across Queensland: The case of 10,000 Steps.

Assessing physical activity in general practice: evaluating the feasibility, reliability and validity of two short instruments within symposia: physical activity and vascular disease in the general practice setting.

Successfully increasing physical activity behaviour after rehabilitation.

Efficacy of a computer-tailored intervention for increasing physical activity in a sequential or simultaneous intervention mode.

SESSION: Joined up thinking—intersectoral collaboration in PA promotion free papers

A partnership approach to joined up thinking—guidance for strategic planning targeting physical activity.

The risks and rewards of creating a contestable investment approach for local government.

Governments in partnership: policy implementation for physical activity promotion.

Developing a physical activity network in the Asia Pacific Region—the challenge.

Be Active Australia: A framework for health sector action for physical activity 2005–2010

Source: <www.sma.org.au/ACSMS/2005/program/podium_presentations.asp#9>

Clearly, from the titles of the papers in the box above, the medical and lifestyle approaches to promoting physical activity are thriving. So what does it take to reframe the physical activity debate? The remainder of this chapter argues that it is essential to adopt mixed method research approaches, promote participation and respect ordinary theory, and develop ecological frameworks arising from intersectoral ways of working.

ADOPTING MIXED METHOD RESEARCH APPROACHES
Social epidemiology

A first step in reframing the physical activity debate is to broaden the scope of existing epidemiological studies beyond those demographic and risk factors favoured by a behavioural model of health promotion. This was able to happen in research that I conducted because I was able to use data from the South Australian Community Health Research Units a community health survey of the southern suburbs of Adelaide, South Australia: framed in an explicit socio-environmental perspective. This meant that there was a large data set that included social and environmental factors as well as the then standard physical activity measure (Baum & Abbott 1989). Both the univariate (simple) and multivariate (complex) statistical analyses confirmed the usual findings about the associations between physical activity, age, sex, and socio-economic status (See MacDougall et al. 1997 for a description of the statistical techniques and these usual findings). When the new social and environmental variables were used in a univariate analysis, results showed that people were more likely to report low levels of physical activity when:

■ their health was fair, poor, or very poor compared with those who rated their health as very good
■ people had fewer social connections
■ men rated their local area negatively
■ people were dissatisfied with recreation facilities.

All the results were then used to find out the significant independent factors associated with low activity by using a logistic regression model, which is regarded as being more powerful than simpler statistics (again see MacDougall et al. 1997 for more details). The significant independent factors predicting lower levels of physical activity included two factors that stimulated research to shift the gaze towards social and environmental factors:

■ men who did not report high social connections
■ people who were not satisfied with recreation facilities.

This shows how epidemiology has moved away from privileging biology and disease and health promotion is increasingly underpinned by social epidemiology, which:

is distinguished by its insistence on explicitly investigating social determinants of population distributions of health, disease, and wellbeing, rather than treating such determinants as mere background to biomedical phenomena (Krieger 2001).

Qualitative methods

We know, however, that epidemiological models can propose associations, but cannot by themselves suggest causal pathways. In the early 1990s, an opportunity arose to form a collaboration of people interested in transforming the physical activity debate in a project known as Supportive Environments for Physical Activity (SEPA).

Case Study 22.3: Serendipity and collaboration in Supportive Environments for Physical Activity (SEPA)

In the early 1990s Cheryl Wright, then director of health promotion at the National Heart Foundation (SA Branch), met with Colin MacDougall from the Department of Public Health at Flinders University to discuss new ways to frame physical activity. The initiative was strongly supported by the leadership of the National Heart Foundation at the time. A collaboration was then formed with the Mayor, Chief Executive Officer, and key staff from the local government area of the City of Marion that resulted in the first of two grants from the (then) Commonwealth Department of Health and Family Services. The collaboration soon extended to include Rick Atkinson, an architect and urban planner at the University of South Australia. The collaboration launched what became known as the Supportive Environments for Physical Activity (SEPA) project in South Australia. It started with a departure from the emphasis in contemporary research on leisure time and organised physical activity towards the view that exercise was a feature of everyday life. Hence the first title of the project: Exercise in Daily Life. However, in order to adopt and reflect an explicit socio-environmental framework, the name was changed to Supportive Environments for Physical Activity.

SEPA produced a report that underpinned many subsequent actions and described ways in which the environment supports or inhibits moderate physical activity and guidelines for local governments wishing to change the environment to promote physical activity (Wright et al. 1996; Wright et al. 1999)

As part of its contribution, the City of Marion decided on a number of actions to address the research findings, for example by developing a set of guidelines to focus the efforts of its key departments to implement these findings (City of Marion 1997, November), involving the SEPA project in the redevelopment of a drive-in theatre to a residential site (City of Marion 1997, 25 July) and in approving the planning of a bicycle track that was suggested by a focus group in the research (City of Marion 1996, 9 April).

SEPA is currently described in Victoria (Australia) as an initiative of the Heart Foundation that aims to focus attention on the factors that either inhibit or encourage people to lead healthy, socially engaged, and physically active lives. The desired outcome is an environment that encourages all people, of all ages and capacities, to be out and about in their neighbourhoods, cities, and towns. SEPA seeks to transform public policy, as well as the urban planning, design, and management processes that support and maintain healthy environments for active living. Such a transformation means a shift towards:

- public policy that supports and strengthens community development, community engagement and the celebration of cultural diversity, through the development of urban forms that offer choices for sustainable and active living
- collaboration between all levels of government, health, and other agencies and communities in the ways we envision, design, develop, and manage our urban environments.

Source: <www.heartfoundation.com.au/index.cfm?page=126>.

An example of intersectoral action is the Victorian Division of the National Heart Foundation's *Healthy by Design: A planners' guide to environments for active living.* It was developed in response to local government requests for practical guidance in designing walkable, and ultimately more liveable, communities. The Guide argues that healthy urban planning is about planning for people. It puts the needs of people and communities at the heart of the urban planning process and encourages decision-making based on human health and well-being. Design considerations detailed in the guide facilitate healthy planning and healthy places for people to live, work, and visit. The Guide was developed by the Heart Foundation (Victorian Division), the Cancer Council Victoria, the Department of Sustainability and Environment, and Crime Prevention Victoria <www.heartfoundation.com.au/downloads/sepavic_healthy_by_design_guide.pdf>.

SEPA principles and processes have re-emerged in South Australia as a local project based again in the City of Marion and involving local government, universities, community health services, National Heart Foundation, the Cancer Council (South Australia), and community groups.

The first part of SEPA's research drew directly on the revised epidemiological work described above that linked such variables as satisfaction with local facilities and perceptions of the environment with levels of physical activity (MacDougall et al. 1997). The qualitative research explored the relationships between environments and physical activity in Marion, a southern local government area of Adelaide with a population of 78,000 people. The qualitative design sampled from groups of people with experience of the social and environmental factors that the epidemiological study associated with lower levels of physical activity. Focus groups, interviews, and field studies were used to elicit people's experiences of these factors. The research (Wright, MacDougall et al. 1996) led to an Australia-wide action research project (Wright, Atkinson et al. 1999). The conclusions immediately pointed to the importance of agencies outside the health sector taking a leading role in policy development and argued that local government, not the health sector, was ideally placed to drive the study's recommendations. The study recommended supportive environments characterised by community spirit, social support, and destinations to which people can walk or cycle safely and where pedestrians and cyclists share the road system with motor vehicles.

PROMOTING PARTICIPATION AND ORDINARY THEORY

The health perspective of SEPA overtly adopted a primary health care approach (World Health Organisation 1978), with community participation as one of its underpinning principles. However, bureaucratic structures frequently do not value community knowledge and seem impenetrable to community members (Putland et al. 1997) so we need research that can influence organisational structure and culture and that values and uses community knowledge. This can only come from research methods that allow the time to distil lay or ordinary theories from in-depth interviews or focus groups (MacDougall 2001a). In Chapter 6 of this book Jennie Popay and Colin MacDougall discuss *lay knowledge*, which is one of the terms used to describe the views of people in the community about health and illness.

The SEPA data set was later re-analysed to ask the questions:

- How do ordinary people theorise about health, physical activity, and con-straints on choices to increase physical activity?
- How do ordinary theories (i.e. lay knowledge) differ from expert theories?
- What are the implications of these differences for the promotion of physical activity?

The results show how ordinary theories (lay knowledge) qualify or challenge expert theories, explore what is reasonable as well as rational, and maintain (rather than reduce) complexity and uncertainty. They deal with unhelpful expert advice. They construct normal stories about chronic conditions. Ordinary theories build from expert theories to suggest new approaches to health promotion. The results suggest that we should consider expert theories as scaffolds, not prescriptions. This helps experts to improve the quality of their advice by developing new theories of health promotion and sorting through the complex links between physical activity, health, and life in general. Why do this? Because experts' consultations and campaigns have a 'multiplier effect' whereby time taken to work with ordinary theories will influence future ordinary theorising leading to new discourses showing the benefits of expert–community dialogue (MacDougall 2003).

WORKING INTERSECTORALLY

In the SEPA project, a local government, the City of Marion, was a partner in the research and subsequently decided on a number of actions to address the research findings: for example, by developing a set of guidelines to focus the efforts of its key departments to implement these findings, involving the SEPA project in the redevelopment of a drive-in theatre to a residential site, and in approving the planning of a bicycle track that was suggested by a focus group in the research.

So why did local government take action? To find out we interviewed the (then) chief executive officer, who argued that there were four factors that were important in the City of Marion's role in taking a lead in developing supportive environments for physical activity: *framing the issue as core business, taking a strategic rather than operational focus, creating open organisational structures*, and *leadership* (MacDougall et al. 2002).

Framing the issue as core business

Providing infrastructure is the core of local government business and the goal of supporting physical activity can be framed as a new way of looking at infrastructure.

Developers and urban planners who negotiate with local government are always seeking new ideas for planning and marketing new housing developments and urban renewal projects.

A strategic rather than operational focus

In order to establish the creation of supportive environments as core business on the local government's agenda, they should be framed as a strategic, rather than an operational, focus. He described an operational focus as when engineers view roads and paths as engineering problems and planners look at planning regulations. A strategic focus asks the questions in a different way, for example: *'How does the infrastructure relate to its surroundings?'*

Open organisational structures

To maintain a strategic focus, the organisation needs a structure to enable it to look across all the various functions and departments, ask the strategic questions and work together to change the way things are done.

Leadership

Leadership is required to enable senior management to believe in and drive these changes, especially by creating the organisational structures, endorsing strategic thinking, and taking a leading role in negotiations. Change does not automatically flow from a plan or structure; it has to be driven by people who champion the cause (MacDougall et al. 2002).

DEVELOPING ECOLOGICAL FRAMEWORKS

Theories, or frameworks, help those involved in health promotion to make sense of the world by explaining patterns from data and making predictions about what could or should happen if a particular policy or intervention is implemented. Theory helps us to develop health promotion as a field of study. Theory—or a story or narrative—is very helpful for communicating with policy-makers, as discussed in Chapter 14 on Healthy Public Policy. The ecological framework described here was developed to synthesise new knowledge from the research methods, collaboration and intersectoral action described earlier in this chapter (MacDougall 2000). The framework reflects a *settings approach*, working from the dictum made famous in the Ottawa Charter that:

> 'Health is created and lived by people within settings of their everyday life; where they learn, work, play and love'. It is carried out by and with people, not on or to people! The Settings for Health approach to health was reinforced by the Jakarta Declaration on Leading Health Promotion into the 21st Century (World Health Organisation 1997).

A setting is where people actively use and shape the environment and thus create or solve problems relating to health. Settings can normally be identified as having physical boundaries, a range of people with defined roles, and an organisational structure.

The ecological framework builds on the themes, described earlier in this chapter, derived from coding of the qualitative research focus group transcripts demonstrating how physical activity was enhanced by supportive environments, characterised by community spirit, social support, and destinations to which people can walk or cycle safely and where pedestrians and cyclists share the road system with motor vehicles. The ecological framework comprises three themes that link human agency and structural and environmental factors: *locating in space, moving through space, and relating to people in space and place*. These factors are defined as:

- *Locating in place* refers to the way experiences of the settings where people live, work, shop, and play (including the facilities and services they use) influence, and are influenced by, experiences and decisions about moderate physical activity. Participants in the studies locate themselves not only in the immediate vicinity of their home (in a geographically defined community) but also (where appropriate) in settings away from their home; including in communities of interest.
- *Moving through space* refers to the way people move around either their immediate environment or geographic community and between locations or communities of interest. Environment and transport systems influenced decisions about incorporating physical activity into movements between locations.
- *Relating to people in place* refers to the way people relate to each other in their immediate environment, in families and social networks, in locations, and as they move between locations. An important part of the presentation of results is an analysis of how, for example, supportive social relationships and concerns about safety influence decisions about incorporating physical activity into movements between locations.

In Figure 22.1, a Venn diagram at the top left portrays the explanation of current ways in which the environment makes it difficult for physical activity. The size of each circle can represent the importance of that element and the positions reflect the relationship between the elements; in the example they intersect because each factor is related. If, however, the analysis suggested that two elements (say locating and relating to people in space) were supportive but one (say moving through space) was not supportive, then the relating to people circle would be larger and separate from the other two. Forces that inhibit moderate activity, risk and difficulty, are included as barriers. Force-field analysis, described in Box 22.2 can be used to propose a vision and to explore what social and environmental changes might make it easier to build moderate physical activity into life.

Box 22.2: Force-field analysis

Force-field analyses are frequently used when planning or managing personal and organisational change, and derive from the force-field theory of Kurt Lewin, which argues that outcomes are the result of equilibrium between driving and restraining forces. Driving forces push one way, restraining forces the other so that an increase in driving forces may increase change, but may also provoke restraining forces. Lewin conceptualised change as involving unfreezing, changing, and refreezing (Stoner, Yetton et al. 1994).

In Figure 22.1, unfreezing involves using the left-hand side to understand current patterns and make a case for change. Changing involves the movement to the right-hand side by developing new approaches and structures, taking into account driving and restraining forces on the diagram. Refreezing involves establishing new arrangements, structures, and partnerships depicted on the right-hand side, involving a vision of what might be, as used in the development of visions for healthy settings (Baum 2002). Forces that support physical activity, purpose and benefit, are enhancers that may involve change in one or more of locating, moving through, or relating in space. There may be multiple options, so in this step it is possible to present alternatives. At the top there is a general force labelled ordinary theory, which acknowledges the principle of respecting ordinary theory in order to promote people's participation in debates about health and policy. At the bottom, there is another general force, convenience

Figure 22.1 Ecological framework for physical activity

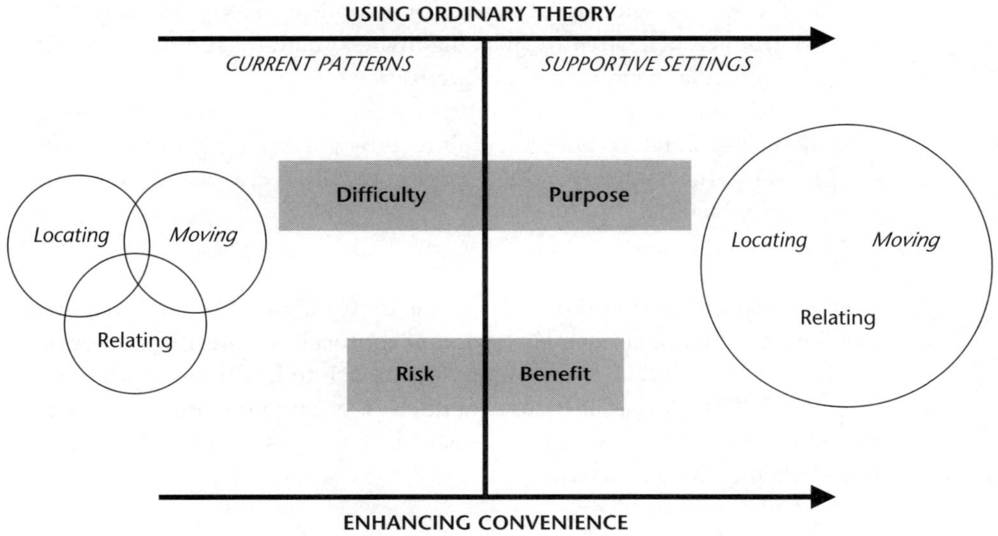

of settings, which reflects the principle of making the healthy choice the easy choice.

In Figure 22.1, change moves from left to right towards a new Venn diagram that supports the choice to increase moderate physical activity. Again, the size of each circle represents the importance of that element and the relative position of each circle reflects the relationship between the elements. The three circles become one to represent a future whereby each element of the setting blends with the other to support physical activity.

Box 22.3: Ecological health promotion

Exercise: Using the ecological framework for physical activity and force-field analysis to explain and predict

■ The purpose of the ecological framework is to help those involved in health promotion to make sense of the world by explaining patterns from data and making predictions about what could or should happen if a particular policy or intervention is implemented.

■ As an exercise, use the framework in Figure 22.1 to draft a force-field analysis of the following commonly described physical activity problems. Suggest a vision for a future in which the settings support decisions to build moderate physical activity into life:

☐ Older women who have been told by their doctors to lose weight but report that they are worried about falling on uneven footpaths and scared of being harassed by young people.

☐ Middle-aged men who live in outer suburbs, work long hours, and drive to and from work every day.

☐ Teenagers who supplement their income at school and university from casual, part-time jobs that make it hard for them to commit to regular training and competition.

☐ Women with young children who have extensive parenting responsibilities and who are urged by governments to find a job.

☐ Children living in rural towns with steadily decreasing populations and facilities.

The ecological framework for physical activity exemplifies the fundamental contrast between the medical and behavioural approaches to health promotion on the one hand, and the socio-environmental approach to health promotion on the other (Baum 2002). That is, it focuses neither on existing diseases in individuals nor the lifestyles of high-risk groups. Instead, it focuses on changing high-risk environments for physical activity.

SUMMARY

The journey towards an ecological model for promoting physical activity illustrates some important theoretical arguments in health promotion: the definition of health and the need for intersectoral action; the evidence that medical and behavioural approaches alone do not and cannot work at a population level; the need to focus on high-risk environments; and for the three common approaches to health promotion to work in harmony.

In Chapters 1 and 2 of this book we presented the debate about whether health is an end in its own right—or a means or resource for living. In this chapter, the quantitative or epidemiological model shows that poor health status is a predictor of low physical activity. The qualitative data, especially the ordinary theories, clearly showed how people (for example with arthritis) needed to take action to improve their physical health in order to engage in physical activity, which in turn increased their social contacts, engagement with society, and enjoyment of life. So both the qualitative and quantitative analyses support the view that health is not on end, but can be a means for increasing physical activity and social contact.

The ecological framework for physical activity and the evaluation of the centrality of local government in networks to create supportive environments all support the statement in the Ottawa Charter that:

> Health promotion is the process of enabling people to increase control over, and to improve, their health. To reach a state of complete physical, mental and social well-being, an individual or group must be able to identify and to realise aspirations, to satisfy needs, and to change or cope with the environment. Health is, therefore, seen as a resource for everyday life, not the objective of living. Health is a positive concept emphasising social and personal resources, as well as physical capacities. Therefore, health promotion is not just the responsibility of the health sector, but goes beyond healthy lifestyles to well-being' (World Health Organisation 1986: i).

As research points physical activity in the direction of supportive environments, it becomes obvious why health promotion represents a comprehensive social and political process. This chapter demonstrates ways in which systematic action can occur to reorient health promotion, including:

1   Broadening the definition of health to include social and economic determinants.
2   Going beyond the emphasis on individual lifestyle strategies to broader social and political strategies.
3   Embracing the notion of individual and collective empowerment.
4   Advocating the participation of the community in identifying and addressing health problems (Robertson & Minkler 1994).

The chapter has also discussed the contributions of the medical, lifestyle, and socio-environmental approaches to promoting physical activity. We now leave it to you to consider how best to change or enhance your practice, research, or teaching about the promotion of physical activity. To do this, it may help to consider the following caveats from Ron Labonte about using these three approaches to health promotion (Labonte 1992):

1   They are complementary, not exclusionary. In other words, a question is not which one is right, but how will they work together? Another question is, which approach dominates the system, and why? So, in relation to the promotion of physical activity, why does the behavioural approach still dominate research and practice? Is there an alternative?

2   Their characteristics are presented in a simplistic, stereotypical fashion. In other words, in the real world, strategies and policies do not faithfully reflect either one of the three approaches in a pure fashion—rather there will be elements of each, often jumbled up. So, in relation to the promotion of physical activity, how and when is it essential to distinguish between the three approaches?

3   The behavioural approach accommodates the medical approach and in turn both are accommodated by the socio-environmental approach. In other words, policy driven by a socio-environmental approach would maintain a role for medical and behavioural approaches when the evidence suggests they are likely to be effective. So, in relation to the promotion of physical activity, what would it take for systems to adopt a socio-environmental model as part of the Ottawa Charter's call to reorient the health system?

PROMOTING HEALTH THROUGH SPORT

23

Berni Murphy

Key concepts

- Sport, whether organised or unstructured, can provide a broad range of opportunities for people to participate in physical activity.
- Partnerships to promote health involving the sport sector must be built on negotiated goals and a shared understanding of roles and responsibilities.
- A systematic approach to capacity-building optimises efforts to promote health through sport.
- The sport sector can accommodate downstream and midstream approaches to promoting health with relative ease and short lead times.
- Upstream approaches to promoting health through sport need more time to evolve, as they invariably involve cultural shifts, organisational change, and/or the development of new policy directions and systems.

Key terms

- Sport
- Partnerships
- Capacity-building
- Multisectoral collaboration
- Upstream
- Midstream and downstream health promotion

OVERVIEW

The physical, mental, and social health benefits of being physically active are well documented in the literature and are compelling (VicHealth 2006a). Physical activity is linked with a reduction in risk of obesity, coronary health disease, stroke, Type II diabetes, osteoporosis, arthritis, some types of cancers, and high blood pressure (DHS 2006; Rowe, Beasley et al. 2004). Bauman et al. (2002) argue that even small increases in physical activity can achieve significant public health gains. Opportunities to be physically active are, however, in decline, as our workplaces, homes, and modes of transport become more automated. In the future, active transport strategies to promote walking and cycling will in all likelihood increase as the obvious environmental and health benefits gain currency (National Public Health Partnership 2001). In the meantime, however, sport can continue to provide a logical access point to physical activity, particularly in sports-mad Australia. 'Sport' refers to informal or unstructured recreational- and fitness-related activities, as well as organised activities that are structured and usually involve rules and competitions (Rowe et al. 2004). This chapter explores what can happen when the sports sector is encouraged to take an interest in health promotion. A fictional scenario—*the bad news story*—is utilised here as a vehicle for exploring the how, what, where, and why of engaging the sports sector in a broader health agenda. This story is deliberately tongue-in-cheek, depicting some of the worst elements that can emerge when a partnership is established without careful consideration of goals, roles, responsibilities, and effective planning processes. Key health promotion concepts introduced in Chapter 2, such as collaboration, capacity-building, and downstream, midstream, and upstream actions to promote health are explored as they relate to the sports sector. Finally, a snapshot of activities that sporting clubs and associations currently implement in contributing to the health agenda provides a *good news story*. These activities have been mapped against the *'Framework for Health Promotion Action'* (Keleher & Murphy 2004).

Case Study 23.1: First, the bad news story ...

(The names and places included in this story are NOT based on fact. Any resemblance to real persons, organisations, or places is purely coincidental.)

Once upon a time in a land far away, a sports organisation was approached by the government of the day and offered significant funding in return for increasing its participation base. The notion was a simple one. The government was concerned that the population was getting too fat and too inactive. People clearly needed encouragement to stop eating and get moving again. Funding would be rolled out over a three-year period, though exactly what the government had in mind with this project remained somewhat unclear at the launch. Details would obviously be clarified down the track. *'Engaging communities'*, *'building capacity'*, and *'collaborative partnerships'* were terms the Minister referred to rather a lot in his speech.

The honeymoon period ...

Enthusiasm was running high. A steering committee was formed comprising representatives from the government and the sports organisation, together with a panel of experts and two community members. They met initially to scope the project and to define the terms of reference (TOR). Essentially, the government would provide *significant funding and strategic support*, while the sports organisation would identify and implement a range of interventions to increase participation rates across a diverse range of age groups, genders, ethnicities, abilities, and locations. A champion within the sports organisation management team emerged, a charismatic person with the vision to conceptualise how it would unfold and the energy to drive it. The steering committee sat entranced as the champion unveiled *the vision*. First, all metropolitan and regional associations would share their knowledge and experiences about what works and what doesn't in attracting and retaining players and volunteers to the sport. Best practice would be recorded and disseminated around the state. The game would be marketed with ingenious campaigns and participation rates would soar. School holiday clinics with a focus on having fun would be oversubscribed and competitions would suddenly boast extensive waiting lists. Adolescent drop-off rates would be arrested with effective strategies, and mature players would be attracted to the sport through *'come and try'* novice skill development sessions. Men and women seeking new ways to keep fit would create a boom in modified rules and mixed competitions. Many would discover the sport for the first time. Some would play multiple times per week. Communities would lobby for new facilities to match this demand. Child care would be made available during women's competitions and attention would be paid to creating space and ambience for social interaction after the game— space to sit and enjoy coffee, a beer, a wine, a chat with friends. Car pools would be organised to ensure better access for those who might otherwise experience transport as a barrier to participation. Costs would be contained through reasonably priced membership subscriptions and more relaxed uniform regulations. The profile of the sport would grow exponentially and success at the elite level would flow from this surge in interest, which in turn would generate even more participation at the grass roots level.

The honeymoon is over ...

It would be fair to say that things did not go according to expectations. First of all the sports organisation realised that they had no accurate data about how many were actually playing their sport. So how would they know if strategies to *increase* participation were actually working? Data management had never really been a priority for this organisation. Like many sports organisations reliant on the goodwill and hard work of volunteers, getting teams on the field of play and running the competitions efficiently had always been the main focus. Up until now there had never been any real incentive to keep accurate records. Insurance brokers had only ever required an estimate, and the national body and other stakeholders had never really queried the accuracy of estimates furnished from time to time when someone in power wanted to know how many people were playing the game. Admitting this problem to the steering committee could lead to a loss of confidence in the sports management team and their capacity to achieve results.

The champion made a decision. The steering committee would not be informed. At least not until the problem had been resolved. All associations and clubs would be asked to immediately conduct a census to determine their participation rates. Once this census was completed, accurate statewide data would quickly be established and stratified according to gender, age groupings, competition types, and locations. The database would henceforth be maintained and multiple-level strategies to build participation rates implemented in accordance with the vision. Progress would be carefully tracked over the three-year period, incorporating process, impact, and outcome evaluation measures, as specified in the TOR. Success stories and other lessons learnt would be shared with other sports organisations at conferences and forums in a spirit of collaboration. The census survey was distributed to associations and clubs across the land.

The fatal blow ...

Headhunted by a global player in the business world, the champion suddenly left. The sports organisation management team called a crisis meeting to plan their next move. Someone would have to pick up the baton and run with it. But no one really knew the champion's game plan. While they had heard brief verbal reports since the project's launch some twelve months ago, and were vaguely aware that a census of current participation rates was underway, documents had never been tabled at their fortnightly meetings. There was no record of the *vision* or of the strategic thinking processes involved. No evidence of a three-year strategic plan. No documented operational plan and budget. No evaluation plan. In fact no roles or responsibilities had ever really been defined. The steering committee had assumed from the enthusiastic meetings that everyone was working from the same page. There was no question of fiscal impropriety since none of the funding provided for this project had actually been spent yet. But the pressure was on to show results. The census data began to dribble in but was often incomplete. Competition managers and clubs did not appear to have the mechanisms in place to furnish such data, and since many of them were volunteers, they were not inclined to spend the hours required to set up such systems at the whim of the central governing body. The sports management team feared that a perception of mismanagement or incompetence could exact a heavy toll on their organisation. The government could threaten to withdraw financial support. Other sponsors could follow suit. The partnership would collapse. The media would have a field day. The image of their sport would be tarnished and potential participants would drift instead to rival sports. The situation was an absolute disaster. Ironically, the terms *'strategic partnership'* and *'capacity-building'* were printed in bold on the cover page of the Memorandum of Understanding (MOU) between the sports organisation and the government. In practice this arrangement was not *'strategic'* and bore none of the hallmarks of a genuine *'partnership'*. Evidence of *'capacity-building'* was also scant. In this instance lofty goals and good intentions were not enough. Next came the blame game and a complete breakdown of goodwill and trust. And we all know it's a long road to re-establish relationships once goodwill and trust have broken down.

UNPACKING LESSONS FROM THIS *BAD NEWS STORY*

Glaring errors of judgement are apparent throughout this narrative (Case Study 23.1). Yet the original intent was good. The government of the day realised that it needed to respond to worrying trends in the burden of disease data. Physical inactivity was known to be a risk factor for multiple health conditions. Concerns about declining physical activity rates called for action. Multiple strategies and settings for action were required. The sports sector was identified as one of those settings already providing opportunities for physical activity and, given more resources, could potentially increase participation rates with consequent health gains, along with other social and economic benefits. A partnership between the government and a large sports organisation would notionally strengthen that organisation's capacity to boost participation. A significant injection of funds as a catalyst for that endeavour would ensure success, wouldn't it? So what went wrong in far-away land? Spend a few moments creating a list of the positives and negatives of this lost opportunity. The negative list will obviously be longer! Then consider how each negative could have been handled differently. For instance, it is clear that the planning processes were poor from the outset. Review Chapter 8 (Health Promotion Planning and the Social Determinants of Health), Chapter 11 (Strategic Communication) and Guidebook 5 (Health Promotion Program Planning and Evaluation) to help you rethink a more strategic approach to planning in this scenario. Consider the problems that emerged because the structure of the partnership and approaches to capacity-building were flawed from the outset. Let's now take a closer look at issues around building effective partnerships.

BUILDING MULTISECTORAL PARTNERSHIPS: MANNA FROM HEAVEN OR A MINEFIELD?

In this story, forming a partnership between key stakeholders was pivotal to achieving increased participation in physical activity through sport. In theory, effective partnerships can offer a range of benefits including:

- an increased capacity to respond to existing and emerging health problems and their determinants
- improved resource allocation and utilisation
- opportunities to strengthen the community's capacity to identify and respond to factors promoting and inhibiting health in the local context
- opportunities to implement innovative upstream approaches leading to infrastructure and systems changes that are likely to have broad and sustained impact.

Source: Murphy 2004

In order for a multisectoral or intrasectoral partnership to be effective in delivering desired outcomes, the partnership must first be established in keeping with several key principles. Good intent is a great starting point but will rarely sustain a partnership through the inevitable challenges that occur along the way. Walker (2000) identifies three stages in building a collaborative partnership. A checklist for this three-stage process is presented in Table 23.1.

Table 23.1 Stages in building collaboration: checklist

STAGES	BUILDING COLLABORATION	CHECK? ☑ OR ☒
Stage 1: Priority setting and problem definition	Shared understanding of problems and goals	
	Shared definition of the problem	
	Shared commitment to the collaboration	
	Identification of resources required to support the collaboration	
	Collective identification of key stakeholders and convenor	
Stage 2: Reaching agreement	Establish the ground rules	
	Jointly agree on the agenda for the collaborative venture	
	Reach agreement on how problems will be solved	
Stage 3: Implementation	Build external support for the solutions agreed	
	Institutionalise/implement agreements reached	
	Monitor the agreement and ensure compliance	

Source: Adapted from Walker 2000

A review of this checklist uncovers areas of concern at every stage for our sports participation partnership. As early as stage 1, a shared understanding of the problems and goals was never clarified. And while funding was allocated to support the program, other resourcing issues (including existing strengths and gaps in personnel, infrastructure, and systems) were never identified. During stage 2, when ground rules should be established and agreements reached about how problems will be solved in an atmosphere of trust, and open communication, our champion instead was making unilateral decisions. By stage 3, when implementation should ordinarily be occurring, the sports participation partnership was instead disintegrating.

BUILDING CAPACITY FOR HEALTH PROMOTION IN THE SPORTS SECTOR

So far, in unpacking this fictional sports participation scenario, we have considered the consequences of failing to set up an effective partnership from the start. You will also have hopefully spent some time reviewing what went wrong with the planning processes along the way (refer to Chapters 8, 11 and Guidebooks 8 and 9 to help you). Now let's turn our attention to the important issue of capacity-building. In Chapter 2 of this text, Helen Keleher contends that *building capacity* at individual, organisational, and systemic levels is critical in addressing social, economic, and environmental factors that lead to poor health. Capacity-building involves developing sustainable skills, organisational structures, resources, and commitment (Health Promotion Strategies Unit 1999). Prior to commencing a new program, a capacity audit would usually be conducted. This involves assessing the *internal* capacity of the organisation in terms of personnel, competencies, technical infrastructure, and financial support mechanisms. Assessing the *culture* of organisation is also important during this stage. To what extent is the culture of the organisation conducive to embracing any organisational changes needed to take on a new program? Widespread resistance to a program or organisational change processes will inevitably make the task of meeting goals and objectives on time and on budget all the more problematic. An *external* audit should also be conducted to assess the capacity of collaborative partners and the community to embrace the program. Table 23.2 depicts a simple capacity-building checklist, adapted from the Department of Human Services *Integrated health promotion resource kit* (2003).

Table 23.2   Capacity-building checklist

STEPS	KEY QUESTIONS	CHECK? ☑ OR ☒
1	Have all key partners agreed on a strategic direction and signed off on it? This should include a vision statement, goals, and objectives.	
2	Have roles and responsibilities within the partnership been clearly defined and agreed on?	
3	Has an operational plan been developed identifying specific strategies to achieve objectives? Have resources, timelines, infrastructure, personnel been specified? Have gaps in resources, infrastructure, and personnel been identified? How will this be resolved?	
4	What are the individual and collective skills and knowledge of the partners? Do staff and other stakeholders such as community members need skill development?	
5	Specifically related to the budget, has there been an open and transparent process in allocating financial resources?	
6	Are senior managers, boards, and governance committees involved, leading, and advocating for the delivery of this program?	

Adapted from Checklist: capacity-building, in *Integrated health promotion resource kit*, DHS 2003: 39

Mapping the sports participation scenario against this capacity-building checklist is a useful exercise as it immediately provides insights into some of the difficulties encountered. If we begin with step 1 of the checklist, we can speculate that the stakeholders in our story were initially captivated by a vision. But were they clear about the goals and objectives of the program, and did they then agree on a strategic direction and all sign off on it? Probably not. Step 2 in the checklist requires roles and responsibilities to be defined and agreed upon. However, in our story a champion emerged, a charismatic leader who single-handedly took up the challenge of conceptualising and implementing the program. A champion can indeed be a powerful force in driving programs and change processes. But in this instance the champion failed to include others in the journey. Rather than *leading* the program he assumed total control of it. When he eventually left the organisation, succession plans to accommodate this sudden and unexpected change were nonexistent. A review of steps 3–6 of the capacity-building checklist indicate that these steps were also largely neglected with inevitable consequences.

PROMOTING HEALTH THROUGH SPORT: THE GOOD NEWS

Clearly, there is much to be learned about the importance of appropriate planning, capacity-building, and establishing effective partnerships if we are to optimise opportunities to promote health through sport. While the *bad news story* was obviously inserted here as an agency for exploring what can go wrong if these aspects are ignored, the news however from the real world is far more encouraging. For instance, the Victorian Health Promotion Foundation (VicHealth) has implemented a *Partnerships for Health Scheme*, and is currently working with State Sporting Associations (SSAs) specifically to increase participation in physical activity for health gain, while also supporting the vitality of sport (VicHealth 2006b). In resourcing the Partnerships for Health Scheme, VicHealth has recognised the important role that SSAs can play in increasing physical activity levels by:

■ Impacting on the culture of sport
■ Influencing the development of healthy sporting environments
■ Assisting clubs to develop strategies to broaden participation in sporting opportunities; and
■ Playing an advocacy and educative role in promoting the synergies between health and sport within sports clubs and the community (VicHealth 2006b).

The Partnerships for Health Scheme is constructed around clear guiding principles. Strategic directions are explicit. Roles and responsibilities are clarified at the beginning. Funding is generous and support ongoing to ensure that capacity is systematically built within the sector to meet specific goals and objectives. Communication between the partners is recognised as being crucial to the process.

Procedures for keeping information flowing both ways are formalised and appear to work well. Opportunities to strengthen these partnerships are constantly under review.

DOWNSTREAM, MIDSTREAM, AND UPSTREAM ACTIONS TO PROMOTE HEALTH THROUGH SPORT

The ways in which the sports sector takes actions that promote health is of interest here. The following case study describes the ways in which one particular SSA has engaged in health promotion action ever since the 1990s. Of particular interest here is the evolution of this association's understanding and implementation of health promotion action in its own context. Unsurprisingly, silo interventions targeting health behaviours were the starting point and are still evident at club level today, but the association is now leading the way in undertaking more integrated and upstream actions that target socio-ecological factors. Some of the more progressive clubs are following suit in adopting policies and practices that create healthier environments for their members and the wider community. Other clubs remain resistant to change for the time being, but the association is optimistic that the shift to promote healthier environments and healthier people will continue to gather momentum.

Case Study 23.2: Promoting health through sport

A Victorian State Sporting Association (SSA), the Victorian Football League, first got involved in health promotion in the 1990s. Health promotion back then usually meant social marketing and education strategies targeting behaviours. Minor changes were made to canteen menus in the name of promoting healthy eating. In the clubrooms the focus was on being smoke-free and on responsible alcohol management. Some time later came efforts to create more welcoming and inclusive environments. Running social events and 'come and try' days for potential members was easy enough, but developing policies and practices that ensured the environment was in fact 'welcoming and inclusive' was much harder. This invariably required a cultural shift, in some instances a break from long entrenched traditions. So what's changed in recent years? This SSA is now offering a more diverse range of competitions to cater for people of different ages, genders, and abilities. Research is conducted periodically to better understand the profile of potential and existing client groups, their needs and expectations, and to inform strategic planning. The organisation's understanding of health promotion continues to evolve. The management team and some staff have attended health promotion short courses in order to build better knowledge and understanding. Talk to the staff now and they will tell you that *midstream interventions* focusing on education and skill development are still the most common health promotion activities at club level. But things are changing. They will also talk about some of the exciting *upstream interventions* involving infrastructure and systems changes. They'll explain how policies and systems have been developed to address a range of issues. They will speculate that in some instances organisational change is being driven from the *top down*, particularly with regard to the broader social issues such as gender equity, racism, and freedom from discrimination. In other instances socio-ecological change is being driven from the *bottom up*. Staff can now trot out the language of health promotion with ease. But that's not really the point. They say they are still in the business of sport. That won't change. However, they realise that their organisation can make a significant contribution to promoting healthy environments and healthy communities without compromising their own goals. In the 1990s this sport's understanding and actions around health promotion were simplistic, mostly midstream, and usually prompted by a funding incentive from outside the sector. Now there is evidence of the sport conceptualising and instigating its own health promotion initiatives, and the focus in coming years is more likely to be on upstream socio-ecological factors rather than on midstream behaviours.

Adapted from a report for the VFL on research into promoting participation; Murphy 2005

A SNAPSHOT OF HEALTH PROMOTION ACTION ACROSS THE SPORT SECTOR

The extent to which the sports sector is undertaking a broad range of health promotion activities was evident during a series of two-day *'Promoting Health through Sport'* workshops conducted by this author. These workshops were auspiced by VicHealth for staff and representatives from over fifty SSAs. The Framework for Health Promotion Action was presented to participants towards the end of each workshop and they were asked to map examples of health promotion action from their own sport onto the grid. Table 23.3 depicts a snapshot of some of the health promotion activities that are currently occurring across the sports sector.

The extent to which workshop participants could describe and categorise health promotion action currently being undertaken by their own sport varied. During this exercise, some sports recognised that their actions were currently anchored in downstream and midstream domains. However, other sports were able to describe upstream actions currently being implemented, even though they may not have previously labelled these activities with the health promotion 'upstream' jargon.

This process of mapping their own sport's contribution to health promotion action was in itself useful, as ideas were debated and shared within the sector. When asked to reflect on emerging trends, several participants reported on a growing interest in upstream action. The need to create better access to sport for socio-economically disadvantaged groups was identified as one of the next big upstream challenges for the sector.

Table 23.3 Snapshot of current health promotion activities across the sports sector

FRAMEWORK FOR HEALTH PROMOTION ACTION		
DOWNSTREAM *PRIMARY, SECONDARY, AND* *TERTIARY PREVENTION*	*MIDSTREAM* *COMMUNICATION AND* *EDUCATION STRATEGIES*	*UPSTREAM* *COMMUNITY DEVELOPMENT AND* *INFRASTRUCTURE/SYSTEMS CHANGE*
Primary prevention: Risk assessment/ risk management at venues Insurance up to date Occupational Health and Safety principles observed First aid equipment maintained and staff qualifications current *Secondary prevention:* Safety practices implemented (e.g. blood rule) Water bottles which limit potential for cross-infection used *Tertiary prevention:* Rehabilitation for injured players consistent with latest scientific evidence	'Come and Try' skill development clinics Posters, flyers, signage to promote healthy messages Newsletters incorporating stories/announcements with a health theme CDs produced to raise awareness and to build knowledge for players, coaches, officials, parents Website to raise awareness and build knowledge Media releases about good news sports stories and health promotion outcomes School visits to increase participation Coaching accreditation Sequential skill development clinics Responsible serving of alcohol program for facilities staff Parent education programs (e.g. about promoting healthy attitudes to sport and competition) Education programs for officials and boards of management (e.g. about racial vilification)	*Community development:* Players' Association with strong player welfare agenda Players' Association media advocacy to raise awareness about player welfare issues such as depression or alcohol/drug misuse *Policies:* Racial vilification policy Inclusion policy Welfare policy for juniors Anti-bullying policy Anti-discrimination policy Heat policy *Legislation:* Mandatory police check for junior coaches Compulsory head protection for juniors Code of Conduct for players and spectators *Organisational change:* Provision of more welcoming environment Culture shifting to be more gender inclusive Attitudes to alcohol, tobacco now more health-promoting Recognition of importance of social connectedness Deliberate push to involve more females in governance roles Rules and protocols specifically modified to accommodate different ethnicities Modified rules to attract new members Relaxed dress code to attract new members and adapt to changing social mores

Adapted from A *Framework for Health Promotion Action*, in Keleher & Murphy 2004: 160.

SUMMARY

The American Obesity Association (2005) argues that less time spent on leisure time activities such as sport is no doubt contributing to upward trends in overweight and obesity. During the 1980s and the 1990s, health promotion in sports settings was often characterised by single-level strategies addressing downstream factors such as injury prevention and midstream factors such as individual knowledge or skills. A snapshot of the range of health promotion initiatives that sports organisations are now instigating points to a growing understanding within the sector of the importance of also addressing upstream socio-ecological factors through infrastructure and systems change. Multisectoral partnerships involving sport, health, and other sectors (e.g. local government, education) are now emerging as excellent exemplars of what can be achieved when partnerships are built on sound principles, including negotiated goals and a shared understanding of roles and responsibilities. The benefits of such collective endeavours are numerous. The sports sector's primary goal will still be about increasing participation, broadening access, and building memberships, while the health sector's goals will be about health outcomes. As these sectors continue to build more sophisticated alliances, they will find new and innovative ways to capitalise on obvious synergies through mutually beneficial collaborations, and in so doing, contribute to creating healthier environments and healthier people.

RE-IMAGINING HEALTH PROMOTION

24

Colin MacDougall, Helen Keleher & Berni Murphy

OUR JOURNEY

Our understanding of health promotion requires us to reframe our knowledge, research, and practice towards social, ecological and environmental approaches, as they are articulated in the WHO Charters for Health Promotion. Such approaches incorporate the best practices of traditional medical and lifestyle approaches, but are neither controlled nor dominated by their ideological substrates.

Our journey is towards the new frontiers of integrated health promotion, health equity approaches, capacity-building, partnerships, collaboration, and leadership. We explicitly underpin our understanding of health promotion with a wholehearted acceptance of the centrality of equity, sustainability, and the socio-economic determinants of health. This leads us to work within a rights framework that involves and engages communities and respects all the people and cultures who work with us.

In our explorations of the languages and cultures of various disciplines and sectors we accept that the determinants of health primarily lie outside the health sector. We therefore find it essential to learn from experts from sectors and disciplines that contribute to the health promotion debate. Often we will need guidebooks to take us on a rapid tour or to understand key ideas rapidly and more deeply. From these experts and guidebooks we aim to learn the languages and customs that we need to form partnerships and collaborations that are essential for community practice and multisector working.

We reaffirm the proposition of the Ottawa Charter for Health Promotion (World Health Organisation 1986) that health is not an end in itself, but a means to life and well-being. This important affirmation leads us to take our place, respectfully, as but one of many sectors and disciplines whose activities similarly are means to life and well-being. Our acceptance of health as a means should also help avoid healthist tendencies such as imploring partners and collaborators to adopt health language and restate their core activities as health outcomes.

Put bluntly, if health is accepted as an end it encourages health promotion to ask partners and collaborators to redefine their activities in terms of health outcomes and agendas. This restricts the scope of collaboration and renders it unlikely that partners will be able to put their core activities on the collaboration table. By contrast, when health promotion accepts health as a means, partners don't have to search for obviously health-related activities. The collaboration table can thus be filled with myriad ideas and programs that are core to each sector and have two important things in common: a concern with underlying social determinants and the eventual aim of well-being, social justice, equity, and sustainability.

However, talk of social justice inevitably brings us to the ideological and political debates and divides that bedevil health and health promotion. We need to understand policy development and analysis, organisational structure, and how to reflect on practice in order to understand, and do something about, the ways in which ideology and politics help or hinder the quest for social justice, equity, and sustainability.

REVISITING THE UPSTREAM METAPHOR

All this leads us to re-imagine a metaphor for health promotion. An enduring classic was coined in 1974 by John McKinlay (McKinlay 1974) when he relayed the following story from a physician friend:

> 'You know,' he said, 'sometimes it feels like this. There I am standing by the shore of a swiftly flowing river and I hear the cry of a drowning man. So I jump into the river, put my arms around him, pull him to shore and apply artificial respiration. Just when he begins to breathe, there is another cry for help. So I jump into the river, reach him, pull him to shore and apply artificial respiration, and then just as he begins to breathe, there is another cry for help. So back in the river again, reaching, pulling, applying, breathing and then another yell. Again and again, without end, goes the sequence. You know, I am so busy jumping in, pulling them to shore, applying artificial respiration, that I have no time to see who the hell is upstream pushing them all in' (McKinlay 1974:9).

McKinlay used this story to argue that a clear majority of health resources and activities are downstream: responding with superficial, categorical tinkering and jumping from health issue to health issue, without solving anything. Wholly downstream endeavours lack sustainability and are ultimately futile. McKinlay's story urged health promotion to refocus upstream where the real problems lie. Such a reorientation would analyse why individuals, interest groups, and large-scale, profit-oriented corporations are pushing people in, only to erect downstream health services to serve the needs they created and for which they ought to assume moral responsibility.

While we use and appreciate the upstream metaphor, we revisit it here because it refers to individual bodies suffering from disease or injury. We need to change the unit of analysis from the individual to the population. The metaphor suggests health promotion actions that are linear and monocausal: for example many versions suggest the erection of a fence upstream. Socially determined health problems, by contrast, usually reflect complex causes and solutions. We also need to consider interventions in ecological and environmental contexts. More crucially for this book, the river metaphor could be interpreted as the health sector moving up one stream, alongside other sectors that move up their own streams.

REJECTING TECHNOCRATIC METAPHORS

In our quest, we have found and rejected another aquatic metaphor that neatly captures the hegemony of technocratic, behavioural approaches. Despite a superficial sprinkling of structural and social determinants language, these approaches privilege individually focused interventions seeking changes in a narrow range of risk factors. In doing so, they are at best selective primary health care approaches that implicitly accept and entrench inequities.

This technocratic metaphor emerges from the argument that in health systems there is a transformation of nature to conform to culturally constructed images of technocratic solutions (Davis-Floyd 1994). This is the 'one-two punch' using the following example:

> Take a highly successful natural process (eg salmon swimming upstream to spawn.)
>
> Punch One: render it dysfunctional with technology (dam the stream, preventing the salmon from reaching their spawning grounds).
>
> Punch Two: fix it with technology (take the salmon out of the water with machines, make them spawn artificially and grow the eggs in trays, then release the baby salmon downstream near the ocean) (Davis-Floyd 1994: 1125–6).

In this way, the 'one-two punch' destroys a natural process then rebuilds it as a cultural process that values science and technology over nature. It does so by using scientific research that separates elements from the whole they compose: of humans from nature, of mind from body, of mother from child in the birthing process. This is no mere accidental by-product of progress: rather the one-two punch accurately reflects the underlying values of a technocratic society (Davis-Floyd 1994).

AN ECOLOGICAL METAPHOR FOR HEALTH PROMOTION

We criticise approaches to health promotion that attempt to place health at the centre of the universe and ignore the big questions and big ideas from the ecological and environmental movements on the one hand, and of politics and economics on the other. To move from critique to action, we revisit the metaphoric solution of simply travelling upstream to see why the bodies fell in to asking fundamental questions about ecology and environment. We draw again on the more recent work of John McKinlay, who argues:

> Global environmental threats, the disruption of vital ecosystems, planetary overload, persistent and widening social injustice and health inequalities, and lack of access to effective healthcare will be among our major challenges in the future (McKinlay & Marceau 2000: 31).

Box 24.1: An ecological metaphor for health promotion

Our ecological metaphor argues:

When we see a health problem downstream, we immediately move our gaze all around: further downstream, upstream, and sideways. We ask what the health problem tells us about the ecosystem, social justice, equity, and the organisation of health services. What patterns of culture, land use, and human settlement have contributed to the problem we see? This takes us to the ecology upstream, to wonder about micro and macro climates that give rise to the state of the river we see in front of us. To wonder about the economy and society that is changing the climate, ecology, and human behaviour. We then consider what changes we need to make to social and ecological determinants to bring about, at the population level, health, well-being, social justice, and a sustainable ecosystem. To do this, we explore other rivers and water cycles that may be just as, or even more, important than the one problem in the one river upon which we have stumbled. At the same time as we work via community engagement, partnerships, collaboration, and advocacy towards determinants of social justice and sustainability, we use our technical health promotion skills to reorient health systems towards the primary health care approach and involve communities in gaining control over the factors that affect health. Good health results from the interplay of these actions.

WHERE TO NOW?

We seek a reflective approach that grapples with the conundrum that if health is determined outside the health sector what can health promotion do about it from within the health sector?

So what does this mean for health promotion? We think the technocratic skills of identifying needs, then planning and evaluating interventions that originate within the health sector are useful and all health promoters should be able to use these skills proficiently. The emerging focus on partnerships and collaboration is promising, albeit tarnished by the potential downside of the healthism within— consciously or otherwise casting health at the centre of life. However, the best planned interventions, delivered by effective and harmonious partnerships, are not enough. Our gaze to the upstream ecology of which the river is a part must not give rise to longings for travel with colonialist or imperialist intent or outcome. While we may wish that our travels do not dam or pollute any river and our actions should not do harm, we must be reflective and realistic enough to know that they probably will.

As we approach the next frontier of health promotion we must beware of individual ideology clothed in the language of social determinants. These versions of health promotion represent the 'one-two punch' of complying in the destruction of natural processes, then of selectively intervening with campaigns and programs that pay mere lip service to social, economic, and cultural determinants of ecological and human health, well-being, and sustainability.

Instead, we need to re-position and re-imagine health promotion as a valuable set of technical skills that are necessarily nested within a bolder approach to theory. A bold approach takes us beyond the travel guide's capacity to help us to survive short visits to new sectors and disciplines. A bold approach helps us take our place with those sectors and disciplines as a respectful long-term resident or frequent visitor—without imperialist or colonialist intentions.

To refresh, renew, and re-imagine health promotion, we must avoid the tendency for over-specialisation in technocratic skills in favour of health promotion practice informed by theory and research placing social determinants on centre stage. This will not be easy, because, as Fran Baum concludes in her book *The New Public Health*:

> Public health has never been noted for its theoretical base. It has appealed to people who like to implement rather than theorise. Effective public health practitioners, however, are likely to be reflective in their practice and use theories from a variety of disciplines in an eclectic way. Their reflection will benefit considerably from the contribution of different professionals working in genuine partnerships with community groups to arrive at creative solutions (Baum 2002: 529).

This is no easy task. Indeed, considerable capacity-building and comprehensive methods of overcoming structural barriers to inequity are necessary to change cultures of practice. But, just as in the technical aspects of health promotion, we know the benefits of stopping and thinking. We must avoid the leap from problem to solution without crafting and evaluating all the options. We need to ask whether, or to what extent, it is really possible for practitioners steeped in the relatively a-theoretical health promotion system to see the world in the same ways as those in the economy and environment systems. Similarly, to what extent can those in the economic and environmental systems see into the health world? Or do they even want to in the first place?

We can be encouraged by the observation that many of the most visionary thinkers in health came to work in health with both qualifications and experience in other disciplines. Maybe we need more of this. We are encouraged also by the trend towards postgraduate health promotion education with multidisciplinary towards perspectives. We note the acceptance of doctoral research jointly supervised from more than one discipline. We see practitioners and researchers from different disciplines working together and look forward to these collaborations producing new theories and knowledge. We have precedents and possibilities with which to work.

For the twenty-first century we need practitioners, researchers, and educators who have the competence and confidence to create a new understanding of health promotion by synthesising evidence-based technical skills with theorising sophisticated enough to engage them in the big debates about how economy, ecology, and society create or destroy life chances, equity, sustainability, and thus health and well-being.

BIBLIOGRAPHY

Abrums, M. 2000, 'Jesus will fix it after a while': meanings and health. *Social Science and Medicine*, vol. 50, pp. 89–105.

Acheson, D. *Independent Inquiry into Inequalities in Health Report-Part 1* <www.archive.official-documents.co.uk/document/doh/ih/part1a.htm> 2 January 2006.

Acheson, D. *Independent Inquiry into Inequalities in Health Report-Part 2* <www.official-documents.co.uk/document/doh/ih/part2k.htm> 2 January 2006

Alford, R. 1975, *Health Care Politics*. Chicago University Press, Chicago.

Alinsky, S.D. 1972, *Rules for Radicals: A Pragmatic Primer for Realistic Radicals*, Vintage, USA.

American Obesity Association: AOA Fact Sheets. <www.obesity.org/subs/fastfacts/obesity_global_epidemis.shtml>.

Anderson, R.M., Funnell, M.M., Butler, P.M., Arnold, M.S., Fitzgerald, J.T. & Feste, C.C. 1995, Patient empowerment: results of a randomized controlled trial. *Diabetes Care*, vol. 18, pp. 943–9.

Andrews, G. J. & Moon, G. (2005) 'Space, place and the evidence base', *World Views on Evidence-Based Nursing*. Second Quarter, pp. 55–62.

Angus, J. 2001, *A review of evaluation in community-based art for health activity in the UK*, Centre for Arts and Humanities in Health and Medicine, Durham City.

Ashton, J. (ed.) 1992, *Healthy Cities*. Open University Press, Milton Keynes, UK.

Astbury, J. & Cabral, M. 2000, Women's mental health: an evidence based review. Department of Mental Health and Substance Dependence, World Health Organization, Geneva.

Australian Bureau of Statistics 2002, *Measuring Australia's Progress*, ABS Canberra.

Australian Climate Group 2004, *Climate Change—Solutions for Australia*. WWF, Sydney.

Backett, K. & Davison 1992 Rational or reasonable? Perceptions of health at different stages of life. *Health Education Journal* vol. 51, no. 2, pp. 55–9.

Banken, R. 2001, *Strategies for Institutionalizing HIA*. Quebec, Canada, European Centre for Health Policy, Health Impact Assessment Discussion Papers. No. 1.

Barnes, R. 2001, *Health Impact Assessment and Inequalities: A Population Focus or an Area Based Approach (Draft Report)*, WHO, European Centre for Health Policy.

Barnes, R., Cooke, A., Ellis, D., Gee, N. & James, S. 2001, *Health Impact Assessment of Regeneration Programmes*, London Borough of Hammersmith and Fulham.

Batterham, R. 2000, *A Chance to Change*. Commonwealth of Australia, Canberra.

Baum, F. 2002, *The New Public Health*, 2nd edn, Oxford University Press, Melbourne.

Baum, F. 1998, *The New Public Health: An Australian Perspective*. Oxford University Press, Melbourne.

Baum, F. & D. Abbott 1987, *A Social Health Perspective*. Report to the community on the 1987 Marion, Brighton and Glenelg Community Needs Assessment Survey. Adelaide, Southern Community Health Services Research Unit.

Baum, F., Fry, D. & Lennie, I. (eds) 1993, *Community Health: Policy and Practice in Australia*. Pluto Press, Leichhardt, NSW.

Bauman, A., Bellew, B., Vita, P., Brown, W. & Owen, N. 2002, *Getting Australia active: towards better practice for the promotion of physical inactivity*, National Public Health Partnership, Melbourne.

Beaglehole, R. & Bonita, R. 1997, *Public Health at the Crossroads*, Cambridge UP.

Berensson, K. 1998, Focusing on Health in the Political Arena, *Eurohealth*, vol. 4, no. 3, pp. 34–6.

Berkman, L. & Glass, T. 2000, 'Social integration, social networks, social support, and health', in Berkman L. & Kawachi I. (eds), *Social Epidemiology*, Oxford University Press, New York.

Berkman, L. & Kawachi, I. 2000, 'A historical framework for social epidemiology', in Berkman L. & Kawachi I. (eds), *Social Epidemiology*, Oxford University Press, New York.

Bero, L. & Rennie, D. 1995, The Cochrane Collaboration: Preparing, maintaining, and disseminating systematic reviews of the effects of health care, *Journal American Medical Association*, vol. 274, pp. 1935–8.

Black, D., Morris, J., Smith, C. Townsend, P. & Whitehead, M. 1988, *Inequalities in Health: the Black Report; the Health Divide*. Penguin, London.

Blau, G. & Mahoney, M. 2005, *The Positioning of Health Impact Assessment in Local Government in Victoria*, Deakin University, Melbourne.

Blaxter, M. 1990, *Health and Lifestyles*. Routledge, London, UK.

Blum, H.L. 1974, *Planning for Health: Development and Application of Social Change Theory*. Human Sciences Press, New York.

Boud, D. & Walker, D. 1990, Making the most of experience, *Studies in Continuing Education*, vol. 12, no. 2, pp. 61–80.

Bourdieu, P. 1990, *The Logic of Practice*. Polity Press, Oxford.

Bowen, C. 2004, 'HIA and policy development in London: using HIA as a tool to integrate health considerations into strategy', in Kemm, J., Parry, J. & Palmer, S., (eds) *Health Impact Assessment, Concepts, Theory, Techniques and Applications*. Oxford University Press, Oxford.

Bowen, S. & Zwi, A.B. 2005, Pathways to 'evidence-informed' policy and practice: a framework for action, *PLoS Medicine*, vol. 2, no. 7, pp. 600–5.

Bowen, S., Harris, E. & Hyde, J. 2001, Capacity Building: Just rhetoric or a way forward in addressing health inequality, *Health Promotion Journal of Australia*, vol. 11 no. 1, pp. 56–60.

Breeze, C. & Lock, K. 2002, 'Health Impact Assessment as part of strategic environmental assessment: A review of concepts, methods and practice to support the development of a protocol on strategic environment assessment as part of the Espoo Convention.' European Union, <www.euro.who.int/document/e74634.pdf>.

Bridgman, P. & Davis, J. 2003, *The Australian Policy Handbook*, 3rd edn. Allen and Unwin, Sydney.

Brown, M.T. 2005, *Corporate Integrity: Rethinking Organizational Ethics and Leadership*, Cambridge University Press.

Brown, P., Zavestoski, S., McCormick, S., Mayer, B., Morello-Frosch & Altman, R. 2004, Embodied health movements: New approaches to social movements in health, *Sociology of Health & Illness* vol. 26, pp. 50–80.

Brown, V.A. (1989) 'Health care policies, health policies or policies for health?' In Gardner, H. (ed), *Health policy: Development, Implementation and Evaluation in Australia*. Churchill Livingstone, Melbourne.

Bunker, S., Colquhoun, D.M., Esler, M.D., Hickie, I., Hunt, D., Jelinek, V.M., Oldenburg, B.F., Peach, H.G., Ruth, D., Tennant, C.C. & Tonkin, A. 2003, Stress and coronary heart disease, psychosocial risk factors. National Heart Foundation of Australia: position statement update. *Medical Journal of Australia*, vol. 178, no. 6, pp. 272–6.

Bunton, R. 1993, 'Health Promotion as Social Policy', in Bunton, R. & Macdonald, G. (eds), *Health Promotion: Disciplines and Diversity*. Routledge, London.

Bunton, R. 1992, More than a woolly jumper: Health promotion as social regulation. *Critical Public Health*, vol. 3, no. 2, pp. 4–11.

Butterworth, I.M. & Fisher, A.T. 2001, Adult Education and the Built Environment, *Adult Learning*, vol. 13, no. 2/3, pp. 10–14.

Cain, C. 2006, Press Release: AMA(SA) releases 'Election Priorities for Health—2006 and Beyond'. AMA (SA) calls for more listening to doctors instead of 'bean-counters' and bureaucrats–for more clinical input into decision-making about the health. December 6.

Carnwall R. & Carson A. 2003, Understanding partnerships and collaboration, in Peckham, S. & Exworthy, M. (eds), *Primary Care in the UK: Policy, Organisation and Management*, Palgrave, Basingstoke.

Catford, J. 2005, Plenary panel presentation at Australian Health Promotion Association 15th National Health Promotion Conference, Canberra, March.

Catford, J. 1997, Social entrepreneurs are vital for health promotion—but they need supportive environments too, *Health Promotion International*, vol. 12, pp. 1–4.

Cauci, S. 2005, 'CSIRO diet book author makes a meal of critics', *The Age*, 30 December.

Chalmers I. 2005, If evidence-informed policy works in practice, does it matter if it doesn't work in theory? *Evidence & Policy*, vol. 1, no. 2, pp. 227–42

Charles, K., Warren, L. & Oberin, J. 2005, Pallert Tooree Larr: Strong Women's Black Camp. Paper presented at the 5th Australian Women's Health Conference, Melbourne. Paper available: www.awhn.org.au.

Cheng, A.S. & Daniels, S.E. 2005, Getting to 'We': examining the relationship between geographic scale and ingroup emergence in collaborative watershed planning. *Human Ecology Review*, vol. 12, no. 1, pp. 28–41.

Cheng, A.S. & Daniels, S.E. 2003, Examining the interaction between geographic scale and ways of knowing in ecosystem management: a case study of place-based collaborative planning, *Forest Science*, vol. 49, no. 6, pp. 841–54.

Choi, B.C.K., Pang, T., Lin, V., Puska, P., Sherman, G., Goddard, M., Ackland, M.J., Sainsbury, P., Stachenko, S., Morrison, H. & Clottey, C. 2005, Can scientists and policy makers work together? *Journal of Epidemiology and Community Health*, vol. 59, pp. 632–7.

Cialdini, R. 1984, *Influence: The New Psychology of Modern Persuasion*. Quill, New York.

City of Marion 1997, Memorandum about the Marion Drive-In Plan Amendment Report, Adelaide, South Australia, 25 July.

City of Marion 1997, Guidelines for environmental support for physical activity, Adelaide, South Australia, November.

City of Marion 1996, Cycling-proposed local area bike plan, Adelaide, South Australia, 9 April.

Clark, M., Hampson, S.E., Avery, L. & Simpson, R. 2004, Effects of a tailored intervention on the process and predictors of lifestyle behaviour change in patients with type 2 diabetes, *Psychology, Health & Medicine*, vol. 9, pp. 440–9.

Cleveland, H. & Luyckx, M. 1998, *Religion and Governance*, Paper to World Academy of Art Seminar on Governance and Civilizations, Brussels. <www.wnrf.org/cms/govern.html> 15 January 2004

Cobb, R.W. & Elder, C.D. 1983, *Participation in American Politics: The Dynamics of Agenda-building* 2nd edn, John Hopkins University Press, Baltimore.

Considine, M. 1994, *Public policy: A Critical Approach*. MacMillan, Melbourne.

Considine, M. & Painter, M. 1997, 'Introduction. Managerialism: The great debate', in Considine, M. & Painter, M. (eds) *Managerialism: The Great Debate*. Melbourne University Press, Melbourne.

Council of Europe 1998, *Gender Mainstreaming: Conceptual framework, methodology and presentation of good practices*. Final report of activities of the Group of Specialists on Mainstreaming (EG-S-MS), Strasbourg.

Craig, D. 2000, Practical logics: the shapes and lessons of popular medical knowledge and practice—examples from Vietnam and Indigenous Australia, *Social Science and Medicine*, vol. 51, no. 5, pp. 703–11.

Cromley, E. & McLafferty, S. (2002) *GIS and Public Health*. Guilford, New York.

Cumpston, J.H.L. 1989, *Health and Disease in Australia: A History* (ed. M.J. Lewis). Australian Government Printing Service, Canberra.

Curran, T. 2006, 'Promoting Health: compliance or empowerment', in *The Chronicle: Publication of the Chronic Diseases network NT*, vol. 9, no. 2, April.

Curtis, S.E. 2004, *Health and Inequality: Geographical Perspectives*. Sage Publications Ltd.

Dahl, R.A. 1961, *Who Governs? Democracy and Power in an American City*. Yale University Press, New Haven.

Dahlgren, G. & Whitehead, M. 1991, *Policies and Strategies to Promote Social Equity in Health*. Institute of Future Studies, Stockholm.

Davies, P. 2005, Workforce development to support evidence-informed public health. Presentation delivered at 'Cutting Edge Debates', VicHealth, Melbourne.

Davis, G. 1997, 'Towards a hollow state? Managerialism and its critics', in Considine, M. & Painter, M. (eds), *Managerialism: The Great Debate*. Melbourne University Press, Melbourne.

Davis-Floyd, R.E. 1994, The technocratic body: American childbirth as cultural expression, *Social Science & Medicine* vol. 38, no. 8, pp. 1125–40.

Davison, C., Frankel, S. & Smith, G.D. 1992, The limits of lifestyle: Re-assessing fatalism in the popular culture of illness prevention, *Social Science and Medicine* vol. 34, no. 6, pp. 675–85.

Deakin University Course Materials (2005) *Health Communication Study Guide*, Melbourne.

deBlij, H.J. & Murphy, A.B. 2003, *Human Geography: Culture, Society and Space* (7th edn). John Wiley, New York.

de Leeuw, E. 1999, Healthy Cities: Urban social entrepreneurship for health, *Health Promotion International*, vol. 14, pp. 261–9.

de Leeuw, E. 1989, 'Health policy: An exploratory inquiry into the development of policy for the new public health in the Netherlands.' *Boekhandel De Tribune*, The Netherlands.

de Leeuw, E. & Skovgaard, T. 2005, Utility-driven evidence for healthy cities: Problems with evidence generation and application, *Social Science & Medicine*, vol. 61, no. 6, pp. 1331–41.

de Leeuw, E., Abbema, E. & Commers, M. 1998, Healthy Cities Project: Second phase policy evaluation. *Final Report*. World Health Organization Collaborating Centre for Research on Healthy Cities, Maastricht

Delaney, F.G. 1994, Muddling through the middle ground: theoretical concerns in intersectoral collaboration and health promotion, *Health Promotion International*, vol. 9, no. 3 pp. 217–25.

Department of Health and Aged Care (DHAC) 1998, *National Health Priority Areas Cardiovascular health: a report on heart, stroke and vascular disease.* Commonwealth Department of Health and Aged Care, Australian Institute of Health and Welfare, AIHW Cat. PHE 9.

Department of Human Services 2006, *Health promotion priorities for Victoria: A discussion paper*, Government of Victoria, Melbourne.

Department of Human Services 2005, *Review of the Health Act 1958*, Government of Victoria, Melbourne. <health.vic.gov.au/healthactreview/>

Department of Human Services 2003, *Integrated Health Promotion Resource Kit*, Government of Victorian, Melbourne.

DHAC, *see* Department of Health and Aged Care.

DHS, *see* Department of Human Services.

Dickerson, K. & Manheimer, E. 1998, The Cochrane Collaboration: Evaluation of health care and services using systematic reviews of the results of randomized controlled trials, *Clinical Obstetrics and Gynecology*, vol. 41, pp. 315–31.

Dobbins, M., DeCorby K. & Twiddy, T. 2004, 'A knowledge transfer strategy for public health decision makers.' *Worldviews on Evidence-Based Nursing*, vol. 1(2), pp. 120–8.

Dooris, M. 1999, Healthy Cities and Local Agenda 21: the UK experience—challenges for the new millennium, *Health Promotion International*, vol. 14, pp. 365–75.

Douglas, C.H. 2001, *Health Impact Assessment for the Salford Health Investment for Tomorrow—The SHIFT Project*, carried out on behalf of the SHIFT HIA Steering Group by the University of Salford, commissioned by the Capital Directorate of Salford Royal Hospitals NHS Trust.

Douglas, M. & Scott-Samuel, A. 2001, Addressing health inequalities in health impact assessment, *Journal of Epidemiology and Community Health*, vol. 55, pp. 450–1.

Douglas, M., Conway, L., Gorman, D., Gavin, S. & Hanlon, P. 2001, Developing principles for health impact assessment, *Journal of Public Health Medicine*, vol. 23, no. 2, pp. 148–54.

Doyal, L. 2003, 'Sex and Gender: The Challenges for Epidemiologists' in *International Journal of Health Services*, vol. 33, no. 3, pp. 569–79.

Duhl, L.J. 2000, *The Social Entrepreneurship of Change* (2nd edn), Cogent Publishers, Putnam Valley, New York.

Duhl, L.J. (ed.) 1963, *The Urban Condition: People and Policy in the Metropolis.* Basic Books, New York.

Duhl, L.J. & Sanchez, A.K. 1999, *Healthy Cities and the city planning process: A background document on links between health and urban planning*, WHO Regional Office for Europe, Copenhagen. <www.who.dk/healthy-cities/Documentation/20020514_1>. 3 March 2004.

Egbutah, C. & Churchill, K. 2002, *An Easy Guide to Health Impact Assessments for Local Authorities.* Luton Borough Council, Luton Health Action Zone, Luton.

Engels, F. 1844, *The Condition of the Working Class in England.* Basil Blackwell, Oxford.

EnHealth Council 2005, *Unflued Gas Heaters*, Department of Health and Ageing, Canberra.

EnHealth Council 2004, *Healthy Homes*, Department of Health and Ageing, Canberra.

Ereut M. 1994, *Developing Professional Knowledge and Competence.* Falmer Press, London.

Esping-Anderson, G. 1999, *Social foundations of postindustrial economies.* Oxford University Press, Oxford.

Eveline, J. & Bacchi, C. 2005, What are we mainstreaming when we mainstream gender? *International Feminist Journal of Politics*, vol. 7, no. 4, pp. 496–512.

Everson, S., Maty, S., Lynch, J. & Kaplan, G. 2002, Epidemiologic evidence for the relation between socioeconomic status and depression, obesity, and diabetes, *Journal of Psychosomatic Research* vol. 53, pp. 891–5.

Ewles, L. & Simnett, I. 1999, *Promoting Health: A Practical Guide*, 4th edn, Scutari Press, UK.

Fauth, R.C., Leventhal, T. & Brooks-Gunn, J. 2004, Short-term effects of moving from public housing in poor to middle-class neighborhoods on low-income, minority adults' outcomes, *Social Science & Medicine*, vol. 59, no. 11, pp. 2271–84.

Federal Provincial and Territorial Advisory Committee on Population Health 1999, Intersectoral action ... towards population health. Minister of Supply and Services, Canada.

Federation of Swedish County Councils Focusing on Health 2005, HIA, Sweden. <www.lf.se/hkb/engelskversion/eb/nghkb.htm>.

Fleay, B. 1997, *The End of the Age of Oil*, Pluto Press, Sydney.

Fleming, B. & Henkel, D. 2001, Community-based ecological monitoring: a rapid appraisal approach, *Journal of the American Planning Association*, vol. 67, pp. 456–66.

Flinders University 2006, *PHCA 8924 Practicum Guide to Learning*, Department of Public Health, Adelaide.

Frankel, S., Davison, C. & Smith, G.D. 1991, Lay epidemiology and the rationality of responses to health education, *British Journal of General Practice*, vol. 41, no. 351, pp. 428–30.

Freire, P. 1970, *Pedagogy of the Oppressed*. Continuum Publishing Company, New York.

Fry, D. & Baum, F. 1992, 'Keywords in community health.' In Baum, F., Fry, D. & Lennie, I., *Community Health: Policy and Practice in Australia*, Bondi Junction, New South Wales.

Gardner, H. (ed.) 1997, *Health Policy in Australia*. Churchill Livingstone, Melbourne.

Garrard, J., Lewis, B., Keleher, H., Tunny, N., Burke, L., Harper, S. & Round, R. 2004, *Planning for healthy communities: reducing the risk of cardiovascular disease and type 2 diabetes through healthier environments and lifestyles*, Victorian Department of Human Services, Melbourne.

Gatrell, A.C. 2002, *Geographies of Health: An Introduction*. Blackwell, Oxford.

Gibson, L. 1994, The Springett Interview, *The Journal of Contemporary Health* vol. 1, pp. 24–5.

Gillespie, J. 1991, *The Price of Health: Australian Governments and Medical Politics 1910–1960*, Cambridge University Press, Sydney.

Goudswaard, A.N, Stolk, R.P., Zuithoff, N.P.A., de Valk, H.W. & Rutten, G.E.H.M. 2004, Long-term effects of self-management education for patients with Type 2 diabetes taking maximal oral hypoglycaemic therapy: a randomized trial in primary care, *Diabetic Medicine*, vol. 21, pp. 491–6.

Goumans, M. 1998, *Innovations in a fuzzy domain: Healthy Cities and (Health) Policy Development in The Netherlands and the United Kingdom*. Maastricht University, Maastricht.

Graycar, A. 2002, Australian Institute of Criminology, *Domains of Crime Prevention*, Paper presented to Crime Prevention Conference, Sydney, 12 September.

Green, L.W. & Kreuter, M.W. 1999, *Health Promotion Planning: An Education and Ecological Approach* (3rd edn). Mayfield, Mountain View, CA.

Gusfield, J. 1996, *Contested Meanings. The Construction of Alcohol Problems*. University of Wisconsin Press, Madison.

Gusfield, J. 1981, *The Culture of Public Problems: Drinking-Driving and the Symbolic Order*. University of Chicago Press, Chicago.

Ham, C. & Hill, M. 1993, *The Policy Process in the Modern Capitalist State* (2nd edn). Harvester Wheatsheaf, London.

Hamer L., Jacobson, B. Flowers J. & Johnstone F. 2003, 'Health equity audit made simple: a briefing for Primary Care Trusts and Local Strategic Partnerships.' NHS Health Development Agency, Public Health Observatories, London.

Hamilton, C., Hinks, S. & Petticrew, M. 2003, Arts for Health: still searching for the Holy Grail, *Journal of Epidemiology and Community Health*, vol. 57, no. 6, pp. 401–5.

Hancock, L. 1999, 'Policy, power and interests', in Hancock, L. (ed.), *Health Policy in the Market State*, Allen and Unwin, Sydney.

Hancock, T. 1990, Developing healthy public policies at the local level. In A. Evers, W. Farrant, A. Trojan (eds) *Healthy Public Policy at the Local Level*, Frankfurt/New York.

Harding, A. 1985, Unemployment policy: A case study in agenda management, *Australian Journal of Public Administration* vol. XLIV, no. 3, pp. 224–46.

Hay, A., Frew, R. & Butterworth, I. 2001, Environments for Health: Municipal Public Health Planning. *Environmental Health*, vol. 1, no. 3, pp. 85–9.

Hayward, K. & Colman, R. 2003, *The Tides of Change: addressing inequity and chronic disease in Atlantic Canada, a discussion paper.* Population and Public Health Branch, Atlantic Regional Office, Health Canada.

Health Canada <www.phac_aspc.gc.ca/ph_sp/phdd/determinants/index.html>.

Health Development Agency 2000, 'Art for health: a review of good practice in community-based arts projects and initiatives which impact on health and wellbeing.' HDA, London: <www. hda-online.org.au>

Health Education Authority 2001, *Making it happen: a guide to delivering mental health promotion*, Department of Health, UK.

Health Inequalities Research Collaboration 2002, *Position Statement*, Department of Health and Aged Care, Canberra.

Health Promotion Forum of New Zealand 2004, *A Review of the use and future of health promotion competencies for Aotearoa–New Zealand.* A report to the Ministry of Health from the Health Promotion Forum of New Zealand. <www.hpforum.org.nz/resources/competenciesreportJan04.pdf>

Health Promotion Froum of New Zealand. 2002. <www.hpforum.org.nz/>.

Hetzel, B. & McMichael, A.J. 1985, *The LS Factor*, Penguin Books, Ringwood.

Heward, S. 2006, 'Organisational Change—Essential for Quality Practice and Functioning Partnerships.' Conference presentation at Australian Health Promotion Association 16th National Health Promotion Conference, Alice Springs, Northern Territory, 23–26 April.

Heward, S., Hutchins, C. & Keleher, H. 2006, Organisational change—a key component of quality practice and capacity building frameworks. Australian Health Promotion Conference, Alice Springs, April.

Hoeijmakers, M. 2004, *Local Health Policy Development Processes*, Maastricht University, Maastricht.

Hoffman, B. 2003, Health care reform and social movements in the United States, *American Journal of Public Health*, vol. 93, pp. 75–85.

Hogwood, B. & Gunn, L. 1984, *Policy Analysis for the Real World*. Oxford University Press, Oxford.

Horne, D. 1988, *Arts Funding and Public*, Australian Key Centre for Media and Cultural Policy, Griffith University, <www.artscouncil.org.uk/publications/docs/socialexclusionreview.doc> 21 October 2002; <www.gu.edu.au/centre/cmp/Horne_OP1.html> 3 November 2002.

Huygens, I. 1988 *Empowering our Natural Communities*. Presentation at XXIV International Psychology Congress, Sydney, Australia.

Hyde, J. 2002, *Dry: In Defence of Economic Freedom*. Institute of Public Affairs, p 168, <www.ipa. org.au/files/2002hyde_dry.pdf.>

Ife, J. 2000, Local and global practice: relocating social work as a human rights profession in the new world order, *European Journal of Social Work*, vol. 4, no. 1, pp. 5–15.

Innes J. & Booher, D.E. 1999, *Indicators for Sustainable Communities: A Strategy Building on Complexity Theory and Distributed Intelligence*. Institute of Urban and Regional Development, University of California at Berkeley, California.

International Society for Equity in Health (ISEqH) 2005, <www.iseqh.org>.

Jackson, N. & Waters, E. and the Guidelines Taskforce (2005) *Systematic reviews of health promotion and public health interventions: Guidelines*. Cochrane Health Promotion and Public Health Field, Carlton South, Victorian Health Promotion Foundation.

Jermyn, H. 2001, *The Arts and Social Exclusion: a review prepared for the Arts Council of England*, Arts Council of England.

Jones, B.O. (1982/1996) *Sleepers, Wake!* Oxford University Press, Melbourne.

Kates, R.W., Clark, W.C., Correll, R., Hall, J.M., Jaeger, C.C., Lowe, McCarthy, J.J., Schellnhuber, H-J., Bolin, B., Dickson, N.M., Faucheux, S., Gallopin, G.C., Gruebler, A., Huntley, B., Jager, J., Nodha, N.S., Kasperson, R.E., Mabogunje, A., Matson, P., Mooney, H., Moore, B., O'Riordan, T. & Svedin, U. 2000, Sustainability Science, *Science*, vol. 292, pp. 641–2.

Kawachi I. & Berkman, L.F. (eds) 2003, *Neighborhoods and Health*, Oxford University Press, New York.

Kawachi, I. & Kennedy, B.P. 1997, The relationship of income inequality to mortality—Does the choice of indicator matter? *Social Science and Medicine*, vol. 45, pp. 1121–7.

Kawachi, I., Subramanian, S.V. & Almeida-Filho, N. 2002, A glossary for health inequalities. (Glossary). *Journal of Epidemiology and Community Health*, vol. 56(9): 647(6), September.

Kegler, M.C., Norton, B.L. & Aronson, A.E. 2003, *Evaluation of the five-year expansion program of Californian Healthy Cities and Communities (1998–2003): Final report*, Centre for Civic Partnerships, Sacramento CA. <www.civicpartnerships.org/files/TCEFinalReport9-2003. pdf> 13 March 2005.

Keleher, H. 2004, 'Public and Population Health: Strategic Responses', in Keleher, H. & Murphy, B. (eds), *Understanding Health: A Determinants Approach*, Oxford University Press, Melbourne.

Keleher, H. 2002, 'Community development in health', in St John, W. & Keleher, H. (eds), *Community Nursing: Theory, Skills and Issues*, Allen and Unwin, Sydney.

Keleher, H. 2001, Why primary health care offers a more comprehensive approach for tackling health inequities than primary care, *Australian Journal of Primary Health*, vol. 3, no. 3, pp. 59–67.

Keleher, H. & Armstrong, R. 2006, *Evidence-based Mental Health Promotion Resource*. Deakin University for VicHealth and Department of Human Services, Melbourne.

Keleher, H. & Marshall, B. 2003, *Strengthening health promotion in community health*, Report for Victorian Department of Human Services Eastern Region, Melbourne.

Keleher, H. & Murphy, B. 2004, 'Understanding Health: An Introduction', in Keleher, H. & Murphy, B. (eds), *Understanding Health: A Determinants Approach*, Oxford University Press, Melbourne.

Keleher, H. & Round, R. 2006, *Evidence-based mental health promotion resource*, Deakin University for VicHealth and Department of Human Services, Melbourne.

Kelly, P. 2004, 'Not for Wimps: Futures Thinking and First Year Engineers', in Inayatullah, S. (ed.) *Causal Layered Analysis Reader*, Tamkang University, Tamsui (Taiwan).

Kelly, P. 1992, *The End of Certainty: The Story of the 1980s*, Allen and Unwin, St Leonards, NSW, Australia.

Kemm, D.J. 2000, Can Health Impact Assessment fulfil the expectations it raises? *Public Health*, vol. 114, pp. 431–3.

Kickbusch, I. 1989, 'Good planets are hard to find: Approaches to an ecological base for public health', in Brown, V. (ed), *2020: A Sustainable Healthy Future—Toward an Ecology of Health*, Proceedings of a national workshop. Commission for the Future, Melbourne, Australia.

Kieffer, C.H. 1984, 'Citizen empowerment: A developmental perspective', in Rappaport, J. & Hess, R. (eds), *Studies in Empowerment*, Haworth Press, New York.

Kingdon, J.W. 1995, *Agendas, Alternatives and Public Policies*, 2nd edn, Harper Collins College Publishers, New York.

Korten, D.C. 1995, *When Corporations Rule the World*, Berret-Kohler, San Francisco.

KPMG Australia, *Ethical Business and Sustainable Communities*, <www.erc.org.au/busethics/kpmg_ethical_bus.pdf>

Krieger, N. 2001, glossary for social epidemiology, *Journal of Epidemiology and Community Health*, vol. 55, no. 10, pp. 693–700.

Krockenberger, M., Kinrade, P. & Thorman, R. 2000, *Natural Advantage: Blueprint for a Sustainable Australia*, Australian Conservation Foundation, Melbourne.

Kuhn, T. 1970, *The Structure of Scientific Revolutions* 2nd edn, University of Chicago Press, Chicago, USA.

Labonte, R. 2005, Plenary panel presentation at Australian Health Promotion Association 15th National Health Promotion Conference, Canberra, March.

Labonte R. 2003, *How our programs affect population health determinants: A workbook for better planning and accountability*. Population and Public Health Branch, Manitoba and Saskatchewan Region, Health Canada.

Labonte, R. 1997, *Power, participation and partnerships for health promotion*, VicHealth, Carlton South.

Labonte, R. 1992, Heart health inequalities in Canada: Models, theory and planning, *Health Promotion International*, vol. 7, no. 2, pp. 119–28.

Labonte, R. & Laverack, G. 2001a, Capacity building in health promotion, Part 1: for whom? And for what purpose? *Critical Public Health*, vol. 11, no. 2, pp. 111–26.

Labonte, R. & Laverack, G. 2001b, Capacity building in health promotion, Part 2: whose use? And with what measurement? *Critical Public Health*, vol. 11, no. 2, pp. 129–38.

Lasswell, H. 1936, *Politics: Who Gets What, When, How*. McGraw-Hill, New York.

Lasswell, H.D. 1930, *Psychopathology and Politics*. University Chicago Press, Chicago.

Lehto, J. & Ritsatakis, A. 1999, *Health Impact Assessment: Main Concepts and Suggested Approach— the Gothenburg consensus paper*, European Centre for Health Policy, WHO Regional Office for Europe, Brussels.

Lennie, I. 1988, Do health departments promote health? If not, what do they do? *Community Health Studies*, vol. 12, no. 4, pp. 404.

Lester, C., Griffiths, S., Smith, K. & Lowe, G. 2001, Priority Setting with Health Inequality Impact Assessment, *Public Health*, vol. 115, pp. 272–6.

Lewis, J.M. 2005, *Health Policy and Politics: Networks, Ideas and Power*. IP Communications, East Hawthorn.

Lewis, M. 1999, *The Culture of Inequality*, University of Massachusetts Press, Amherst.

Lewis, M.J. 2003, *The People's Health: Public Health in Australia 1788–1950*, Praeger Publishers, Westport, Connecticut.

Lewis, M.J. (ed.) 1989, *Health and Disease in Australia: A History* by J.H.L. Cumpston, Australian Government Publishing Service, Canberra.

Liedtka, J. 1988, Linking strategic thinking with strategic planning', *Strategy and Leadership*, October, no. 1, pp. 120–9.

Limerick, D. & Cunnington, B. 1993, 'The New Organisation: key issues, opportunities and challenges', in *Managing the New Organisation: A Blueprint for Networks and Strategic Alliances*, Business and Professional Publishing, New South Wales.

Lin, V. & Gibson, B. 2003, *Evidence-based Health Policy: Problems and Possibilities*. Oxford University Press, Melbourne.

Lindblom, C. 1959, The science of muddling through, *Public Administration Review*, vol. 19, no. 2, pp. 79–88.

Lomas, J., Culyer, T., McCutcheon, C., McAuley, L. & Law, S. for the Canadian Health Services Research Council (2005) *Conceptualizing and combining evidence for health system guidance*, Final report, Canadian Health Services Research Foundation, Ontario.

London's Health Commission resources at <www.londonshealth.gov.uk/hia.htm#Top>.

Lovelock, J. 1988, *The Ages of GAIA*. Oxford University Press, Oxford.

Lowe, I. 1994, *Performance Measurement*. Proceedings of the Fenner Conference, Canberra, November.

Lowe, I. 1993, 'Towards a new sunrise—Prospects for renewable energy.' *Consuming Interest*, p. 11, January.

Lupton, D. 1994, 'Analysing new coverage', in *The Fight for Public Health: Principles and Practices of Media Advocacy*, BMJ Publishing Group, London.

Macdonald, G. & Davies, J. 1998, 'Reflection and vision: proving and improving the promotion of health', in Davies, J. & Macdonald, G. (eds) *Quality, Evidence and Effectiveness in Health Promotion: Striving for Certainties*, Routledge, London.

MacDougall, C. 2003, Learning from differences between ordinary and expert theories of health and physical activity, *Critical Public Health*, vol. 13, no. 4, pp. 369–87.

MacDougall, C. 2001, Thoughts on barriers and enablers for incorporating ordinary theorising into the community participation in health debate, *Australian Health Review*, vol. 24, no. 4, pp. 30–3.

MacDougall, C. 2000, *Public Policy and Physical Activity*, School of Medicine. PhD Thesis, Adelaide University.

MacDougall, C. 1985, Lifestyle change and health promotion, in Baum, F.E., *The New Public Health: The South Australian Experience*, Wakefield Press, Melbourne.

MacDougall, C., Cooke, R. et al. 1997, Relating physical activity to health status, social connections and community facilities, *Australian and New Zealand Journal of Public Health*, vol. 21, no. 6, pp. 631–7.

MacDougall, C., Wright C. & Atkinson, R. 2002, Supportive environments for physical activity and the local government agenda: a South Australian example, *Australian Health Review*, vol. 25, no. 2, pp. 178–84.

Macintyre, S. & Petticrew, M. 2000, Good intentions and received wisdom are not enough.' *Journal of Epidemiology and Community Health*, vol. 54, pp. 802–3.

Mahoney, M. & Morgan, R. 2001, Health Impact Assessment in Australia and New Zealand: an exploration of methodological concerns, *Education and Promotion*, vol. 8(1):8–11.

Mahoney, M., Durham, G., Townsend, M., Reidpath, D., Wright, J. & Potter, J.L. 2002, Health Impact Assessment: a tool for policy development in Australia.' Report for Commonwealth Department for Health and Ageing, Deakin University, Melbourne.

Marmot M. & Wilkinson R. 1999, *Social Determinants of Health*. Oxford University Press, Oxford.

Marshall, B. 2004, 'Health promotion in action: Case studies from Australia', in H. Keleher, and B. Murphy (eds), *Understanding Health: A Determinants Approach*, Oxford University Press, Melbourne.

Matarasso, F. 1997, *Use or Ornament? The Social Impact of Participation in the Arts.* Comedia, Stroud, UK.

Mays, N., Pope, C. & Popay, J. 2005, Systematically reviewing qualitative and quantitative evidence to inform management and policy-making in the health field, *Journal of Health Services Research and Policy*, vol. 10 (Suppl 1), pp. 6–20.

Mazmanian, D.A. & Sabatier, P.A. 1989, *Implementation and Public Policy. With a New Postscript.* University Press of America, Lanham/London.

McCombs, M. & Shaw, D.L. 1993, The evolution of agenda-setting research: Twenty-five years in the marketplace of ideas, *Journal of Communication*, vol. 43, no. 2, pp. 58–67.

McElduff, P. & Dobson, A.J. 2000, Trends in coronary heart disease—has the socio-economic differential changed?' *Australia and New Zealand J.Public Health*, vol. 24, pp. 465–73.

McKinlay, J.B. 1974, *A Case for Refocussing Upstream: The Political Economy of Illness. Applying behavioral science to cardiovascular risk*, American Heart Association, Seattle, Washington.

McKinlay, J.B. & Marceau, L.D. 2000, 'To boldly go ...', *American Journal of Public Health*, vol. 90, no. 1, pp. 25–33.

McQueen, D.V. 2001, Strengthening the evidence base for health promotion, *Health Promotion International*, vol. 16, pp. 261–8.

McQueen-Thompson, D. & Ziguras, C. 2002, *Promoting Mental Health and Wellbeing through Community and Cultural Development: a Review of Literature focussing on Community Arts Practice*, The Globalism Institute, RMIT, Melbourne, Oxford University Press, Melbourne.

Metcalfe, A. 1993, Living in a clinic: the power of public health promotions, *Anthropological Journal of Australia*, vol. 4, no. 1, 291–7.

Mezirow J. 1997, Transformative Learning: Theory to Practice, *New Directions for Adult and Continuing Education*, vol. 74, pp. 5–12.

Mezirow J. 1985, 'A critical theory of self-directed learning', in S. Brookfield (ed.), *Self-directed learning: From Theory to Practice*, Jossey-Bass, San Francisco.

Milburn, K. 1996, The importance of lay theorising for health promotion research and practice, *Health Promotion International*, vol. 11, no. 1, pp. 41–6.

Milio, N. 1988, Making healthy public policy; developing the science by learning the art: an ecological framework for policy studies, *Health Promotion International*, vol. 2, no. 3, pp. 263–74.

Milio, N. 1987, Healthy Public Policy: Issues and Scenarios, Unpublished paper prepared for a Symposium on Healthy Public Policy, Yale University, 5 October.

Milio, N. 1986, *Promoting Health Through Public Policy*. F.A Davis Co., Philadelphia.

Milligan, C., Gatrell, T. & Bingley, A. (2004) '"Cultivating health": therapeutic landscapes and older people in Northern England.' *Social Science and Medicine*, 58, pp. 1781–93.

Mills, D. 2003, Art and Wellbeing; Securing the connections—integrating policy and practice, *Artwork Magazine*, Issue 57, December.

Mills, D. & Brown, P. 2004, *Art and Wellbeing*, Australia Council for the Arts, Sydney.

Millward, L.M., Kelly, M.P. & Nutbeam, D. 2003, *Public Health Intervention Research-The Evidence*, London, Health Development Agency.

Mindell, J., Hansell, A., Morrison, D., Douglas, M. & Joffe, M. 2001, What do we need for robust, quantitative health impact assessment? *Journal of Public Health Medicine*, vol. 23, no. 3, pp. 173–8.

Ministerial Summit on Health Research (2004) The Mexico Statement on Health Research: Knowledge for better health: Strengthening health systems (from the Ministerial Summit on Health Research, 16–20 November, Geneva, WHO. <www.who.int/rpc/summit/agenda/Mexico_Statement-English.pdf> 14 September 2005

Mintzberg, H. 1994, *The Rise and Fall of Strategic Planning*. Englewood Cliffs, New Jersey, Prentice Hall.

Mittelmark, M. 2004, 'How to influence policy', in Moodie, R. & Hulme, A. (eds), *Hands-on Health Promotion*, IP Communications, Melbourne.

Mohan, T., McGregor, H., Saunders, S. & Archee, R. 2004, 'Intercultural Communication Competence in Business and the Professions.' In *Communicating as Professionals*, Thomas, Melbourne.

Mouffe, C (ed.) 1992, *Dimensions of Radical Democracy: Pluralism, Citizenship, Community*, Verso, London.

Mulgan, G. 2005, Government, knowledge and the business of policy making: the potential and limits of evidence-based policy, *Evidence & Policy: A Journal of Research, Debate and Practice*, vol. 1, no. 2, pp. 215–26.

Murphy, B. 2005, *Footy Rocks: A report for the VFL into promoting participation for young women*, Deakin University, Melbourne.

Murphy, B. 2004 'In search of the 4th dimension of health promotion', in Keleher, H. & Murphy, B. (eds), *Understanding Health: A Determinants Approach*, Oxford University Press, Melbourne.

Naidoo J. & Wills J. 2000, *Health promotion: foundations for practice*, 2nd edn, Balliere Tindall, London.

National Aboriginal Health Strategy Working Party 1989, *A National Aboriginal Health Strategy*, NAHSWP, Canberra.

National Public Health Partnership 2005, *Be Active Australia: A Framework for Health Sector Action For Physical Activity 2005–2010*, NPHP, Melbourne.

National Public Health Partnership 2002, *Guidelines for the Development, Implementation and Evaluation of National Public Health Strategies in Relation to Aboriginal and Torres Strait Islander Peoples*, NPHP, Canberra.

National Public Health Partnership 2001, *Promoting Active Transport: A Portfolio of Interventions*, NPHP, Canberra.

National Public Health Partnership 2000, *Public Health Planning and Practice Improvement: A Planning Framework for Public Health Practice*, NPHP, Canberra.

National Research Council [of USA] 1999, *Our Common Journey—a Transition Toward Sustainability*, National Academy Press, Washington.

National Training Information Service (NTIS) (2006). <www.ntis.gov.au>.

Nature, Editorial 2005, 'A recipe for trouble.' *Nature* 438:1052.

Navarro, V. 1976, *Medicine under Capitalism*, Croom Helm, London.

Nordlinger, E. 1981, *On Autonomy of the Democratic State*, Harvard University Press, Cambridge, Massachusetts.

NPHP, *see* National Public Health Partnership.

NRC, *see* National Research Council.

NTIS, *see* National Training Information Service.

NSW Health 2004, *Four Steps Toward Equity: A Tool for Health Promotion Practice*, NSW Health Promotion Director's Network, NSW Health, Sydney.

NSW Health 2001, *A Framework for Building Capacity to Improve Health*, Health Department, Sydney, NSW.

NSW Health 1999, *A Framework for Building Capacity to Improve Health*, Health Promotion Strategies Unit, Sydney.

Nutbeam, D. 1998, Health Promotion Glossary, World Health Organisation, Geneva. <www.who.int/hpr/archive/docs/glossaryu.html>

Nutbeam, D. & Harris, E. 2004, *Theory in a Nutshell: A Guide to Health Promotion Theory* 2nd edn, McGraw-Hill, Sydney.

O'Dwyer, L.A., Palmer, C., Baum, F. & Ziersch, A. 2004, Conceptions of neighbourhood, Public Health Association of Australia 36th Annual Conference, Perth, 25–28 September.

O'Dwyer, L. A., Baum, F., Kavanagh, A. & MacDougall, C. (under review) 'Do area based interventions to reduce health inequalities work? A systematic review of evidence.' *Critical Public Health*.

Office for Women and University of Adelaide 2006, *Gender Analysis: Implementing a South Australian model*, Government of South Australia.

Office for Women and University of Adelaide 2005, *Gender Impact Assessment: Implementing the Netherlands Model*, Government of South Australia.

Ogilvie, D., Hamilton, V., Egan, M. & Petticrew, M. 2005, Systematic reviews of health effects of social interventions: 1. Finding the evidence: how far should you go? *Journal of Epidemiology and Community Health*, vol. 59, pp. 804–8.

Ogilvie, D., Egan, M., Hamilton, V., Petticrew, M. 2004, Promoting walking and cycling as an alternative to using cars: systematic review.' *British Medical Journal*, vol. 329, pp. 763.

Øvretveit, J & Gustafson, D. 2002, Evaluation of quality improvement programmes, *Quality and Safety in Health Care*, vol. 11, pp. 270–5.

Pal, L. 1997, *Beyond Policy Analysis: Public Issue Management in Turbulent Times*, Nelson, Ontario.

Palmer, G. & Short, S. 2000, *Health Care and Public Policy: An Australian Analysis* 3rd edn, Macmillan, Melbourne.

Palmer, G.R. & Short, S.D. 1994, *Health Care and Public Policy: An Australian Analysis,* 2nd edn Macmillan, Melbourne.

Parry, J. & Palmer, S. 2001, *Health Impact Assessment, Concepts, Theory, Techniques and Applications,* Oxford University Press, Oxford.

Parry, J. & Stevens, A. 2001, Prospective health impact assessment: pitfalls, problems and possible ways forward, *British Medical Journal,* vol. 323, pp. 1177–82.

Patterson, E. 2006, 'Health teaching', in St John, W. & Keleher, H. (eds), *Community Nursing Practice,* Allen and Unwin, Sydney.

Patton, M.Q. 2002, *Qualitative Research and Evaluation Methods* 3rd edn, Sage, Thousand Oaks, California.

Pawluch, D., Cain, R. & Gillett, J. 2000, Lay constructions of HIV and complementary therapy use, *Social Science and Medicine,* vol. 51, no. 2, pp. 251–64.

Pederson, A. P. 1988, *Coordinating healthy public policy: An analytic literature review and bibliography,* Health and Welfare Canada, Health Services and promotion Branch Working Paper. Ottawa.

Peel, M. 1995, *Good Times, Hard Times: the Past and the Future in Elizabeth,* Melbourne University Press, Melbourne.

People's Health Assembly 2000, *The People's Health Charter,* <www.phmovement.org> 6 September 2005.

Perkins, D.D. & Zimmerman, M.A. 1995, Empowerment theory, research and application, *American Journal of Community Psychology,* vol. 23, pp. 569–79.

Peterson, A.R. 1994, *In a critical condition: Health and power relations in Australia,* Allen and Unwin, Sydney.

Petticrew, M., Whitehead, M., Macintyre, S.J., Graham, H. & Egan, M. 2004, Evidence for public health policy on inequalities: 1. the reality according to policy makers, *Journal of Epidemiology and Community Health,* vol. 58, pp. 811–16.

Pickin, C., Popay, J., Staley, K., Bruce, N., Jones, C. & Gowman, N. 2002, Promoting Organisational Capacity to Engage with Active Lay Communities: Developing a Model to Support Organizational Change For Health, *Health Service Research and Policy,* vol. 7, no. 1, 34–46.

Popay, J., Thomas, C., Williams, G., Bennett, S., Gatrell, A. & Bostock, L. 2003, A proper place to live: health inequalities, agency and the normative dimensions of space, *Social Science and Medicine,* vol. 57, no. 1, 55–69.

Posner G. 1989, 'Why and how should you reflect on your field experience?' in *Field experience. Methods of Reflective Teaching,* 2nd edn, Longman, New York.

Prochaska, J.O. & DiClemente, C.C. 1982, Transtheoretical therapy: Toward a more integrative model of change, *Psychotherapy: Theory, Research and Practice,* vol. 19, no. 3, pp. 276–88.

Putland, C. Baum, F. & MacDougall, C. 1997, How can health bureaucracies consult effectively about their policies and practices? Some lessons from an Australian study, *Health Promotion International,* vol. 12, no. 4, pp. 299–309.

Quiggin, J. 1999, 'Rationalism and rationality in economics.' *On Line Opinion,* November 15, 1999, <www.onlineopinion.com.au/view.asp?article=1376> accessed 17 January 2006.

Raeburn, J. & Corbett, T. 2001, Community development: How effective is it as an approach in health promotion? Paper prepared for the *Second International Symposium on the Effectiveness of Health Promotion.* University of Toronto, 28–30 May.

Raftery, J. 1995, 'Health policy development in the 1980s and 1990s', in Baum, F., *Health for All: The South Australian Experience*, Wakefield Press, Adelaide.

Raphael D. 2002, *Poverty, Income Inequality and Health in Canada*, CSJ Foundation for Research and Education, Toronto.

Raphael D. & Farrell S. 2002, Income inequality and cardiovascular disease in North-America: shifting the paradigm, *Harvard Health Policy Review*, vol. 3 no. 2.

Raphael, D., Anstice, S., Raine, K. & McGannon, K.R. 2003, The social determinants of the incidence and management of type 2 diabetes mellitus: are we prepared to rethink our questions and redirect our research activities? *International Journal of Health Care Quality Assurance*, vol. 16, no. 4/5, pp. x–xx

Rappaport, J. 1987, Terms of empowerment/exemplars of prevention: Toward a theory for community psychology, *American Journal of Community Psychology*, vol. 15, no. 121–48.

Ratzan, S. 2001, Health literacy: communication for the public good, *Health Promotion International*, vol.16, no. 2, pp. 207–14.

Reid, P. 2006, 'Challenging Ourselves.', Keynote presentation at Australian Health Promotion Association, 16th National Health Promotion Conference, Alice Springs, Northern Territory, 23–26 April.

Reader, R. 1996, *The National Heart Foundation of Australia and Heart Disease in Australia: An Account of the Foundation's First Twenty Years*. National Heart Foundation, New South Wales.

Reeves, H. & Baden, S. 2000, Gender and Development: Concepts and Definitions, *BRIDGE Report No 55*, IDS, Sussex: 2–3 <www.bridge.ids.ac.uk/reports/r55%20con&defw2web.doc>.

Reppucci, N.D. 1990, 'Ecological validity and the deritualization of process', in Tolan, R., Keys, C., Chertok, F. & Jason, L. (eds), *Researching Community Psychology: Issues of Theory and Methods*, American Psychological Association, Washington DC.

Reynolds, C. 1995, *Public Health Law in Australia*. Federation Press, Sydney.

Reynolds M. 1998, Reflection and critical reflection in management learning *Management Learning*, vol. 29, no. 2, pp. 198–200.

Rifkin S.B. 2003, A framework linking community empowerment and health equity: is it a matter of CHOICE, *Journal of Health, Population and Nutrition*, vol. 21, no. 3, pp. 168–80.

Robertson, A. & Minkler, M. 1994, New public health movement: A critical evaluation, *Health Education Quarterly*, vol. 21, no. 3, pp. 295–312.

Roe, M. 1984, *Nine Australian Progressives: Vitalism in Bourgeois Social Thought 1860–1960*, University of Queensland Press, St Lucia.

Rootman, I., Goodstadt, M., Potvin, L. & Springett, J. 2001, 'A framework for health promotion evaluation' in Rootman, I., Goodstadt, M., Hyndman, B., McQueen, D., Potvin, L., Springett, J. & Ziglio, E. (eds). *Evaluation in Health Promotion: Principles and Perspectives*, WHO Regional Office for Europe, Copenhagen.

Rose, G. 1985, Sick individuals and sick populations.' *International Journal of Epidemiology*, vol. 14, no. 1, pp. 579–603.

Rosen, G. 1985, *A History of Public Health*, MD Publications, New York.

Rosenkrantz, B. 1972, *Public Health and the State: Changing Views in Massachusetts, 1842–1936*, Harvard University Press, Cambridge MA.

Round, R., Marshall, B. & Horton K. 2005, *Planning for effective health promotion evaluation*, Victorian Government Department of Human Services, Melbourne.

Rowe, N., Beasley, N. & Adams, A. 2004, Sport, physical activity and health: Future prospects for improving the health of the nation, <www.sportdevelopment.org.uk/dupfuture2.pdf> 3 April 2006.

Rummel, R.J. 1976, *Understanding Conflict and War: Volume 2 The Conflict Helix*, Sage, Beverley Hills, California.

Sackett, S.L., Rosenberg, W.M.C., Gray, J.A.M., Haynes, R.B. & Richardson, W.S. 1996, Evidence-based medicine: what it is and what it isn't, *British Medical Journal*, vol. 312, pp. 71–2.

Sallis, J.F. & Owen, N. 1999, *Physical Activity and Behavioral Medicine*. Sage, Thousand Oaks, California.

Schön D. 1987, 'How a reflective practicum can bridge the worlds of university and practice', in *Educating the Reflective Practitioner*, Jossey-Bass, San Francisco.

Schön D. 1983, *The Reflective Practitioner*, Temple Smith, London.

Scott, K., McInerny, M. & Tye, M. (1999) *Mentoring for Women: A Guide to Finding and Using Multiple Mentors*. The Australian Federation of Business and Professional Women Inc (BPW Australia), Swan Hill, Victoria.

Scottish Needs Assessment Programme (SNAP) 2000, *Health Impact Assessment: Piloting the Process in Scotland*, Scottish Needs Assessment Programme Network.

Scottish Needs Assessment Programme 2000, *Health Impact Assessment of the City of Edinburgh Council's Urban Transport Strategy*, Scottish Needs Assessment Programme.

Scotton, R.B. 2000, Medibank: from conception to delivery and beyond, *Medical Journal of Australia*, vol. 173, no. 1, pp. 9–11.

Scott-Samuel, A. 1996, Health Impact Assessment, an idea whose time has come, *British Medical Journal*, vol. 313, no. 27, pp. 183–4.

Sen, A. 2001, *Development as Freedom*. Oxford University Press, New York.

Senge, P. Kleiner, A. Roberts, C. Ross, R. Roth, G. Smith, B. 2002, *The Dance of Change: The Challenges of Sustaining Momentum in Learning Organizations*, Nicholas Brealey Publishing, London.

Sheldon, T. 2005, Making evidence synthesis more useful for management and policy-making, *Journal of Health Service Research Policy*, vol. 10 (Supplement 1), pp. 1–5.

Signal, L. & Durham, G. 2000, Health Impact Assessment in the New Zealand Policy Context, *Social Policy Journal of New Zealand*, no. 15, pp. 11–26.

Sim, F. & Mackie, P. 2003, Health Impact Assessment-a science and an art, *Public Health*, vol. 117, pp. 293–4.

Simpson, S., Harris, E. et al. 2004, Health impact assessment: an introduction to the what, why and how, *Health Promotion Journal of Australia*, vol. 15, no. 2, pp. 150–5.

Sindall, C. 1997, Intersectoral collaboration: the best of times, the worst of times, *Health Promotion International*, vol. 12, no. 1, pp. 5–7.

Skok, J.E. 1995, Policy issue networks and the public policy cycle: A structural-functional framework for public administration, *Public Administration Review*, vol. 55, no. 4, pp. 325–32.

Sloan, A. (2005) *Washington Post*. 6 September. Accessed via CorpWatch: <www.corpwatch.org/article.php?id=12608>.

Smith F.B. 1979, *The People's Health 1830–1910*, Croom Helm, London.

Smith, K. 2000, 'Implementing health inequalities impact assessment in Bro Taf, (Case study 8.1.1)', in Ison, E. (ed.) *Resource for Health Impact Assessment*, vol. 1 *(The Main Resource)*, NHS Executive, London.

Smyth, John 1989, Developing and Sustaining Critical Reflection in Teacher Education, *Journal of Teacher Education*, March-April (2), 2–9.

SNAP, *see* Scottish Needs Assessment Programme.

Sorenson, G., Emmons, K., Hunt, M.K. & Johnston, D. 1998, Implications of the results of community intervention trials, *Annual Review of Public Health*, vol. 19, pp. 379–416.

Springett, J. 2001, Appropriate approaches to the evaluation of health promotion, *Critical Public Health*, vol. 11, no. 2, pp. 139–51.

Sprinks, N. & Wells, B. 1997, Intercultural communication: a key in global strategies, *Career Development International*, vol. 2, no. 6, pp. 287–92.

State of the Environment Advisory Council 1996, *State of the Environment Australia 1996*, CSIRO Publishing, Collingwood.

Steed, L. Lankester, J. Barnard, M. Earle, K. Hurel, S. & Newman, S. 2005, Evaluation of the UCL Diabetes Self-Management Programme (UCL-DSMP): A randomized controlled trial, *Journal of Health Psychology*, vol. 10, pp. 261–76.

Stone, D. 1997, *Policy Paradox. The Art of Political Decision Making*, W.W. Norton, New York/London.

Stoner, J.A.F., Yetton, P.W. et al. 1994, *Management*. Sydney, Prentice Hall.

Swedish National Institute of Public Health 2003, National Public Health Policy Report: <www. hi.se/templates/Page_6720.aspx>

Syme, L. 2003, 'Social determinants of health: the community as empowered partner.' Paper presented at Communities in Control Conference convened by Our Communities and Catholic Social Services, April, Moonee Valley Racing Club.

Syme, S.L. 1996, 'To prevent disease: The need for a new approach', in Blane, D. &. Brunner, E., *Health and Social Organisation*, Routledge, London.

Taylor B 2000, 'Types of reflection', in: *Reflective Practice. A Guide for Nurses and Midwives*, Allen and Unwin, Sydney.

Teeple, G. 2000, *Globalization and the decline of social reform*, Aurora, Garamond.

Tesh, S. 1988, *Hidden Arguments, Political Ideology and Disease Prevention Policy*, Rutgers University Press, New Bruswick, NJ.

Thame, C. 1974, 'Health and the State: The Development of Collective Responsibility for Health Care in Australia in the First Half of the Twentieth Century', PhD Dissertation, Australian National University, Canberra.

Theobald, S., Elsey, H. & Tolhurst, R. 2004, Gender, Health and Development 1: Gender Equity and Sector Wide Approaches, *Progress in Development Studies*, vol. 4, no. 1, pp. 59–64.

Thiele, M. & Marsden, S. 2003, *Engaging Art: The Artful Dodgers Studio*, Jesuit Social Services, Richmond, Vic.

Thomson, H., Hoskins, R., Petticrew, M., Ogilvie, D., Craig, N., Quinn, T. & Lindsay, G. 2004, Evaluating the health effects of social interventions, *British Medical Journal*, vol. 328, pp. 282–5.

Thomson, H., Petticrew, M. & Morrison, D. 2002, *Housing improvement and health gain: a summary and systematic review.* MRC Social and Public Health Sciences Unit; <www.msoc-mrc.gla. ac.uk/Publications/pub/PDFs/Occasional-Papers/OP005.pdf> 15 September 2005

Thomson, N. 2003, *The Health of Indigenous Australians*, Oxford University Press, Melbourne.

Thornley, L. & Langford, B. 2001, Unpublished report on a Health Impact Assessment of the Draft Integrated Transport Strategy, Public Health Advisory Committee, New Zealand.

Tilmouth, W. 2006, 'Social Determinant: The Tangentyere Story.' Keynote presentation at Australian Health Promotion Association 16th National Health Promotion Conference, Alice Springs, Northern Territory, 23–26 April.

Tobias, M & Jackson, G. 2001, Avoidable Mortality in New Zealand 1981–97, *Australia and New Zealand Journal of Public Health*, vol. 25, pp. 12–20.

Tones, K. & Green, J. 2004, *Health Promotion: Planning and Strategies*, Sage Publications Ltd, London.

Torjman, S. 1998, *Partnerships: the good, the bad and the uncertain*, Caledon Institute of Social Policy, Canada.

Travis, C & Compton, J. 2001, Feminism and health in the decade of behavior, *Psychology of Women Quarterly*, vol. 25, pp. 312–23.

Trosa, S. 1997 'The era of post managerialism', in Considine, M. & Painter, M., *Managerialism: The Great Debate*, Melbourne University Press, Melbourne.

Tsouros, A. 1995, *The WHO Healthy Cities Project: State of the art and future plans. Health Promotion International*, vol. 10, pp. 133–41.

Tunstall, H., Shaw, M. & Dorling, D. 2004, Glossary: places and health, *Journal of Epidemiology and Community Health*, vol. 58, pp. 6–10.

Turrell, G., Oldenburg, B., McGuffog, I. & Dent, R. 1999, *Socioeconomic determinants of health: towards a national research program and a policy and intervention agenda*, Queensland University of Technology.

Twiss, J. & Duma, S. 2003, Interview with the Director of the Californian Centre for Civic Partnerships, Sacramento, October.

UNEP, *see* United Nations Environment Program.

United Nations Environment Program 1999, *Global Environmental Outlook 2000*, Earthscan Publications, London.

VicHealth 2006a, *Sport and Active Recreation Fact Sheet*, February 2006, Melbourne.

VicHealth 2006b, *Partnerships For Health* <www.vichealth.vic.gov.au> 4 April 2006.

VicHealth 2005a, *The Short Course: Promoting Mental Health and Wellbeing*, Victorian Health Promotion Foundation, Carlton South.

VicHealth 2005b, *Mental Health Promotion Plan 2005–7*, Victorian Health Promotion Foundation, Carlton South.

Vic Health 2005c, *The partnerships analysis tool: for partners in health promotion*, <www.vichealth. vic.gov.au/rhadmin/articles/files/Partnerships.pdf> 21 September 2005.

VicHealth 2003a, *Creative Connections: Promoting Mental Health and Wellbeing through Community Arts Participation*. Learnings from the Community Arts Participation Scheme funded under the Victorian Health Promotion Foundation's Mental Health Promotion Plan 1999–2002: 8–12.

VicHealth 2003b, *Partnerships Analysis Tool*. Victorian Health Promotion Foundation, Carlton South.

Victora, C., Wagstaff, A., Schellenberg, J.A., Gwatkin, D., Claeson, M. & Mabicht, J. 2003, Applying an equity lens to child health and mortality: more of the same is not enough, *Lancet*, vol. 263, pp. 233–41.

Walker, R. 2000, *Collaboration and Alliances: A Review for VicHealth*, Melbourne.

Wallerstein, N. 2006, *What is the evidence on effectiveness of empowerment to improve health?* WHO Regional Office for Europe, Copenhagen <www.euro.who.int/Document/E88086.pdf> February 2006.

Wanless D. 2004, *Securing good health for the whole population* Final report, HM Treasury, UK.

Wass, A. 1994, *Promoting Health: The Primary Health Care Approach*, Harcourt Brace, NSW.

Weick, K.E. 1984, Small wins: Redefining the scale of social problems, *American Psychologist*, vol. 39, pp. 40–9.

White, K. 1996, 'The Social Origins of Illness and the Development of the Sociology of Health', in Grbich, C., *Health in Australia. Sociological Concepts and Issues*, Prentice Hall, Sydney.

Whitehead M. 1990, *The concepts and principles of equity and health*, World Health Organisation, Europe Regional Office.

WHO, *see* World Health Organisation.

Wildridge, V., Childs, S., Cawthra, L. & Madget, B. 2004, How to create successful partnerships—a review of the literature, *Health Information and Libraries Journal*, vol. 21, pp. 3–19.

Wilkinson, R. 1996, *Unhealthy Societies: The Afflictions of Inequality*, Routledge, London.

Wilkinson, R.G. & Marmot, M. (eds) 2003, *Social Determinants of Health: The Solid Facts*, 2nd edn, World Health Organisation, Geneva.

Williams, D. 1995, *Creating Social Capital: a study of the long-term benefits from community based arts funding.* Community Arts Network of South Australia, Adelaide.

Williams, A. (ed.), 1999, *Therapeutic Landscapes: The Dynamic Between Place and Wellness.* University Press of America.

Williams, B. 2001, Developing critical reflection for professional practice through problem-based learning, *Journal of Advanced Nursing*, vol. 34, no. 1, pp. 27–34.

Wise, M. & Signal, L. 2000, Health promotion development in Australia and New Zealand, *Health Promotion International*, vol. 15, no. 3, pp. 237–48.

Wolff, T. 2003, The Healthy Communities movement: A time for transformation, *National Civic Review*, vol. 92, no. 2, pp. 95–111.

Wolff, Young, Beck et al 2004.

Woolley, J. 2005, Recent Advantages of Lower Speed Limits in Australia, *Journal of the Eastern Asian Society for Transportation Studies*, vol. 6, pp. 3652–73.

World Health Organisation 2005a, The Bangkok Charter for Health Promotion in a Globalized World: Sixth Global Conference on Health Promotion. <www.who.int/healthpromotion/conferences/6gchp/bangkok_charter/en/>.

World Health Organisation 2005b, *Action on the social determinants of health: learning from previous experiences*, Commission on the Social Determinants of Health, WHO, Geneva. Available: <www.who.int/social_determinants>.

World Health Organisation 2004, *Healthy Cities and Urban Governance*, WHO, Geneva. <www.who.dk/healthy-cities>.

World Health Organisation 2000, Health Promotion: Bridging the Equity Gap: Fifth Global Conference on Health Promotion, WHO, Geneva. <www.who.int/healthpromotion/conferences/previous/mexico/en/index.html>.

World Health Organisation 1999, *Assessing the Health Impact of Integrating in the European Union*, WHO, Geneva.

World Health Organisation 1997, *City planning for health and sustainable development.* Copenhagen: WHO Regional Office for Europe. <www.who.dk/document/wa38097ci.pdf> 1 March 2004.

World Health Organisation 1995, *Twenty Steps for Developing a Healthy Cities Project* (2nd Edn.). Copenhagen, Denmark: World Health Organization Regional Office for Europe. <www.who.dk/healthy-cities/Documentation/20010918_14>. 3 March 2004.

World Health Organisation 1986, Ottawa Charter for Health Promotion, *Health Promotion*, vol. 1, no. 4, pp. i–v.

World Health Organisation 1978, Primary Health Care: Report of the International Conference on Primary Health Care, Alma Ata, USSR, September.

Wrong, D.H. 1996, *Power. Its Forms, Bases and Uses,* Transaction Publishers, Somerset.

Yeatman, A. 1997, 'The reform of public management', in Considine, M. & Painter, M., *Managerialism: The Great Debate*, Melbourne University Press, Melbourne.

Zolberg V.L. 1990, *Constructing a Sociology of Art*, Cambridge University Press, Cambridge, UK.

Zoller, H. 2005, Health Activism: Communication Theory and Action for Social Change, *Communication Theory*, vol. 15, November, pp. 341–64.

INDEX